Gone the Way of the Dodo Bird

Gone the Way of the Dodo Bird

Bret Kissinger

Dedication

This book is dedicated to the broken and the missing, and to the Lost Generation. Let their voices never go silent. I also dedicate this book to my grandparents. You're missed for a myriad of reasons, but how I wish I could ask you about life before, during, and after the two World Wars.

Special Thanks

To author and Chicago Mafia expert John Binder for fielding questions on the Chicago Outfit during Prohibition. His book "Al Capone's Beer Wars" is a detailed account of that time, one which skillfully separates fact from fiction.

Chapter List

Goma's Burial Service

It's suffering.

Those words came to Johnny every day. Sometimes, they came late at night as he tried to fall asleep, staring at his ceiling. Other times, they crept up on him during his morning shower, as the water massaged his scalp and ran down his broad shoulders. Those words always came whether his mind was idle or preoccupied. They came to him unerringly, snapping him out of the tranquil facade of an occupied mind. No matter when they came, they always brought him back to that day.

It was damn hot outside, and stifling inside the black Sedan. It was like being a roast that had been left inside an oven all day. It was impossible to be in a good mood, and anyone who smiled in this heat was looney and deserved to be dragged away by men in white coats.

Chicago was nicknamed The Windy City. But where was the damn wind? If Lake Michigan offered any breeze that first day of July, it did not make it through the towering skyscrapers. Though it hadn't been living up to its moniker, Chicago had lived up to its reputation as a place where a *no one* could become *someone*. The Midwestern Giant was a place where a man could make something of himself. Where he could rise above and beyond what he could have been had his parents stayed in the old country. There was a place for every race and creed in America. But as it is in nature, so it was in the city—the wolves dictated the order of things. But in Chicago, you got to choose if you were a wolf or a sheep. The rise was limitless if you were willing to clench your fist and fight for it. Some say success is only for a few, and most people have to learn their place at the bottom of the totem pole. But that is the talk of sheep blending into the flock. Every mighty oak started in the dirt, fighting for the sun. The ladder was available to everyone, but most people want an elevator. They expect the easy, comfortable way up. The ladder was malicious, missing steps, coated in grease, teetering like a buoy. The further you rose, the more precarious it became. Most called it too risky, saying that standing on a wobbly, makeshift ladder only resulted in one thing—a fall to the bottom. But most failed to realize they were there already.

In Chicago, success was ubiquitous. It was available around every corner, in every speakeasy, every casino, and every brothel.

Men who sold liquor illegally could make as much in a month as they had in a year working their "legal" jobs. Capone's South Side outfit raked in just short of two million a week. And Chicago had plenty of places to put that kale back into the economy. And Johnny was there to ensure the money got transferred to the right people at the right time.

Johnny removed his pearl-gray fedora and wiped the sweat from his forehead. Tomato, hunkered down in the driver's seat, was even more miserable, looking like someone had pissed in his morning coffee.

He was approaching forty summers in Illinois and knew what to expect, but that didn't mean he liked it. In addition to being older, Tomato was also heavier than Johnny, aided by a dying metabolism and a love of pasta, making him more vulnerable.

Seated in the back, arms spread over the seats and head tilted back, was Hotsy. He was a few years younger than Johnny, and significantly more care-free than Tomato. He had been blessed with a smooth chin and a grin that made the fathers and husbands of Chicago's women pump shells into their shotguns.

"Good God. How long are we going to sit here and bake?" Hotsy asked.

He ran his hand through his black, slicked-back hair with an accompanying undercut. It was kept long on top, so it constantly fell over his eyes. It drove the girls mad when he flicked back the locks with a jerk of his head, and as a result, the gesture had become an unbreakable habit.

"We were told to talk to Goma, so that's what we're going to do," Tomato said.

"Not if we die first," Hotsy muttered.

Hotsy had been born and raised in Chicago. He complained about the snowy winters. He complained about the hot summers. He complained about the rainy springs. He complained about the crisp, windy autumns. His ideal and only acceptable weather was seventy degrees and sunny with a slight breeze. Anything else was unlivable.

"Can't you just sit back there and not complain every five minutes? Maybe just shut up for a while," Tomato snapped.

"I could, but I like reminding myself that I'm still alive," Hotsy replied smoothly.

"Dear God, you're intolerable."

"Listen, all's I'm saying is that if I were a piece of meat, you'd of took me off the grill twenty minutes ago. I'm charred leather back here."

"You don't gotta tell me how hot it is in the car. I'm in here with you."

"Yeah, but you're up front."

"What?"

"What *what*?"

"What do you mean I'm up front?"

"I mean you're sitting in the driver's seat, Tomato. Jesus, keep up."

3

Tomato closed his eyes and exhaled a stream of smoke, like a dragon. "I realize I am in the driver's seat—the steering wheel is in front of me. Why. Does. It. Matter?"

"It's hotter in the backseat. Hot air travels backwards. Everyone knows that."

Tomato rubbed his hands together, then squeezed them to signal his annoyance. "Hot air does not travel backwards. Hot air rises."

Hotsy shrugged, with a phony smile of surrender. "Sure."

Tomato looked to Johnny for an ally. But Johnny was neutral. If Hotsy truly thought hot air traveled backwards, bless his heart. But Hotsy winked when he saw Johnny's eyes in the rear-view mirror.

The heat only seemed to intensify in the ensuing silence. Seconds trudged by like hours. They had been told to make sure it wouldn't happen again. Sometimes, that meant harsh words, other times, it meant onomatopoeic words like *crunch, knock, pop, and pow,* followed by groans, moans, whimpers, and, sometimes, eternal silence. But one thing was for certain—Johnny was going to break something for having to stew in this furnace.

"Where is that pudgy bastard?" Tomato asked after a while.

"Supposed to leave at five," Johnny said.

"Yeah, well it's twenty past," Tomato said. "I'd like to break a toe or finger for every minute we sit out here. One more minute, and I'll have to break something else."

"Maybe he was born with an extra toe," Hotsy said.

Tomato turned and glared at him. "Shut up."

"There he is," Johnny said, pointing to a mound of a man locking up a shop.

"Thank Christ. Let's go," Tomato said.

Johnny had to peel himself off the seat. His pants and shirt had welded to his skin.

Something was definitely going to be broken.

Tomato and Johnny crossed the street shoulder-to-shoulder while Hotsy, in the middle of a deep yawn, lagged behind.

4

"Al, you made us wait in that hot box for over twenty minutes!" Tomato yelled before they were even across the street.

Al's eyes lit up like two firecrackers, his mouth formed a gaping "O" capable of stuffing back a donut in two bites. Something that, judging by his size, he did quite often.

"Tomasso, I didn't know you were waiting," Al said. "I had a little trouble with the books, and some bloke puked in the urinal. It was truly awful, horrible! We're talking Old Testament level destruction."

Tomato flipped up Al's drooping fedora so he could see his eyes. Tomato's eyes were bloodshot from a late night and an early wakeup call, and must have looked downright demonic to Al.

"You know what day it is, Al?" Tomato asked.

"July 1st," Al answered.

"The day of the week, wise guy," Tomato said.

"… Thursday?" Al replied.

"Thursday. That's right, Al. Good job. What happens on Tuesdays?" Tomato asked.

"Pick up."

"The pick up! Great job, Al! You're on a roll," Tomato said.

Al shrugged, smirking even though he knew he shouldn't.

Hotsy leaned toward Johnny. "If Al were on a roll, he'd eat himself."

"You're not lying," Johnny whispered back.

"Johnny, did you get money from Al on Tuesday?" Tomato asked.

"Not a dime," Johnny replied.

"Hotsy, what about you? Did Al give you the money he owes?"

"No, sir. I would even think him being late is an attempt to avoid us. I'm not a sentimental man, Al, but that hurts my feelings. I know you do business with us, but I thought we was friends first," Hotsy said, sounding as sincere as when he promised to call his dates the next day.

"You know you can count on me as a friend, Quintu," Al said, looking worried now.

"Friends don't hide and not pay, Al. For how stringy you are, I would of thought you a Jew," Tomato said.

"He ain't eating kosher," Hotsy said.

"Guys, I'm sorry—"

"Why are you late, Al?" Johnny asked. It was too hot for bullshit.

"I had my daughter's birthday last week. The big nineteen. The money pool was a bit shallow," Al said.

"Why did you have to do that, Al?" Tomato asked. Al's words had killed his playful manner.

"Do what?"

"Lie."

"I didn't."

"Come on Al," Hotsy said, squeezing the back of Al's thick neck, "your daughter had her birthday two months ago."

"You know how we know?" Tomato asked.

"… Vencini gave a birthday gift," Al said, eyes widening from the realization.

"You use your daughter to lie? That's something I can't respect. You keep your family out of your business," Tomato said, pushing his index finger into Al's chest. On a fit man, Tomato's finger would have pressed against a sternum. On Al, it got lost in his cleavage.

Every respectable gangster followed the rule that women and children were not part of the business. Any retaliation was aimed at the man, away from his family. A rule Al Capone of the South Side and Hymie Weiss and George "Bugs" Moran of the North Side followed, and enforced. And to Tomato, it was scripture.

Tomato pulled out a billy club from inside his suit. Hotsy did the same. Johnny's was hand-constructed from a piece of hardwood with iron studs hammered into the tip. The ends of the nails were bent, a faded silver absent of sheen, with strands of hair woven in between and stained with dried blood. He tapped it against the side of his leg. Hotsy smacked his into his open hand.

6

Al put up his hands in surrender, fear looming large in his eyes. "What are you guys gonna do?"

"Al, this is a dangerous part of town. You need friends. All sorts of things can happen. Like smashed windows, busted walls, destroyed goods," Tomato said.

"Think of us as insurance salesmen. We're here to protect you from natural disasters," Johnny said.

He smashed the glass door of the shop. The words "Goma's Burial Services" in white lettering shattered into a hundred pieces. Hotsy and Tomato drove their clubs against the glass-paneled windows. They stepped inside, the glass crunching under their boots. Al's shop had everything a grieving family needed in order to put a loved one to rest in style and class. He had coffins, urns, and funeral wreaths. But buried beneath the floorboards was where the dead came back to life. Al hosted some of the best parties in Chicago. Parties well-stocked with whiskey from Canada, rum from the Caribbean, beer brewed in Milwaukee and Chicago, and wine from the holiest of churches and synagogues. All with the invisible watermark of Al Capone, Vencini Valcoro, and the South Side.

Valcoro and Johnny "The Fox" Torrio had known each other for years. After Torrio had stepped away from running the South Side a little more than a year earlier in 1925, Capone had allowed Valcoro to stay on in his current role. Valcoro wasn't a threat because he had never lusted after world domination or even Chicago domination. His world was The Moonlight, and he was perfectly content ruling over it and sharing the profits with a businessman of Al Capone's caliber.

But Vencini Valcoro also liked to know his "partners" could think on their feet and keep a silent tongue in front of police and prohibition agents. There was always the potential for a loose tongue at a speakeasy. A man who had been turned down by a woman and gotten laughed at for it. Some dame or dork who had gotten too zozzled and faced the wrath of God the next morning and bought into the propaganda that alcohol was the devil's drink. Johnny had seen enough in his life to spot a talker too. It was in the eyes. Men who would fold under the softest interrogation. Johnny didn't know which of the above had applied to the night the police had come snooping at Al's. But thanks to some quick thinking on Al's part, what the police descended the steps to had been a funeral celebration. The Negro band had switched from upbeat jazz to melancholic church music in one note. Al served his drinks out of wooden pints or copper cups, so it was impossible for the police to tell what was inside them. It was this sort of quick thinking that made Al a desirable "partner"… except for his missed payment.

Hotsy ran his club along the ledge full of urns, sending each one onto the floor, creating his own musical crescendo, while Johnny smashed his club onto the shelves, splintering them in half. Then Hotsy raised his club to bludgeon the wooden caskets in an effort to dent the immaculate hand-made boxes, but Johnny covered them with his hand and shook his head.

Johnny had no desire to end up in a box. It wasn't that he had illusions of immortality, far from it. Those had left him years ago. He wanted his body burned to ash. There was something innately terrifying about coffins and caskets. It made him think of everyone he had loved lying inside one. While most were naïve to what happened once the body was put in the ground, Johnny had seen every stage of decomposition and the fetidness that came with it. But despite his hatred for coffins and caskets, he could not deny that Al added grace and beauty to them with hand-carved roses and crosses in the mahogany and walnut. The taffeta and velvet gave a sense of comfort, something that made loved ones truly feel their dearly departed could be at eternal rest. A fate not afforded to many. Sometimes, there was no intricate carving or padded bedding. Sometimes there was no coffin at all.

Anxiety swooshed through him like a gust of flame. Sheer panic consumed him. He tried to counter it with two deep breaths, but that failed. He closed his eyes, but that only made it worse. And then, it felt like he was inside one of those coffins.

His hand on the hardwood, Johnny was transported back to that place. His breath shortened. His heart raced. A cold sweat ran down his neck. The air he gulped in offered no relief. He was a thrashing fish out of water.

The damn attack was back.

"You okay?" Hotsy asked.

Johnny nodded dismissively.

Breathe. Breathe. Breathe.

It should have happened without thinking and without command. Babies did it automatically, yet here he was at thirty-two, having to manually command his lungs to inflate and deflate. He snapped his eyes open, staring at the world outside the broken windows, drawing that fresh albeit thick, muggy air into his lungs. It took twelve sobering breaths before the curse of the coffins passed.

Al fell to his knees, horrified at the damage to his shop. "I'm finished."

"No, you're not," Tomato said. "These accidents happen, Al. You are a prized member of Valcoro's and, in extension, Al Capone's extended family. They take care of their own. You didn't pay your premium this week, and unfortunately for you a natural disaster landed on your business. But Valcoro forgives. He extends a hand to help you back on your feet."

Tomato offered Al his hand. Al's face contorted in bewilderment. His mouth drooped low enough that saliva threatened to spill out.

"I don't understand…" he managed to say eventually.

"Don't be late with your payments. It's that simple," Johnny said.

He was ready to step outside into the sunlight. Each second that passed was a shovel-full of dirt burying him alive. Every casket and coffin stared at him, reminding him of his fate and the fate of all men.

"Or you may end up in one of your own boxes," Hotsy added.

"I can't repay you," Al said. "Take a look around. I can't file a police report and blame it on someone else. They'll take a look downstairs. They'll write me up for violation of the Volstead Act, I'll be in prison—"

"Al, Al! Calm down. Take a deep breath," Tomato said, slapping Al on the back as if the man had been choking on a piece of steak. "Go home. Get some sleep. When you come back tonight, this place will look like it did on the day you opened shop."

Al looked like he was still confused, but at least he knew better than to keep asking questions.

"What happens to your rates after you file a claim?" Tomato asked.

"They go up," Al answered.

"Like hot air," Tomato flashed a look at Hotsy. "They go up. Thirty percent now, up from twenty-five. But it's a necessary evil. You could think of dropping the insurance all together. But you'd be risking an awful lot. Natural disasters can happen at any moment," Tomato warned.

"Yeah, like next Tuesday," Hotsy said.

It wasn't the subtlety Tomato had been going for. Hotsy was not one to catch on quickly, so he liked to go all hit-the-nail-on-the-head with his threats.

"Thank you… I owe you guys, I really do."

"You remember that next Tuesday," Hotsy said.

"Or it won't be porcelain, glass, and wood we'll break. It'll be bone," Johnny said.

Al nodded like a bobble head.

"Get out of here," Tomato said.

Al waddled out of his shop, taking one last look before closing his eyes and putting his faith in God and "the insurance agents."

"Something about being stuffed in a box that ain't right," Hotsy said.

"It's not like you're alive for it," Tomato said.

"Still. You burn me and put me in one of those nice vases before you put me in that hunk of wood," Hotsy said.

It very well could have been the first time Hotsy had contemplated his own death.

"Urn," Tomato corrected him.

"Earn what?" Hotsy asked.

"Not earn, *urn*. They're called urns, not vases. You put flowers in vases. You put ashes in an urn," Tomato said.

"What if you put my ashes in a vase and put some roses in there too?" Hotsy asked.

"You have a morbid mind," Tomato said, stepping out of the building.

Hotsy and Johnny followed him to the car.

Hotsy had been on his own since he was a teen, and ever since they had started working together in 1919, Tomato had taken it upon himself to share whatever wisdom he had with the boy through small "teachable moments."

The car sped forward, and Johnny removed his fedora to let the wind cool his steaming head. It was so ungodly hot in the car that the sweat couldn't even drip off his forehead. It just boiled and evaporated. But when he caught his piercing blue eyes in the side mirror, he put his fedora back on. He rested his hand on the open window, blocking the mirror from reflecting his eyes.

Tomato fought off a yawn and rubbed his eyes.

"Tired?" Johnny asked.

Tomato had been rubbing his red eyes all morning. Red eyes that told of *minutes* —and not *hours*— of sleep.

"Lorraine rode into me all night," Tomato said.

"The good way or the bad way?" Hotsy asked, leaning forward from the back seat.

"What do you think?" Tomato snapped back.

"True. If it had been good, you would of said, 'rode me for twelve seconds,'" Hotsy said, suppressing a smirk.

"Same reason?" Johnny asked, ignoring Hotsy.

"Same reason," Tomato answered, disappointment coloring his voice.

"I tell you all the time, Tomato, you need to shower that off. Those girls wear all that perfume for a reason," Hotsy said.

"Nah, she can just sense it. I walk in the door with a hundred pounds of guilt."

"They don't mean anything though."

"They mean something to her."

Johnny stayed silent, enjoying the lake breeze wafting through the cracks of the skyscrapers. The rush of wind was sobering. It calmed his breathing and subdued worries of another attack.

Tomato intentionally took the long way, driving alongside the lakeshore, so they could enjoy the temporary relief it brought. Johnny drank in the fresh air like he had found water in a desert, tilting his head back so the wind traveled down his neck. The water was imaginary. The desert was real.

"When do you think I should tell Al I slept with his daughter in one of those caskets?" Hotsy asked.

Johnny burst out laughing, and even Tomato couldn't contain himself.

"I made her squeal with zeal!" Hotsy shouted.

The Moonlight Hotel was one of many hotels frequented by Al Capone. But ever since Big Bill Thompson had lost his reelection bid for mayor, and the incorruptible William Emmett Dever had taken the seat, Capone spent most of his time at The Hawthorne Hotel in Cicero. Valcoro had shown he could bring in profits through alcohol, gambling, and prostitution, so Capone let Valcoro be as long as the profits continued and Valcoro didn't get greedy.

The hotel had an actual name, perhaps belonging to a hotel chain or named after a business mogul—Johnny couldn't recall. And when he thought on it, he wasn't even sure if he had ever known the hotel's true name. All of Chicago knew it as The Moonlight. First, because it was a beacon for lost souls wandering in the dark, and second, because it was a place where a man could unleash his inner beast. A place where all manner of vices could be met. A place to gamble and lose everything and descend into poverty or a place to win big and ascend into the one percent. A place to fulfill sexual fantasies with strangers or a place to ruin a marriage. A place to share drinks and create unforgettable memories or a place to consume in excess to forget it all. The dichotomy of The Moonlight was part of its appeal. It had it all. Something for everyone, and to be used at the guest's discretion.

Valcoro lived and operated out of the seventh floor and spent his nights in the hotel lobby, gambling halls, and ballroom. In the five years since Johnny had worked for him, he'd never seen Valcoro leave the hotel. A streak of confinement that, according to Tomato, had begun well before then.

Presently, the lobby was quiet and empty, not rare for the time of day. But Johnny knew that once the clock struck five, the drinks were served, and the band filled the hall with music, Dr. Jekyll transformed into Mr. Hyde.

It wasn't just gangsters and blue collar men looking for drink and dame at The Moonlight. It was police officers, prohibition agents, and politicians, all as dirty as the bathroom floor. Each thought that by leaving early, they could avoid the walk of shame. But Johnny made sure to stare each one down, even ramming his shoulder into the lower-ranking cops, so they would know they weren't ghosts passing through undetected. Some kept their heads low, not high enough on anyone's payroll to make a fuss, but there were some who were high enough that nothing could be done to them. Captains, detectives, even men who worked for former mayor Big Bill Thompson. Thompson himself was a well-acquainted guest of the hotel, trying, these days, to enlist support for another run at being mayor. Selling booze had certainly been easier under a "sympathetic" and "understanding" mayor. Dever was hated by many, including Tomato and Hotsy, but Johnny respected him. Maybe even admired him. He disagreed whole-heartedly with his policies about booze, but what he respected was that the man had made an oath and upheld it. A lot of people said alcohol brought out the worst in men. Did men beat their wives in drunken rages? Yes. Would they do it sober? Yes. Vermin are vermin, with or without alcohol.

Besides, it wasn't Dever who had made the sale and consumption of alcohol illegal. That was the 18th amendment ratified by forty-six of the forty-eight states. Only Connecticut and Rhode Island had had any common sense and rejected the amendment. President Wilson had vetoed the bill, but the House of Representatives immediately vetoed to override the veto, and the Senate followed suit the next day. And once again, a few had made the law for the masses.

Presently in the lobby, the scurrying pigs switched back their wedding rings to the proper hand. Johnny hoped none of them would take Hotsy's advice and shower off the strong perfume that clung to their bodies like ticks. They may be untouchable at The Moonlight, but that immunity did not extend to their homes and their infuriated wives.

Getting Albert Goma back on his payment schedule and informing him of his increased rate earlier that morning had been yesterday's orders. They had to wait for new orders from Valcoro, but he wouldn't wake for at least two-and-a-half hours. And no one dared wake him up. Not even an alarm clock.

The Moonlight had some of the best lunches and dinners in the city, but their breakfast was hardly noteworthy: a menu limited to eggs—fried or scrambled—toast—butter or jam—and bacon strips and sausage links. In the mornings, most guests fled the hotel, like rats from a sinking ship, after a night of gambling, booze, and women. And that's exactly how The Moonlight wanted it, giving guests no reason to linger until eleven a.m.—their mandatory check out time. After eleven, when new guests had checked in, The Moonlight was quicksand, doing everything it could to hold on to you and your money.

Johnny, Tomato, and Hotsy ordered and ate breakfast, and then played four games of three-handed cribbage—a routine for when they needed to kill time.

"Nineteen," Tomato said, throwing his cards on the bar.

Nineteen was impossible to get in cribbage, meaning Tomato had a dreaded zero-point hand. Hotsy counted his two runs and pair and advanced his wooden peg eight places.

Johnny tossed down a pair of sixes and eights. The king that had been cut did jack for his hand.

"He gets all the cards," Tomato said, nodding at Hotsy.

"I make something out of my hands," Hotsy said.

"What do you mean you make something? You get what you get," Tomato said, the saliva in his mouth turning to steam.

"I would of turned your hand into at least five points," Hotsy said.

"You would of turned my hand into at least five points? Like a magic trick?"

"Don't be ridiculous, Tomato. I would of stratergized better."

"First thing. It's strategized, not stratergized—"

14

"While you corrected my grammar, I was skunking you, making my hand better than it should of."

"You. Can't. Change. The. Points. The. Cards. Are. Worth."

Hotsy shrugged, granting Tomato a victory. "Sure."

Tomato's veins continued to swell in anger, since he knew Hotsy's conceding was as authentic as the Trojan horse was a gift.

Hotsy winked at Johnny. Before Tomato could yell further, the phone behind the bar rang. The bartender answered.

"Mr. Valcoro will see you now.

Judge, Juror, and Executioner

No expense had been spared in making The Moonlight a spectacular and ritzy mansion. London had the Buckingham Palace, Paris had the Palace of Versailles, and Chicago had The Moonlight. The carpet was burgundy with swirling designs that looked like liquid gold. It was the place royalty and celebrities wished to stay in but couldn't because of the scandal that would follow them. The elevators were coated gold with real gold flakes mixed in. Rumor stated they were worth more than most schmucks made in a year. They were immaculate but for a small scratch Valcoro had been meaning to fix. A drunken guest who had lost all his money at the tables had tried scraping off the gold with a fork. He had been stopped, thrown into the back of a car, and was never seen at The Moonlight nor anywhere else again.

Johnny, Tomato, and Hotsy piled into the elevator, the heat rising with them floor to floor before spilling out onto the seventh floor where the lift stopped. Hoagie, a man nearing three-hundred twenty pounds, sat in front of the entrance. Like a quarter lost in a sofa, somewhere beneath the glutinous man was a stool. They exchanged pleasantries before Hoagie let them through.

Valcoro's suite was so large it could have been separated into four rooms. The suite was usually spotless, but empty booze bottles were strewn about the floor and food was scattered over the kitchen counter.

Valcoro was seated at the kitchen glass table in front of the long windows showcasing the city of Chicago. His feet were on the table, the morning *Tribune* covering his face. He folded it down when the three approached.

"Grand mornin', ain't it?" he said, a cigar stub dangling in the corner of his mouth. His bathrobe was untied, leaving nothing to the imagination.

"Al's going to need a cleaning and a repair. We got through to him though. He'll pay next week," Tomato said.

"Good, good, good," Valcoro said, looking puzzled.

He didn't even remember Al hadn't paid, and most likely, didn't even know who Al was. He only remembered names like Jefferson, Washington, Grant, Cleveland, Hamilton, and Franklin and only when they were printed below portraits on green paper.

Two nude women—one blonde and the other a redhead—scampered out from his bedroom across the hallway, trying to conceal themselves as they scavenged the floor for their clothes. Hotsy eyed them up with a smirk, while Johnny and Tomato tried to be less obvious with their glances. The blonde returned Hotsy's smirk.

"Gee, Mr. Valcoro, you didn't have to get us breakfast," Hotsy said.

Tomato discretely punched him for the comment.

"Get out of here," Valcoro said, slapping the blonde on the ass for her hesitation.

Using the same physical flexibility that made them such favorites, the women pulled their dresses on without breaking stride.

"I hope we didn't rush you," Tomato said.

Rush? We waited in the lobby for two hours.

Valcoro shrugged the comment off, having already forgiven the offense.

"Samuel Derby, the name light any bulbs?" Valcoro asked.

"Kentucky? He worked for the West Side O'Donnells until he was killed," Johnny said.

"That's right, blue eyes. You know who pulled the trigger?" Valcoro asked.

"Everyone knows it was Diamond," Hotsy said.

"Everyone knows. But *no one* would go on the stand. Chicago amnesia," Tomato said.

"The amnesia has passed," Valcoro said with a secretive smile.

"Who the hell grew a pair of iron nuts?" Tomato asked.

"We have a witness to the whole thing. George Dillert, goes by the nickname 'Dilly Dawdle.' He was hiding around the corner when Mickey Diamond put a bullet in Sam 'Kentucky' Derby's head."

"And this schmuck is going to go on the stand and look Mickey Diamond in the eyes and tell the court that's the man who killed Kentucky?" Tomato asked.

It was one of those too-good-to-be-true stories about heroes who didn't exist in the real world.

"A few presidents may have helped talk him into it," Valcoro said, then laughed through a deep, phlegm-filled cough.

"If Diamond finds this out, he's going to go after him," Tomato said.

"If Diamond finds out, he'll hunt him and kill him," Johnny corrected.

"You have to admire the set on this guy," Hotsy said.

"Courage, like anything else, can be bought," Valcoro said boastfully, as if his bribing was more courageous than Dillert testifying.

In Johnny's experience, that statement couldn't be further from the truth.

"You're right, Diamond won't take this news too good. That's why you're here," Valcoro said.

"What do you need from us?" Tomato asked.

18

"You're going to Northbrook and keep tabs on him," Valcoro said. He grabbed a sheet with a Chicago police emblem from the table. "He's staying at his mother's. Here's the address."

Tomato took the paper. "How'd you manage to get a hold of this?"

"Prohee named Nash, with some help from his friend in the Chicago police department," Valcoro answered.

"Shouldn't there be police watching the place?" Johnny asked.

"I don't trust the police, Johnny. I bought that paper, which means the police are up for auction," Valcoro said.

"We'll see it done," Tomato said, waving the paper.

Valcoro sipped his orange juice, nodding annoyingly. Then he went back to the newspaper, and his enforcers headed to the elevator.

"Fantastic, we get to sit in the oven again," Hotsy said when they were back inside Tomato's Cadillac.

It was kinder language than what Johnny had spewing in his mind. None of them were thrilled with the idea of sitting in a baking car for something that was little more than babysitting. The thirty miles to Northbrook brought the cool breeze from the lake into the car, reducing Johnny's temperature from scalding to hot. But cooler was cooler.

Derby's body had been found on Roosevelt Street by a group of women on their way to shop. It had made the papers, and though nothing concrete had been printed, even the press knew it was Diamond. But none dared print this or they'd see their name go from the front page to the obituaries.

"Maybe Dillert will be at a swimming pool," Hotsy said from the back seat.

"I can tell you where *you* won't be—in the bed of anyone in that city," Tomato said.

"Like any good detective, I go where the investigation leads," Hotsy said.

Tomato shook his head, suppressing a laugh. Johnny smirked, too hot to completely smile. But as they drove into the heart of the affluent suburb, Johnny's smirk turned to a hateful sulk. The homes stretched out before them with perfectly landscaped green lawns and washed windows were large enough that, in Chicago, they would have housed twenty. But here, they were considered to be of "adequate size" for families of only four or five. The lawns were long enough that only Ruth and Hornsby could hit one out.

"What's the address?" Tomato asked.

Johnny took the note from Tomato and scanned it. "1403 Cherrywood Lane."

Tomato was one of those people who always knew where they were going. Hotsy was awful with directions. So much so that he still got lost inside The Moonlight. Johnny fell somewhere in between, but Tomato always knew how to get somewhere and a dozen ways to leave.

The house built on 1403 Cherrywood Lane was modest in comparison to its neighbors, only because Dillert's mother hadn't spent money on the upkeep. It wasn't run down by any means, but she hadn't flaunted her wealth with bird baths, flag poles, and flowers like her younger neighbors had.

"Hold up. He knows we're coming right? He ain't going to shoot us the moment he opens the door?" Hotsy asked.

"I don't know. That's why you're knocking," Tomato answered.

"I'll knock," Johnny said.

They stepped out of the car, deliberately tramping in full view of the living room bay window, hoping a paranoid Dillert was peeking through the blinds. Johnny knocked on the door and took a step back. Hotsy stood off to the side.

"Coward," Tomato said.

"Says the guy who let Johnny knock," Hotsy countered.

"I didn't *let* him knock, he said he'd knock."

"Sure, Tomato, whatever you say."

"Kid, I swear if Dillert doesn't shoot you, I will."

Johnny knocked again. Tomato scanned the bay window to gauge if there was any movement inside. After a while, he shook his head.

Johnny tried the doorknob. It turned. That wasn't surprising, considering the apparent halo of safety surrounding the town.

20

"George, we work with Valcoro, we're here to check up on you," Johnny called into the house.

When no response came, he pushed the door open further and stepped inside. He repeated himself loudly enough that if George was anywhere in the house, he'd hear him.

Nothing seemed to be out of sorts in the living room. In fact, it seemed that Dillert's mother was a slave to organization, going as far as categorizing her books alphabetically by author.

"Nice place," Hotsy said.

Tomato and Johnny rounded the corner and stepped into the kitchen.

"Oh, shit…" Tomato said.

Hotsy dashed to them. "What is it? Oh, shit."

Dillert's mother sat at her kitchen table, face-down in her bowl of soggy oatmeal. Blood, now coagulated, had dripped from the bullet hole in her head and tainted the milk in her bowl. Bits of her brain and skull on the wall had ruined what had been a comforting undertone of white.

"I thought she was out of town?" Hotsy asked.

"This isn't right. You leave the family out of it," Tomato said.

He rubbed his forehead, shaking his head at the horror and monstrosity of it all.

Johnny disappeared to check the other rooms and came back shaking his head. "Tomato, we have to find Dillert."

Tomato nodded and then bent his head in prayer. "God be with you, and let him welcome you into his kingdom."

Tomato and Hotsy followed Johnny back outside.

"Guns out. But for the love of Christ, Hotsy, please don't shoot at the breeze," Tomato said.

"Fat chance, Tomato. There ain't no breeze," Hotsy said.

The boy had never spoken truer words.

Johnny's light gray vest had turned dark gray from sweat. If it was possible to shoot at the breeze, Johnny would have mowed it down with a Thompson submachine gun and put one in its head to make sure it stayed dead.

Johnny pulled his M1911 pistol from his shoulder holster. He thought of Tomato and Hotsy as his brothers, but the M1911 had been the most reliable thing in his life for the last eight years.

They could only keep their weapons out for mere seconds before people were piling out of their homes. Had they seen them leave the Dillert house? A house that in a few short hours would be an active crime scene of a murder? But the Northbrook citizens paid no attention to them. They were flocking someplace else. Instinct told Johnny something unusual was happening in the idyllic suburb.

"Let's see what all the fuss is about," Johnny said.

They followed the small crowd to two streets over. It was filled with what looked like every citizen Northbrook had. Flashing red and blue lights spun around the neighborhood.

Johnny, Tomato, and Hotsy pushed their way through the crowded street of gasping, horrified people. The police were there, commanding the crowd to back up and not intrude into the crime scene.

"Jesus, is Louie Armstrong putting on an outdoor show?" Hotsy asked.

Johnny led the way. He was the tallest and broadest, and the townsfolk were either going to make room for him to pass or be rammed by his boulder-like shoulders.

"I think we found him," Johnny said.

Tomato gawked at the scene in front of him. "Jesus Christ."

Dillert hung from a noose strung up over the tall maple tree branch hanging over the road. None of the three had ever met George "Dilly Dawdle" Dillert, but all three knew that it was he who swayed with the breeze, his face blue, eyes bulging. His feet hung mere inches above the road. It was entirely possible his tippy toes had scraped against the asphalt as he died. They knew it had been a deliberate move on the part of his murderer—to further toy with his victim. It

22

was a windless day, but his body swayed left and right like a swing set in an abandoned playground.

"Look at his knees," Johnny said.

It didn't take a doctor to know Dillert's knees were broken. The kneecaps were off to the side and nearly at shin level.

"That bastard O'Malley," Tomato said.

Johnny nodded.

It was a truly horrific sight, but Johnny was fixated on something else. Something worse. It wasn't because he had seen sights like that before. No, his indifference was because of the King of Diamonds protruding out of Dillert's breast pocket. Hotsy and Tomato saw it too, and like Johnny, they knew what it meant.

But that wasn't all. Inches away from falling into the sewer grate was a folded piece of paper. Johnny bent down and picked it up.

"Cops will be looking for unfamiliar faces," Tomato warned.

Johnny nodded, and they pushed past the crowd, trying to leave as quickly and unnoticeably as possible. It was the sort of neighborhood where everyone knew each other and no one knew Johnny, Tomato or Hotsy. A good cop would have at least interrogated them. A bad cop would have stuck all three of them with a murder charge and saved himself a barrage of questions, evidence, and a demand for answers from both the press and public.

They rushed into the car, and Tomato, intuitively knowing the quickest way out of the suburb, drove with haste.

"What's on the paper?" Hotsy asked.

Johnny unfolded it. "It's a poem."

"A poem?" Tomato asked.

"You know poetry, Tomato. Romantic stuff. Rhymes about flowers and sunshine," Hotsy said.

"I know what a poem is—"

"You asked," Hotsy said, shrugging.

"Just shut up, will you? I didn't expect to find a poem. What's it say?" Tomato asked.

Johnny read:

> *Heroes Stand, Cowards Lie*
> *I was the latter so now I die*
> *Warriors face the gun*
> *Cowards hang from a rope*
> *Either way I have no fun*
> *I'll be buried in the ground*
> *To rise in heaven I can only hope.*
> *Goodbye world, goodbye wife, goodbye sky*
> *I leave all three to a better man than I.*

"He's a real Van Gogh," Hotsy said.

Tomato let it slide. There were more important things at hand than informing Hotsy that Van Gogh was a painter, not a poet.

Johnny scrunched the note. "These murders make both sides look bad. If word gets out this was a gang killing, Dever will have all of Chicago on his side."

"Yeah, but if it does, maybe Weiss will take his rabid dog out back and kill it. This isn't right, Johnny. Going around killing a civilian… and a woman at that," Tomato said.

"Tomato's right. We should plant that note by Mrs. Dillert. Sign his name to it," Hotsy said.

"Mickey Diamond's death or arrest is not going to be worth us losing millions. Capone won't take that deal," Johnny said.

Tomato grumbled but knew Johnny was right. Their ability to use their judgement was one of the reasons their pay was higher than the average gunman. While most took in fifty to one hundred dollars a week, Johnny, Tomato, and Hotsy (by association) took in a hundred and fifty a week. They had never lost a shipment of alcohol, never had a delivery taken by the police, and weren't afraid to get their hands dirty (bloody).

As they drove alongside the lakeshore, the vision of Dillert hanging lifelessly flooded Johnny's thoughts. Money was certainly part of the reason Dillert would have testified. But maybe he had decided to do it because it was the right thing to do. Diamond had killed his friend, and that was worth dying for.

The suburbanites liked to think their idyllic neighborhoods were safe from the horrors of the big city. There were children in the crowd. Parents had done their best to shield their eyes, but even if they didn't see, they would hear about it. In the city, it would have been forgotten about in a week, but here it was a horrific event that would still be talked about twenty years later. But Johnny's sympathy was short lived. Why should the rich be cushioned from the horrors of the real world? Money doesn't stop that. It wouldn't be fair if it did. Certainly, he didn't want children to see such a gruesome sight. But fourteen or fifteen, that was different. Uncle Sam wouldn't have any problem sending them to slaughter less than a handful of years down the line. Best to have some idea of the horrors of death before leaving.

"Let me tell Vencini," Tomato said when they walked back into The Moonlight.

"This wasn't your fault," Johnny said.

"No, but if you speak, he'll focus on you," Tomato said.

"Yeah, might want to keep those blue marbles closed, Johnny," Hotsy said, putting his arm around Johnny's shoulders.

"We'll blame it on Hotsy. We'll say he was stupid, impulsive, and incompetent. We'd get no rebuttal on that," Tomato said.

"Yeah, yeah, you keep singing, Tomato," Hotsy said.

The sun had set, and the oncoming evening had transformed the unassuming men of Chicago into precarious, gambling, drunken, sexually charged monsters. The music from the band's trombones and saxophones hit their ears as soon as the doors opened. The dance floor was packed, and the tables covered in white cloth and sumptuous spreads of food. Waiters expertly navigated the space. Some of the paying customers listened intently to the music while others flirted, discussed politics or listened to jokes or farfetched stories.

"I need a drink before we head up," Tomato said.

"Let's make this quick," Hotsy said, his eyes catching every attractive woman in the hotel—and with standards like his, it was nearly every woman.

"Gin Rickey, French 75, and a whiskey Old Fashioned Sweet," Tomato ordered.

Hotsy preferred the Gin Rickey because of the seltzer. He was prone to stomach aches and heartburn. Tomato had first tried the fearsome French 75 in Paris. It was a mix of gin, champagne, lemon juice, and two dashes of simple syrup. It was named after the forest-clearing, body-blasting 75 mm field gun. As for Johnny, the whiskey Old Fashioned had been the only love in his life for a while. Just a sip sent waves of relaxation washing over him.

The men who lined the bar were annoyed, even angry, that Tomato was served within seconds. But Johnny dared them to say something with a fierce glare. Intimidation is a silent word, a physical demonstration. A lion often only needs to make eye contact with a fellow beast for it to scamper off, tail tucked between its legs. The bar was lined with sheep, and Johnny enjoyed the hunt.

There were three different things that Johnny, Tomato, and Hotsy did every day without fail. Tomato fought with his wife, Hotsy took a woman to bed, and Johnny enjoyed an Old Fashioned. Johnny's was a comfort and love that never disappointed.

Tomato raised his glass. "To the Dillerts."

Hotsy and Johnny raised their glasses and drank in honor of the fallen.

They turned, their backs resting against the dark-walnut bar, and faced the band. They were a staple at The Moonlight. Each member was well-skilled, but the pianist played like he had fifty fingers.

"Guy could please a dozen women with fingers like that," Hotsy said in awe.

They sipped their drinks as the song went on. It seemed that for every note played, ten more people flooded inside. By the time the song ended, fifty more people had piled in.

"What kind of bite does Valcoro have?" Hotsy asked.

Johnny and Tomato looked at each other, dumbfounded.

"You know, size?" Hotsy tried clarifying.

"What in God's name are you talking about?" Tomato asked.

"I want to know how big his bite is, so I'll know how much of my ass I'll have left," Hotsy said.

Tomato and Johnny could only shake their heads.

"Alright, let's go get our asses chewed," Tomato said.

The lobby, ballroom, and gambling rooms were beyond capacity, and it always made Johnny wonder if the fire department had been paid off too. The gambling rooms housed Black Jack, roulette, craps, and poker. Striding through the crowd, gamblers cheered and cursed in equal measure. The hotel's women exiting the gambling rooms smiled at Johnny, Tomato, and Hotsy, reaching for their hands or crotch.

"Not yet, but soon. Go dance, you're going to need to be limber," Hotsy cooed at them.

The elevator was at three-quarter capacity, filled with men taking women to one of the pleasure rooms. The men moved their wedding rings to their right hands, and one of the newly naked left hands reached for a button below seven.

"You hit that button, I'll break your hand," Johnny said.

The man looked taken aback, his hand paralyzed.

"He ain't lying," Hotsy said.

The man flung his hand back. The doors *pinged* and then opened. Hoagie was still seated, and it was testament to the stool's craftsmanship that it was still intact.

After a quick greeting, Hoagie nodded them through.

Valcoro stood in front of the glass panels, looking out at the city stretched before him like a sea of shining stars. At this height, it was impossible to not feel that the entire universe was sprawled out in front of you for the taking. He had an empty glass in one hand and rubbed his dark eyes with the other.

"Mr. Valcoro," Tomato said.

But Valcoro either didn't hear or ignored him. Tomato repeated himself and only after a third time did Valcoro react.

27

"Sorry. I was… deep in thoughts," he said.

Thoughts? Johnny had only ever known Valcoro to have basic thoughts—including deciding what he was hungry for, if he truly had to go to the bathroom or if it could wait, and what ethnicity of woman he was lusting after. But the way he had said "thoughts" signified something deeper and far more worrisome.

"I'm afraid we have some bad news," Tomato said.

"Dillert's dead," Valcoro said, still staring out at the city.

"Yeah…" Tomato said.

Valcoro looked as though he would disappear back into his thoughts. Hotsy was too oblivious to know what was coming, and Tomato had taken the responsibility of telling Valcoro they had failed to protect George "Dilly Dawdle" Dillert. So, even if it was best Johnny didn't speak, he did.

"There could be a chance he gave you up," Johnny said.

Valcoro laughed. It wasn't uncommon for him to do so anytime Johnny spoke. It was a way to make him feel worthless. But there was nothing funny about his laugh now. It was one filled with pain and grief.

"Follow me."

The Body

The entirety of the elevator ride to the fourteenth floor, Valcoro had his head turned toward the ceiling. When the doors opened, the hallway was vacant except for two men in gray fedoras and double-breasted hem vests of the same color, standing guard outside room 1426. They stepped aside and opened the door as Valcoro lumbered down the hallway. A strong odor wafted out of the room. It was a smell recognized but never welcome. It sent a hot stream of bile into Johnny's chest. Years ago, he would have vomited from it.

But not now.

The origin of the horrendous smell was the bed. Atop the bed was a body, stripped of its clothes with only a King of Diamonds playing card in its left hand. The man on the bed was roughly the same age as Valcoro, approaching the back nine of his forties, but—having abused their bodies for the last three decades—they both looked a decade and a half older than that. The man had been a staple of the hotel, seen at the bar, in front of the stage, and in numerous bedrooms. His name was Antonio Varelly. He had bootlegged at the onset of Prohibition in 1920, bringing whiskey down from Canada along the Wisconsin coast of Lake Michigan. But Varelly was an old man in a young man's game and had been on the way out when Johnny came to Chicago.

Varelly's eyes were open in a disturbing way, and like the *Mona Lisa*, no matter what angle, it seemed that he was staring right at you.

"Mickey Diamond," Tomato said.

Valcoro nodded and sat at the foot of the bed.

"There was one by Dillert's body," Hotsy said, pointing at the King of Diamonds.

The King of Diamonds was Mickey Diamond's calling card. He had shown a considerable amount of brass by placing his signature on the body. But there was little proof for police to convict. You can't sentence a man to prison with just a playing card.

"Was there a poem too?" Valcoro asked.

"There was," Tomato replied.

Valcoro pulled a crumpled note from his pocket and held it out for Tomato. He took it and read:

> *Let this man stand as a lesson*
> *Let this be the fate of all weasels and rats*
> *Your class is now in session*
> *Rats are rats, no matter Republicans or Democrats*
> *You try me again, you'll never be found*
> *You'll disappear*
> *Deep into the ground*
> *Better believe you have much to fear*

"Can we get a goddamn blanket on him?" Valcoro asked, his voice growing louder with each word.

The other men moving in and out of the room hurried to find one.

"Two Shits and me, we grew up together. Been out of the game for years. Just wanted to live out the rest of his days with booze and dames," Valcoro said.

"Why would Diamond want him dead?" Hotsy asked.

"Two Shits did one last job for me," Valcoro said.

"He got you Dillert's address," Johnny said. The reference to rats hadn't been a term of endearment.

Valcoro nodded, regret wrinkling his leathered face.

The fact that Mickey Diamond had personally entered The Moonlight, a headquarters for not only Vencini Valcoro and his crew, but a place frequented by Al Capone himself, showed a level of fearlessness few possessed and even fewer flaunted. It had to be Mickey Diamond himself who had killed Antonio "Two Shits" Varelly. If he had ordered the hit, there would be no King of Diamonds in Two Shits' cold hand and no poem. He only placed that playing card when he had personally ended the life of his victim. It was a "duty" most men in his position would have passed off to a subordinate and then left town for a few days in order to secure an airtight alibi. But not Mickey Diamond.

There was a knock on the door. A man in his mid-fifties and dressed in a red suit stepped into the room. Out of habit, he insured his suit was free of any wrinkles and that his slicked-back jet-black hair was in place.

"Cardinal, thanks for coming," Valcoro said.

The Cardinal. The man everyone under Valcoro, himself included, went to for advice.

The Cardinal nodded and went to the bed. He bowed his head and made the sign of the cross. The Cardinal had known Two Shits. The two had run jobs together, dined together, and gone on whiskey trips to Canada.

Valcoro, The Cardinal, and Two Shits had started off in much the same way Johnny, Hotsy, and Tomato had. Johnny didn't hold much love for Valcoro, but watching him sit on the edge of the bed and gaze upon a dead man he had considered a brother was hard.

"Cared about two things—booze and women," The Cardinal said.

"Both left him broke and queasy," Valcoro added.

The Cardinal waved away the two men who had finally found a blanket to cover the body. They looked to Valcoro who gave them an annoyed glare as if he had never asked for the blanket in the first place. The two men backed up

31

and stood there awkwardly with the blanket sprawled open. They were two guys trying to work their way up and prove they could add something. Unfortunately for them, in Valcoro's eyes, they had failed at the simple task of getting a blanket and now were just being rude.

The Cardinal and Valcoro reminisced about their friend and their shared history—a history that spanned decades. Listening to them and seeing the love for their friend in their eyes transported Johnny in time. Some day he, Hotsy or Tomato would be dead, and the surviving two would remember the fallen. The thought poisoned his mood further.

"I'll get this cleaned up. I want every one of you downstairs. We're going to drink in honor of our fallen friend," Valcoro said.

Johnny, Tomato, and Hotsy followed The Cardinal out of the room, Valcoro swearing at the two men still holding the blanket to cover Two Shits' body. Johnny knew they would get no love from Valcoro as both were far from Italian. Polish or Irish perhaps. It was likely they'd be changing out the toilet paper rolls in every room tomorrow.

"I take it you heard about Dillert?" Tomato asked when they were in the elevator.

The Cardinal nodded. "And his mother. This life we live… it is dangerous. But most of us acknowledge there are rules… Diamond… he doesn't follow rules. He's a wild animal."

"We took the poem he left by Dillert," Johnny said.

"That was the right call," The Cardinal said. "If this war stays between gangsters, Chicago belongs to us. If the public starts getting killed, it will be the end of us all."

"Maybe this would of forced Weiss' hand. And he would of gotten rid of Diamond himself," Johnny said.

"Johnny, Diamond's a mythical creature. Like a werewolf. We need to keep his existence a rumor," The Cardinal said.

"I heard he shot a guy at a bar sitting at the far end. Just to prove he could hit him," Hotsy said.

"Yeah and his first wife, her dog, and the poor bloke delivering the mail who decided to talk about the weather," Tomato added.

"Maybe his death is worth a million," Johnny said.

"I have to tell you, Cardinal. The fact this werewolf's feeding off civilians doesn't sit well with me," Tomato said.

"You did the right thing," The Cardinal said.

Johnny nodded his appreciation of the comment. "Somehow, Diamond knew who got the list of names for Vencini."

"He got the name from a prohibition agent," The Cardinal said.

"It was a prohee who gave Two Shits the list," Johnny said.

"Same one," The Cardinal said.

"Nash?" Johnny asked.

"So that prohee betrayed him?" Tomato asked.

"The agent called in a favor with a friend of his in the Chicago Police," The Cardinal said.

"That's why we shouldn't trust them. Those bastards with badges are cowards and will roll over first chance they get," Hotsy said.

"We offered Nash money. Mickey Diamond offered him his life," The Cardinal said.

Johnny knew that Tomato thought Nash should have stood his ground. Hotsy thought so too but only because Tomato did. But Johnny couldn't blame Nash for what he had done. They played an illegal game—the rules changed, and no one could say someone had cheated. The North and South side gangs had too many differences to count. Chief among them was that in the North, people came and went. But if you joined Al Capone's gang, you didn't join for a month or a year, you joined for life. Nash playing both sides may seem like a betrayal to Tomato and Hotsy, but to most, it was leaving one company for another with better pay and incentives.

The elevator door opened with the familiar *ping*. Music and conversation flooded in. The lobby was packed elbow to elbow. A new, more upbeat band had taken the stage now that dinner was over. Couples danced to the Charleston, laughing and smiling as they swung their arms and swiveled their heels.

The bar was lined with people holding out empty glasses or dollars bills. The women of the hotel stalked the dance floor looking for men with overfilled glasses and fat wallets.

"You staying for that drink?" Johnny asked.

"No," The Cardinal answered. "You know me. Besides, when is it ever one drink with Vencini?"

Johnny nodded. It was always one drink. One long drink extending from glass to glass.

"Vencini better get down here for that drink because there are many a fine dames on that dance floor," Hotsy said.

"You know there is a man lying dead upstairs?" Tomato said.

"No better reminder that we have to keep living," Hotsy said.

Even though Hotsy was only a few years younger than Johnny, he had the maturity of a sixteen year old. He didn't view death as a permanent thing, more of a "you got me this time." But it had always been a game of tag. You put a hit on one of ours, we put one on yours. "Ours" had never been anyone who was more than an acquaintance. Hotsy had seen killings but not at the same rate as Tomato and Johnny.

The hotel's women strolled past, their sweltering gazes lingering on Hotsy in particular.

"The beast in me is raging," Hotsy said.

Some of the prostitutes Johnny had seen before, both publicly and privately, and others he was seeing for the first time. Valcoro always made sure he had fresh "attractions." There was a woman for every strain of desire. Hair colors ranged from silvery blonde to fiery red to raven black. There was the tall and thin, the short and stocky, the well-endowed and the willowy. Every man had his own taste, and The Moonlight had the cuisine to satisfy his palate.

"I'm going to sneak out before Vencini has me pumped so full of giggle juice that I'm out on the dance floor," The Cardinal said.

"That's the point!" Hotsy said.

"God forgives all sins except for my dancing," The Cardinal said.

In the years Johnny had known him, The Cardinal had never been one for the parties. His consumption of alcohol was limited to his bi-weekly embrace of the Blood of Christ.

The Cardinal disappeared out of the revolving front door just as Valcoro stepped to the bar. Every bartender stopped what they were doing to take his order of a round of whiskeys—a shot for every person at the bar, thirty some in all. Some had known Two Shits—they had listened to his bullshit stories or had slept with him or lost money to him in card games—while others only wanted the free shot.

Valcoro raised his glass. The bar followed. "I knew Two Shits since we were in Sister O'Callaghan's second grade class," Valcoro started. "His knuckles had scars from that Irish nun smacking them with a ruler so often. Mine, sure they got hit, I mean what else brings a nun joy but beating a kid's knuckles?"

There was a smattering of courtesy laughter.

"But my knuckles should look a hell of a lot worse than what they do. Two Shits took the blame for everything. It continued that way for forty years and ended today when he died taking the ruler for me again." Valcoro's voice faltered and cracked. "… Antonio, may God take you, keep you in his arms. I love you brother. As you stand before God, I make this solemn vow, vengeance rides on a pale horse. May God bring you peace."

While the others drank, Valcoro held his glass out a little longer, savoring the memories more than the drink.

The room temperature whiskey (meaning whiskey a few degrees shy of Hell) burned Johnny's throat on the way down, but damn, it was the best burn. It brought a wave of relaxation and a craving for an Old Fashioned. No night was complete without a half-dozen or so of that delectable poison. The muddled orange, maraschino cherries, and crushed sugar cube mixed into a nectar of the Gods. Like all alcoholic drinks it was against the law. Forbidden. But Adam and Eve had broken the one rule God had given them. If they had sacrificed

35

immortality and a perfect world for an apple, Johnny could break man's law for an Old Fashioned. He ordered one and took the liberty of ordering a French 75 for Tomato and a Gin Rickey for Hotsy. Both took them with an appreciative nod, promising to catch the next round. Tomato's promise was truth. Hotsy's was always a kind gesture never carried out.

"Mr. Valcoro, you going to get us dessert or do we need to go scrounging in the dumpsters?" Hotsy asked.

"We have honored Two Shits with a drink, and now we honor him with dames," Valcoro said.

He waved the hotel's women over. The man had complete control over everyone and everything in the hotel. It was his own personal Wild West.

Valcoro wrapped his arms around as many of the women as he could, and it just so happened his reach ended on the backside of a blonde named Betty. He ran his fingers along it like it was braille.

"Tomato, you take Ruth. Here's a room key for you," Valcoro said.

Ruth was a tall blonde in an emerald dress that revealed private details like a diary. Tomato finished his French 75 and took the offered key with the number 215 etched on the golden key chain.

Ruth grabbed Tomato's hand and led him to the elevator.

"What to do with Hotsy Totsy?" Valcoro said, tapping his fingers on Betty's backside.

"Let me take these women off your plate," Hotsy offered. His eyes fell on each and every one of them, first on their breasts, then hips and lips, and at last, their eyes.

"Donna, Kat, get this kid out of here," Valcoro said, slapping both their butts and then tossing the room key for Hotsy. "And be sure to spank his ass like his momma should have!"

There were three women left next to Valcoro, meaning one of them should have been meant for Johnny. But Valcoro was greedy and way too confident in his skills in the bedroom. He was also no longer short of being sloshed. He was fast adrift on tumultuous waves of intoxication, and Johnny knew that the lightning flashing in his eyes would soon be followed by thunder. He was like a tornado in an open field, and Johnny was the only object to destroy.

Johnny took a drink of his Old Fashioned and waited for Valcoro and his third-grade ridicule.

Just get it over with.

"Go upstairs to room 518. You'll find a nigger up there for you, you half-breed," Valcoro said.

Whether out of drunken clumsiness or actual intent, his slap across Johnny's shoulders was anything but gentle. Johnny couldn't even look him in the eye, for Johnny's cobalt-blue eyes were nothing but targets. Instead, he grabbed the key and, keeping his eyes on the gold-swirled burgundy carpet, stormed to the elevator. Once inside, he drove his fist into one of its walls. He didn't even know why he hit the fifth floor button. Where he longed to go was the lakeshore, and hopefully get some remnants of a breeze. The elevator *ping* had become an annoyance, and if he could have found the origin of the sound, he would have driven his fist into that too. If Valcoro wanted to talk about knuckles, Johnny's were covered in perpetual bruises and had delivered permanent facial disfiguration to over a dozen men.

He pushed through the elevator doors before they were fully opened, smacking his shoulders against them. Something that only increased his anger. He swore at the annoying *ping*. He took a left, cursing under his breath.

"Whore! Trying to overcharge me!" a man shouted as he stormed down the hallway, his shoes and homburg hat in his hands.

He looked like he was nearing both his fifties and the limit on a weighing scale. His red hair was balding on top except for a narrow strand bridging together the two continents of hair. Was he a bootlegger? Doubtful. Congressman? Possibly. Some rich prick from the suburbs whose old lady was sick of his flatulent, overweight ass? Most likely.

The number on the door was 518. Johnny peeked into the room. The woman inside clutched her nightgown close to her chest, alarmed at what had happened.

"That dew dropper short change you?" Johnny asked her.

"Don't worry about it, everything's Jake," she said.

Not everything is fine. Far from it.

Johnny would worry about it. Not that he truly cared… just that it gave him an excuse for driving his fist into somebody's face and not be reprimanded for it. Unless the man did turn out to be a politician or police captain. But anger didn't think of tomorrow. Anger thought of now. And it demanded action. Truthfully, Johnny had had a strong urge to punch somebody all day. It had started in the oven-hot car, intensified among the coffins and caskets, and maxed out about two minutes ago with Valcoro's insult. The timer on the bomb was up. That cheap bastard scurrying down the hallway was the punching bag Johnny needed. He stormed after him like a thunder cloud, his eyes flashing lightning.

The man tried to jog while putting his shoes on at the same time, something far out of his skill set. Obviously, it had been decades since he had last been able to reach his toes. Johnny grabbed him by the back of his shirt and slammed him against the wall. He waited for the man to see his face before he drove his fist across his. Punching somebody had always been an enjoyable pain, like tugging on a loose tooth.

"You owe the girl her cut," Johnny said.

"I gave her what's she's worth. I gave her more than what she's worth," the man said, panting, his teeth covered in blood.

Johnny slammed him against the wall again and drove his fist into the man's flabby stomach. The woman from room 518 stepped out, her arms covering her breasts, clearly uncomfortable with what was playing out.

"Let him go. It's not worth a scene," she said.

"Did you have sex with her?" Johnny asked.

"No," the man answered.

The blows to his face and head had left angry bruises and swellings that would blossom into throbbing pain.

Johnny's grip was vice-like. The man couldn't escape even if he squirmed like a fish. He could only answer and hope Johnny believed what he said.

Johnny turned his head to look at the woman. "Is he telling the truth?"

"I'm telling the truth!" the man said.

Johnny pointed a menacing finger at him, and even though it wouldn't fire a bullet, it was more threatening than a gun. "You shut your mouth. You talk when I tell you to talk. Understand?"

The man nodded frantically.

"Do you understand?" Johnny asked, slamming him against the wall.

"I understand," the man said, shaking so hard with fear that his stomach jiggled like gelatin.

"Is that true?" Johnny asked, turning his gaze back to the woman.

"Yes… he wanted a finger," the woman replied, both embarrassed and unsure if she should answer.

"Alright, you finger her. That's half a dollar. Pay up," Johnny said.

"The finger wasn't for me…" the woman said.

Johnny looked at her for clarification.

"He's been in my room for close to an hour. The only thing that got hard was the mattress. I asked him what was wrong, and he exploded," the woman said.

It was hotel policy that what happened in a Moonlight room stayed in a Moonlight room. Many adulterous policemen, prohibition agents, judges, city councilmen, and even congressmen believed that. Now, they all did Al Capone's bidding for free. Some men came clean, but those who preferred the company of other men risked scandal and ruined careers.

"Listen to me, cake eater," Johnny said, rounding back on the man, "you can either give her fifty cents or I can get a pair of pliers and pull the silver fillings from your teeth. Doesn't matter to me. Either way, the woman's getting her silver."

The man frantically reached into his pocket and removed two Standing Liberty quarters and, with shaking hands, held them out for Johnny to take.

"You pay the lady," Johnny ordered.

He shoved the man in the right direction, nearly knocking him over.

The man gave the woman the two quarters, looked to Johnny, and after receiving a nod, bounced off to the elevators like a bowling ball careening off the gutters.

"You shouldn't have done that," the woman said.

"Yeah, maybe not. But you got your money, didn't you? Valcoro doesn't keep girls around that don't get paid," Johnny said.

"I mean thank you for getting me the money. But you didn't have to do *that*," she said.

"Yeah, well it's been a long, hot day," Johnny said with no hint of an apologetic tone.

"Well, I have an antidote for that. Care for a drink?" she asked.

Valcoro had seen Johnny storm to the elevators. If he went down now, there would surely be a juvenile joke with words like "quick" or "premature."

"Sure," Johnny said.

He followed her into the room. The woman took a puff of a fresh cigarette, Lucky Strike by the name on the pack, and set it against the ashtray, then went into the bathroom. The faucet ran for several seconds and then shut off again. She came out drying her hands with a red towel embroidered with a golden M. Her laced black kimono robe sparingly covered her smooth flesh, a color somewhere between beige and caramel. The sight was lethal enough to dethrone the katana as Japan's most dangerous weapon.

He had intended to take in a quick photograph of her body, but his eyes had ended up drawing a sketch. He looked away, hoping she hadn't noticed.

"And who is this knight in a fedora standing in front of me?" she asked, taking a puff of her Lucky Strike and closing the door.

Johnny removed his fedora and held it in front of him as he took in the room. "They call me Johnny."

"They *call* you? That's not your name?" she asked.

"No," Johnny said.

The woman, somewhat annoyed with his fidgeting, took his fedora from his hands and set it on the table.

"Do I need to beat your real name out of you?" she asked.

"I don't hear you giving me yours," Johnny said.

"I don't hear you asking me for it."

"What's your name?"

"Paris Dawson."

"Like the city?"

"Like the city."

"Giovanni De Luca."

"Johnny? That's as creative as they could get? What, don't they like you?"

Johnny was quiet, awkwardly diverting his attention to the room before bringing it back to Paris.

"What about you? You don't look like a normal negro," Johnny said.

"*I don't look normal.* Wow. It's a good thing you're paying for this conversation," Paris said.

"I mean you aren't nearly as dark as some."

"And most of you Italians around here don't have blue eyes, yet, here we are."

But immediately after, she was worried about what she had said, unsure of how he would react.

"Sorry," Paris said.

"Nah, don't worry about it. I deserved it… Wait, did you say you are charging me for the conversation?" Johnny asked.

"Unless you're planning on moving to the bed?"

Johnny shifted his gaze from Paris to the bed. Half-made, damp with sweat, and God only knew what else. Twenty minutes ago, a closet fag had been there, wanting a finger jammed into his ass. It would be a pass for him. But, truthfully, that wasn't the only reason. Those caskets and coffins at Al's had stuck with him all day, and if he was entirely honest, they had stuck with him far longer than that. He hadn't had an attack since Al's, meaning he was due. Having it happen in the middle of the act would be cringe-worthy. And the heat…

"Nah, do you care if we just talk?" Johnny asked.

"Talk… boy, you sure know how to order off menu," Paris said.

She sauntered to the dresser and scooped what little remaining ice there was into a glass, poured whiskey into it, and handed it to Johnny.

"None for you?" Johnny asked.

"No," Paris answered.

Johnny took a sip and nearly gagged from the tainted, liquid fire he had swallowed. That wasn't whiskey. The alcohol in his glass was overpowering and had no taste of the sugar maple charcoal process it should have and far from the balance of sweet and oaky he knew and loved.

"You want the real stuff, you'll have to go to another room," Paris said.

Johnny abandoned the glass on the counter. There was not a chance in hell he would finish that skunk piss.

"Want water?" she asked.

"I don't know. Is it the same quality as that whiskey?" Johnny asked.

"No of course not… It's fresh from the toilet."

Johnny chuckled. "You sold me."

Paris took his glass and then strutted into the bathroom. The toilet flushed.

"Just joshing you," she assured.

She stepped out, the glass of water out-stretched for him to take. He took it and thanked her.

"So why do they call you Johnny?" she asked, taking a seat on the edge of the bed.

Johnny's eyes flashed to her smooth legs, further revealed now with her nightgown hugging tightly above her thighs.

"Giovanni is Italian for John. Valcoro nicknamed me Johnny as a permanent reminder I'm not full blooded."

"That matters?"

"To some."

"Your mother or father Italian?"

"My father. He met my mother on the boat over here."

"Where was she from?"

"Schönfeld, Germany."

"You're a Hun. Should I call you Kaiser?"

Johnny smirked. "If it pleases you."

"So your mother and father… love at first sight?"

"I don't know about love at first sight. She was seventeen. He was twenty. They left with a couple of suitcases between them—"

"And arrived with a baby in her belly."

Johnny nodded.

"Make sure you thank her for those eyes."

"These eyes aren't a gift."

"Why?"

"Because any chance of me blending in is gone."

"That's not a curse, Giovanni. That's a blessing. Wear it like armor."

He hadn't been called Giovanni in years. Hearing her say his birth name brought back memories of his parents and his grandmother. To some, nostalgia was a light breeze. To Johnny, nostalgia was a hurricane.

And here it came.

He took a sip of his water, closing his eyes. His face flushed with color, and he became overly aware of how damn hot it was in the room. His breathing escalated. He focused on the window and the bright lights outside instead of the memories flashing before him.

And then it was gone.

"What about you? You wear yours like armor?" Johnny asked.

"My black skin and your blue eyes are not on the same scale, handsome. Plenty of white folks with eyes like yours, maybe not as fierce but same color," Paris said.

"You know the secret behind my eyes. Spill yours."

"Maybe another time."

"You're getting paid to be my company. Or should I ask for a finger too?"

"How's this one?" she asked, holding up her long middle finger.

Johnny smiled. He had always been drawn to feisty women.

43

"Easy bearcat," Johnny said, holding his hands up in surrender.

Paris scoffed and leaned against the counter.

"How'd you get involved in this?" he asked.

"What are you, the police? I feel like I'm being interrogated," Paris said.

"Sorry. I've never done this before."

"Done what? Been alone with a woman?"

Johnny laughed nervously. "No, I've been with a woman. I mean just talking."

Don't stare into my eyes or it will come back.

He took a drink, trying to escape the awkwardness that hung in the room like heavy smoke. Chatting was not a skill he possessed.

"So, then why are we?" she asked.

"Vencini sent me up here, if I go down too soon…"

"You won't be a real man."

Johnny nodded.

"What were you planning on paying me?" she asked.

"Depends on how satisfied I am when I leave this room."

Paris seemed to consider his response as she walked to the window. She took a drag from her Lucky Strike, exhaling a perfect ball of smoke toward the ceiling. Her shiny, oil black hair was styled in finger waves, keeping its true length a mystery. Johnny's eyes ran the length of her body before fixating on the way she rubbed her fingers on her cigarette.

"My grandmother was a slave," Paris said, staring out at the city. "In Georgia… a city called Eden. She had worked the cotton fields when she was younger and then moved into the house when she was fourteen. A relationship began with the white man that owned her. He was married, handful of kids. I don't know if it was consensual. I like to imagine it was. War broke out. She got pregnant. He gave her freedom and put her on a train heading north along the Mississippi to Missouri. From there, she went to Milwaukee… had my mother. My mother was involved with a white man… my father… quite the scandal. There's the reason for the cream in my chocolate."

44

"How'd you end up in Chicago?"

"I bounced around city to city. Minneapolis, St. Louis, Indianapolis, Atlantic City, New York. Got on a bus and stayed on until the last stop."

"Don't want to set up roots?"

"I guess I'm searching for something I haven't found."

Johnny nodded. She had no idea how relatable that was. He stood and joined her by the window. She studied him to see if he had changed his mind about moving to the bed. But his eyes were on the city stretching out in front of them.

"You got a piece of real estate down there?" he asked.

"An apartment on Dearborn and 23rd. I've got a great view," Paris said.

Her eyes went to the clock.

The gesture wasn't missed, and Johnny finished his water and set the glass on the dresser.

"Thanks for the conversation," Johnny said.

He dug into his pockets, removed a five and some ones, and tossed them on the dresser.

"This isn't necessary," Paris said, grabbing the money from the dresser and holding it out for him.

"Take the rest of the night off… See you later, half-breed," Johnny said.

He put his fedora back on and tipped it out of respect.

"Good night half-breed," Paris said.

The Nettesheims

Johnny left The Moonlight and its monsters behind. He had always enjoyed solitary drives. They helped him unwind and go over things—things from that day, that week. But the longer the drive, the deeper and further back into his past his thoughts took him. It was as if his brain was a maze, the minor annoyances of a day were easy to find. But deep in the center, surrounded by dead ends, were his most vulnerable thoughts. No matter how hard he tried to change the maze so that they were kept hidden and unfindable, he always found the center. Cicero was the perfect drive in terms of distance for Johnny. It was enough time to navigate through the outer layers but not enough time to hit the center and the thoughts he tried to keep buried and caged there.

The town itself had become a second Chicago for Al Capone and the South Side since Dever had become mayor. A home to casinos, brothels, and breweries, it was the wettest town in America. On 22nd street was the Hawthorne Hotel, Hawthorne Smoke Shop, and the Anton Hotel. All three silently screamed "vice." But even though the vices were ever present, it was the type of idyllic town people thought of when they heard the word "Midwest." Johnny preferred Cicero over the Northern suburbs of Northbrook, Lake Forest, and Glenview. The people here worked for everything they got. They weren't like the affluent and entitled who populated the North Shore.

Johnny's business dealings with Valcoro and Capone had brought him to the city nearly a hundred times. It was late, perhaps too late for a visit. Johnny decided, on his march up the stoop to the beaten-down tan apartment building, that he would slide the envelope under the door. But after taking a quick eye count of the money inside the white envelope, it was clear that it wouldn't fit. Not even with the unevenness of the floor and the chipped door. A mouse could squeeze through. But a mouse could bend and twist, and although cash was crooked, it couldn't contort.

Johnny knocked on the door of apartment four. There was a good chance it would go unanswered. He checked his watch—9:30. He hesitated and debated knocking a third time. He turned to leave. The door opened, and a woman stood behind it, her dark blonde hair disheveled from sleep.

"Johnny," she said.

"Sorry for such a late visit, Cilly," Johnny said.

"It's okay," she whispered. She looked behind her, apprehensive. "I just don't want him to wake up."

Footsteps came from behind the door. Cilly closed her eyes tightly.

"Sorry," Johnny mouthed.

"Who is it mom?" a boy's high-pitched voice asked.

"It's Johnny," Cilly answered.

She stepped aside, and a young boy with shaggy chestnut brown hair, patted down in spots and sticking straight up in others, came into view, his sleepy face brightening up with excitement.

"Johnny!" he nearly shouted.

"Hey Wally, how you doing?" Johnny asked.

"You know, living," the nine year old said, with the air of a person seven decades older.

"Yeah, living. It will be easier when it's forty degrees colder."

"For sure, it's so goddamn hot out."

"Wally! You excuse yourself!" Cilly said, her face blushing with embarrassment.

Johnny tried his best to not smile or it would ruin Cilly's attempt to control Wally's language.

"Excuse me… but everyone says it, mom," Wally said.

"Well, do you want to grow up to be a gentleman?" Cilly asked.

"I didn't mean no offense by it, Johnny," Wally said.

"Any… you didn't mean *any* offense," Cilly corrected.

Johnny nodded and tried not to return Cilly's half-formed smirk.

"Did you want to come in for something to drink?" Wally asked.

"It's late," Johnny said.

"Not really, besides it's too hard to sleep in this da… in this heat," Wally said, catching himself.

"We have milk, I'm sure you don't want coffee," Cilly said, nodding for Johnny to enter.

Johnny stepped in. The apartment was modest, and that was putting it politely. It was a horribly kept building, but Cilly wasn't in a position to complain about the holes in the wall and the faulty furnace, at least not until winter. Artificial heat was the last thing on anyone's mind. The couch was a relic, the springs threatening to poke through in spots. The nicest piece of furniture was a black leather high point wing back armchair in front of the window.

"I'll just take water, thanks," Johnny said.

Milk was too thick in this heat, and its cost, twenty-eight cents for a half-gallon, was too high for Cilly to waste on Johnny. Wally's growing bones needed the calcium.

Cilly disappeared into the kitchen and, as Wally took a seat on the couch, Johnny put the envelope on the nightstand beside the door. Living below the poverty line wasn't limited to a small percentage of people like Cilly. While some enjoyed the perks of the Roaring Twenties, over sixty percent of the country was deprived of them. Mostly farmers, Negros, immigrants, coal miners, ship builders, and textile workers—employment fields that had seen huge spikes during the war. Now because of prohibition, barley demands had dropped ninety percent. The Nettesheims were not farmers nor were they coal miners, ship builders, or textile workers. They belonged to a much worse demographic—the hereditary poor. Poverty had been passed down in Cilly's family like green eyes or a widow's peak.

Johnny didn't need to look in the fridge or cupboards to know they were as barren as dirt fields.

"I've been talking to mom about getting a job," Wally said.

"A job? Don't you want to play all summer?" Johnny asked.

"I would start in September. Instead of going back to school."

"Why, don't you like school?"

"It's ok, but they don't teach me anything useful. I mean, I hear all the men talk about factories, cars or the stock market, and I don't know none of…I mean *any* of that stuff."

"There's other jobs than just those."

"But those jobs can have apprentices. That's the only way I'll learn. My dad can't teach me anything."

"Sorry it took so long," Cilly said, holding out a glass of water. "It takes a while for the pipes to clear from the hot water."

"It's no problem," Johnny said.

He downed the water like it was his first glass after a long exodus across the desert, leaving only a sip or two—enough that Cilly wouldn't have to ask if he wanted a refill. But instead of looking at his emptying glass, her eyes had caught the white envelope on the stand beside the door.

"Johnny, you don't have to," she said.

Johnny raised his hand to stop her. "Don't mention it."

She clearly wished to mention it further, but bit her lip. A gesture that made Johnny wish he would have at least attempted sliding the money under the door. Guilt was not something he had intended to cause.

"Well, young man, I think it's time you go back to bed," Cilly said.

A mumbled noise came from the kitchen. A man stumbled out, his arms pressed back, causing his chest to blow out awkwardly. It looked as if he was attempting to walk for the first time in his life. His nearly-black hair flopped to the sides but did little to hide his bulging eyes. Eyes that were so black that his pupils were indistinguishable from the irises. He groaned indecipherably before falling flat on his face. Johnny motioned to help him, but Cilly beat him to it.

"Come on honey, let's go back to bed. It's just Johnny saying hello," Cilly said.

"Hi there, Clarence, how are you?" Johnny asked.

He felt stupid for even asking that much. Since Johnny had known him, Clarence hadn't spoken a word.

"I'll see myself out, Cilly. Thanks for the water. Take care, Clarence," Johnny said.

With a strength that did not match her frame, Cilly pulled Clarence to his feet. It was surely a muscle memory learned through repetition. No doubt there had been times when Cilly had been unable to lift her husband from the cold, hard wood floor. Times she could only cry and place a pillow under his head and sleep by his side.

She had her arm wrapped around his back and half-dragged half-carried Clarence back to their bedroom.

Wally's face was beet-red, his eyes glued to the floor. "I'm sorry," he mumbled.

"Nothing to be sorry for, unless you broke wind. Did you fart, Wally?" Johnny asked.

Wally broke into a fit of laughter. There was nothing funnier to a nine year old than the word *fart*. After his laughter came to an end, a silence fell, as short as Wally himself.

"She cried yesterday," he said.

The tone had shifted drastically in seconds, but to children, seconds are more like minutes. Time moves slower when you're young.

"How come?" Johnny asked.

"I think sometimes… it just hits her, you know?" Wally said.

Johnny was quiet, unsure of what to say.

Wally looked down the hall, his face contorting with some unspeakable expression from the abyss of his thoughts.

"She showed me some of my dad's medals," Wally said.

"What did you think of them?"

"I can't ask him about them. I can't ask how or why he got them. So I don't know, you know?"

"Life is cruel sometimes."

"Did you get medals?"

"A couple. Not as many as your dad though."

"What for?"

"For being a big enough idiot to go."

"You were in France?"

Johnny nodded. "Do you know where that is?"

"Europe."

"Can you name a city?"

"Pa—"

"Besides Paris."

"Cantigny."

"Where's that?"

"France," Wally said, failing to hide his pleasure at his quick wit.

"Lip like that and your teachers will slap you."

Wally gave a polite chuckle, but it was clear he hadn't found the joke funny and was only being kind. Children are the toughest critics.

"Mom said that's where my dad was," Wally said.

"He was part of the first battle that America fought over there," Johnny said.

"Is that where you fought?"

Johnny shook his head. "No. I was in Montfaucon-d'Argonne and a few others."

51

"Is that near Paris?"

"Sort of. Northeast of it."

"My mom said my dad wrote every chance he got. She tells me he was brave."

"He *is* brave," Johnny said.

Wally was silent.

Johnny rose from the couch and offered his empty glass to Wally. "I'm heading for the hills, bud."

"You coming back soon?" Wally asked, rising from the couch too.

"You know I'll be around." He rubbed Wally's head.

"Can you name a city in Germany?" Wally asked.

"Ber—" Johnny started.

"Besides Berlin," Wally said with a smirk that would have made his mother wonder what mischief he had gotten into this time.

"Schönfeld."

"Where's that?" Wally asked, clearly not expecting an answer.

"Germany," Johnny answered.

Wally smiled genuinely, granting Johnny a small victory for matching his wit.

"Where my mother was from. I'll see you later, buddy," Johnny said.

"See you, Johnny," Wally said. He checked over his shoulder to see if his mother was nearby. Seeing that the coast was clear, he added, "Good luck beating this goddamn heat."

He beamed with a victorious smile, and Johnny was powerless to do anything but shake his head and return it.

Burning the Booze

L egend states when a werewolf transforms back into a man, he wakes up naked and confused in a strange place, unable to gather what had transpired hours ago or how he had arrived at such a place in such a condition. The Moonlight lived up to such lore. Men woke next to unknown women, checking their wallets, trying to remember if they had spent too much on booze, women, and gambling or if they had been robbed. Most of the time, it was both. The premier customers were off limits, though there were daring women who risked the retaliation. But if the man was a nobody with no titles like "agent," "officer," "councilman," or "commissioner," there was a strong chance he'd wake with a skinny wallet. Not completely broke, that kind of word of mouth would prevent men from returning. It was five or ten bucks here and there.

Tomato was at the bar rubbing his temples, most likely praying to God for his headache to go away, when Johnny walked in at ten to eleven.

"I didn't go home last night. Lorraine is going to serve me for Thanksgiving dinner," Tomato said.

"Your wife's a good cook, but you're not exactly tender meat. I think you'll be alright," Johnny said.

"No... I keep blowing it, Johnny," Tomato said.

He glared at his naked wedding-ring finger; the ring was on his other hand. He shamefully switched it back. Before Johnny could say more, Hotsy plopped down on the stool beside them, a massive all-consuming grin on his face.

"Christ, are you going to have another bastard running around?" Tomato asked.

"I am a gentleman, Tomato. I don't disclose my personal relationships," Hotsy said.

"No? Well your neck does. Did you get sucked on by an octopus?" Tomato asked.

"I didn't get a name for your information," Hotsy said in a way that made it seem like he thought he had won the argument.

"You're unbelievable," Tomato said.

He shook his head. A grimace followed immediately—his prayer to God had gone unanswered.

"Women like to be called baby, sweetie or sexy. Who wants to be called the same name their ma or pa call them? Like that'll get a girl going. Maybe I'll ask for their confirmation names too," Hotsy said.

Tomato put both hands up, looking like a cop stopping traffic. "You could shut up... please? For like five minutes?"

He went back to rubbing the sides of his head, trying to massage away the headache.

"No can do. Vencini wants to see us," Hotsy said.

Tomato grabbed his toast and chomped two-thirds of it, washing it down with some coffee. It was all he could do to keep the toast down.

Hotsy knew the struggle taking place and did not hide his smile. He was impervious to the effects of booze. He swore it was because he "danced" the booze out of his system. Youth was certainly on his side, but some people have the ability to ingest the delicious poison and only experience the highs. Tomato was not among the blessed.

He smacked Hotsy across the back of the head for his cocky grin, then turned to Johnny. "Where'd you disappear to last night?"

"The Nettesheims," Johnny answered.

Hotsy shook his head disapprovingly. "You still donating to that charity?"

"She just needs a bit of help," Johnny said.

"It ain't your responsibility," Hotsy said.

"Hey, Cilly's old man fought," Tomato said, "Any man who fought over there has my respect. You don't understand the burden Cilly's got. Uncle Sam isn't looking out for him. Johnny's being a stand-up guy."

The crooked Warren Harding had vetoed the Soldier's Bonus Bill, arguing that the budget took precedence over the nation's debt to its veterans. That was September of 1922, but in March of 1924, President Coolidge had vetoed a two-billion-dollar Soldier's Bonus Bill that would have given veterans $1.25 per day for service overseas and $1 per day for domestic service. His explanation for the veto? "Patriotism... bought and paid for is not patriotism." Good to know the former and current presidents of the United States appreciated the sacrifice of its young men. Thank God, the Senate and House overrode Coolidge's veto. They promised to pay the veterans of the Great War their bonus... in 1945.

"And speaking of responsibility, why don't you send some kale your children's way?" Tomato asked.

Hotsy shrugged. "Half of 'em are born to rich families."

"And those that aren't?" Tomato asked.

"I'm teaching 'em self-reliance," Hotsy said.

Johnny shook his head. Being a father was not on his to-do list, but he couldn't say exactly what he'd do if it did happen. He'd like to think he'd be like Tomato rather than Hotsy, but those pledges are empty until proven.

"I ain't a father. I never had one. And look how I turned out," Hotsy said.

"My point exactly," Tomato said.

"I don't know how to do any of that."

"Any of what?"

"You know… the parenting stuff."

"You know how to throw a ball?"

"Yeah."

"You teach him to throw."

"What if it's a girl?"

"You teach her to throw. You know how to read?"

"Yeah."

"You teach them how to read. When I taught Gretch and Mary to read… I remember how excited they were when they read that first sentence. And now? Christ, they've read a dozen books this summer already… Bottom line is you be there for them. It should be that easy."

The advice may have been verbally directed at Hotsy, but silently, Tomato was speaking to himself. And in that moment, it wasn't the hangover that made him look queasy, it was his own guilt—guilt for not having had breakfast ready for his girls that morning and for not having listened to the synopsis of the books they were reading. And for a moment, Tomato could forget about the hangover. Guilt and remorse were a far greater pain than an overworked liver.

They left the bar and trudged to the gold elevators. Johnny hit the button, and because it was the quiet time of the day at the hotel, the door opened instantly with that annoying *ping*.

"What's the matter, Tomato?" Hotsy asked, smiling innocently.

The jerk of an elevator always brought on a temporary queasiness, but for Tomato, it was as if he had drunk another pint of beer.

"Someday, kid… someday," Tomato said.

He kept his eyes closed, most likely trying to imagine he was outside in the fresh air.

Hotsy smiled at Johnny. Johnny could only shake his head with a suppressed laugh. The doors of the elevator opened. *Ping.* Hoagie was seated at his stool.

Tomato only lifted his hand to wave. A nod would hurt too much. Valcoro was at his kitchen table, his bathrobe open a disturbing amount and revealing parts of his body he had to pay women to see.

We have to do it for free.

He had his morning cigar in his mouth, a cup of freshly squeezed orange juice in his hand, and the *Tribune* sprawled open on the table.

"How was the night boys?" he asked.

"Tell 'em Tomato," Hotsy said.

Tomato cast him a look that only priests witnessed during exorcisms.

"The hair of the dog, my friend. It gets worse every single day," Valcoro said.

"Toast's working a bit," Tomato said.

A lie.

Valcoro chugged the rest of his orange juice and took a long puff of his cigar before rubbing it out on the ash tray. Then he clapped his hands. Tomato grimaced from the loud noise. Valcoro rose to his feet and retied his bathrobe.

Thank God.

"Let me deal with this shit before we deal with the other shit," Valcoro said.

He went into his bathroom, left the door open, and unleashed a foul hell—smells and sights that wiped Hotsy's smirk from his face. Johnny kept his gaze trained at the city, but the glass was cruel and reflected the horrific sight behind him.

"Johnny, throw me a roll, will ya?" Valcoro shouted through a grunt.

Tomato cast an apologetic, sorrowful look at Johnny. Johnny had zero reservations about Tomato's loyalty. He'd take a bullet for him. But hand-delivering toilet paper to a man exorcising the devil's beast was something else.

How long would it take Valcoro to reach the ground if he was thrown out of the window? Johnny let that question fill his mind as he clomped over.

He bit down on the inside of his mouth until it almost bled. He took a deep breath and held it as he stepped into the bathroom to retrieve a roll of toilet paper. He would rather pass out than inhale the poisonous air. Those deleterious panic attacks he suffered were never welcome, always coming at inconvenient, embarrassing times. But if there was a time for an attack to take him, it was now. But of course there was no such respite.

He reached into the cupboard, grabbed a roll, and set it on the counter next to Valcoro. Then he immediately dashed out like he had left behind a live grenade. Valcoro finished his business, flicked the toilet handle to send his abomination into the abyss of Chicago, rose from the seat, and strutted out of the bathroom.

"About this other shit," he said.

He grabbed a cigar from his kitchen table and struck a match, sucking on the end of the cigar until the embers lit. "Diamond runs a distillery."

"The one on Wabash?" Tomato asked.

"That'd be the one," Valcoro said.

Mickey Diamond had his hand in several South Side distilleries and breweries, but he ran only one. But it was untouchable. At one point, it had been more heavily guarded than the White House, and even if the security had lessened of late, no one dared make a move on it. It had the reputation of a haunted house, and the facade of something truly awful that kept people away. Everyone had heard the stories about Diamond. And even if they were embellished—each drunkard taking pride in adding a new adjective or verb, crossing the lines of fact and fiction—there was still a terrifying truth to all of them.

Tomato, Johnny, and Hotsy exchanged glances. Wabash was not only the street Diamond's distillery was on, but mere blocks away from the Schofield flower shop—owned and operated by the late Dean O'Banion. Now it was the headquarters of Hymie Weiss, a bigger wild card than O'Banion ever had been. Diamond and Weiss shared a Polish ancestry and an affinity for violence. It was said that he did his thinking with a tommy gun. Weiss had shot his own brother, for heaven's sake. He and Diamond probably loved detailing past kills in gruesome, gory detail over a drink.

"… That's the heart of the North Side," Tomato said.

Even with Valcoro never leaving The Moonlight, there was no possible way he didn't know that. If Weiss simply saw the pearl gray fedoras Capone's men wore, he would open fire—without warning, without questions.

"I want Diamond's distillery out of commission," Valcoro said.

"If he's not there, he'll get a minor fine, maybe a couple of nights in the slammer, but nothing huge. It'll be back up and running in days," Hotsy said.

Though not usually one for common sense, Hotsy had a completely valid point.

"I don't want it called in. I want in burned to the ground. Do you understand me? I want the fires of hell to lick the heavens," Valcoro said.

Tomato and Hotsy glanced at Johnny but not quickly enough to go unnoticed.

"What are ya looking at him for? I give the orders, not this Fritz meatball," Valcoro said.

"We'll get it done," Tomato said.

"Yeah, ya will. Now get outta here," Valcoro said, pointing to the elevator.

Hoagie already had the elevator button pushed before they got there and gave them an apologetic frown when they passed through.

Once the doors were shut, the thin veil of calm between them dissipated.

"That crazy old bastard!" Tomato said.

"He's doing it because of me. I've always been his punching bag," Johnny said.

"Nah, he's doing it because of Two Shits," Hotsy said.

"But he chose us because of me. I'll do this… alone," Johnny said.

Ping. The elevator doors opened.

Tomato gave Johnny one of his artillery-caliber piercing glares. When they were outside of The Moonlight and its many eavesdropping ears, he rounded on Johnny.

"Look at me. You're my brother. Understand? I don't care if you're German or Swedish or Asian or Indian. I trust you. And I trust Hotsy. No one does this alone. You hear me?"

"You've got a family," Johnny argued.

"Listen to me. No. One. Does. This. Alone."

Johnny reluctantly nodded.

Hotsy leaned forward. "You know I was thinking—"

"That's scary," Tomato said.

"It's so hot out, maybe the distillery will catch fire on its own," Hotsy said.

Hot was an understatement. Even breathing felt like swallowing invisible flames. The sweat started immediately, first in the armpits and then the lower back until it was everywhere. Hotsy sprawled his arms out in the back seat, and Johnny and Tomato took the passenger and driver seats.

"How many men can we expect in there?" Tomato asked.

"Fifteen? It's a Sunday so maybe less," Johnny said.

"Yeah, it's Church day, right?" Hotsy asked.

"More commonly known as the Sabbath," Tomato said.

Johnny smirked.

"Might be a good time to say a prayer," Tomato said.

"So how are we playing this one, Johnny? Run in, guns blazing?" Hotsy asked.

That was always Hotsy's first idea. But he spoke like a man who had never been in a gunfight. Shooting at someone sounds easy. Getting shot at is something entirely different. And killing someone is something you can't fathom until you've done it.

"No. There'd be too many witnesses," Johnny answered.

"So, what do we do?" Hotsy asked.

Tomato and Hotsy did not like his answer. Hell, Johnny didn't like his answer either. It required waiting. Valcoro wanted the distillery out of commission now, so they couldn't hang around and wait at The Moonlight until darkness descended. But they had a small shopping list of ingredients to acquire for Johnny's plan, and their greatest ally wouldn't arrive until approximately 8:29—darkness.

Tomato decided to risk being cooked by his wife, and the three stopped by at his home for a light lunch.

"You promise to save me if she goes for a knife?" Tomato asked when they were in front of his apartment door.

"No. Lorraine's a sweet gal for the most part. But she's got some crazy in her too," Hotsy said.

Tomato unlocked the door and stepped inside.

"Hello? It's me... and Hotsy and Johnny," he said.

"You came back," Lorraine called out, standing halfway between the kitchen and the living room. Her umber brown hair curled around her face, looking disheveled from the morning chores. She stared daggers at Tomato.

"Things ran late last night. I was a mess, Lorraine. I almost puked all over Tomato's shoes. He had to carry my sorry carcass to my room—" Hotsy said.

"Don't lie for him," Lorraine said with a stern voice.

Hotsy gave Tomato a discreet look—*You're on your own.*

"I was in no shape to drive," Tomato said.

Lorraine nodded, but she didn't believe a word he said. His lies were always shrouded in insignificant truths.

"Where are the girls?" Tomato asked.

"Mary's brushing Gretch's hair," Lorraine said.

Tomato stepped forward, carefully checking if he could give his wife a peck on the cheek. Men had swum with sharks without as much hesitation.

She allowed him to kiss her cheek but gave him a push that was a seventy–thirty blend of rough and playful. But her final push made it eighty–twenty.

"Girls!" Tomato called.

A small stampede echoed down the hallway from the bathroom and in charged his daughters. Mary Louise was thirteen and was handling the onset of womanhood gracefully—no acne or awkward growth spurt. She was a doppelgänger of her mother with olive green eyes. Gretchen leapt into her father's arms. Half her hair was combed, the other half was frizzy and sprawling. She was two years younger than Mary Louise (sixteen months and thirteen days to be exact, as she was sure to point out.)

"You missed breakfast!" she said.

61

"I know, baby girl."

"Doesn't your watch work? You know what time it is?" Gretchen asked.

Tomato smiled. "It's our time!" he and his two girls cried out together.

"I like your hair, Gretch. Going for a new style?" Hotsy teased.

She playfully pushed him. "Hi, Johnny."

"Morning, Gretch," Johnny answered.

Mary greeted them both with a big hug and a bigger smile.

"I was just telling Hotsy and Johnny about how many books you've read this summer," Tomato said.

"I wasn't that impressed," Hotsy said.

"Really?" Gretchen asked, knowing he wasn't serious.

"Really. I mean twelve books in two months… I don't know. I was expecting more," Hotsy said, shrugging.

"Coming from someone who can't read," Mary teased.

"I can read," Hotsy said.

"Can you?" she asked.

"Sure. I mean it depends," he said.

"On what?" Gretchen asked.

"Are there pictures?"

The girls broke out into a fit of laughter.

"Johnny and I hosed this bozo off this morning. You wouldn't believe what we found in his hair," Tomato said.

He had a dollar bill in each hand and held them out for his daughters to take.

"Money's dirty," Lorraine said.

"That money's *filthy*," Johnny corrected.

"Maybe later when I'm at work, you can take your mother outside into the bright sun, so her face melts," Tomato joked.

Lorraine looked like she did not want to smile. Oh, how she tried not to smile. She shook her head, allowing only a smirk to escape her lips. But when Tomato pulled her into a hug, the smirk changed to a radiating smile.

They would always have their differences, but Mary Louise and Gretchen Marie were the intersecting circles of their Venn diagrams. Tomato was a great father, no question. He was hard on himself for his shortcomings. But when Tomato was at home, he was a different man. Their two girls were the most important entity in Lorraine's life, so seeing them smile when their father was home led her to forgive much.

But not all.

"Are you boys hungry?" Lorraine asked.

"Come on, Lorraine. With your cooking, I always leave some space," Hotsy said.

"That'd be great, thanks," Johnny said.

Hotsy was comfortable in any environment. It was an envious trait. Hell, Johnny would even call it an ability. Birds flew. Chameleons changed their skin. Starfish regenerated. Spiders spun webs. And Hotsy fit in *anywhere.*

Tomato sat on the couch, a daughter on each side, listening to what he had missed from the night before and that morning, and then hearing all about the two books they were reading. Gretchen was in the middle of *The Story of Doctor Doolittle,* a story about a man who could speak to and understand animals. Mary Louise was nearing the end of *Emily of New Moon,* a book about a young orphan being raised by relatives after her father dies of an illness.

"Oh!" Gretchen exclaimed; a thought had come back to her. "I was going to ask… what is tuber-cool-o-sis?"

"Use it in a sentence, sweets," Tomato said.

"Her father died of tuber-cool-o-sis."

"*Tuberculosis.* It's a lung disease," Tomato gently corrected.

"Is it something I can get?" she asked.

"No, not at all."

"When did people first start getting it?"

"I'm not sure, sweets."

Children always want to know the oddest things, not knowing their parents are not encyclopedias.

"Are you sure I can't get it?" Gretchen asked again.

"Honey, I promise you will not get tuberculosis," Tomato said.

Half an hour later, Lorraine announced that lunch was ready. She had made sandwiches, taking the time to personalize each one. Johnny hated mayonnaise, while Tomato loved it. Gretchen liked pickles, while her sister despised them. She had even cut the crusts off the sandwiches for Gretchen, Mary, and Hotsy. After lunch, they listened to the radio while Hotsy and the girls played "Go Fish." Johnny sat on the couch, feeling the effects of the bread expanding in his stomach. Tomato napped on and off, waking when his snoring reached high decibels.

"You cheat, Hotsy!" Mary yelled.

"I didn't cheat. I simply used bait," Hotsy said.

The two girls playfully tackled him to the floor. Hotsy retaliated by tickling them.

"Daddy!" Gretchen called out.

Tomato woke from his slumber and smiled. They thrashed about, their laughter echoing.

And then, it happened again.

Breathe. Breathe. Fight it. Don't let it consume you.

The laughter changed, morphing into something dark and morbid. Screams. Screams of pain, screams of terror, screams for help, screams for God, screams for it all to end.

That invisible bag pressed over his nose and mouth. He closed his eyes, taking a deep breath but the sensation of choking was still there. Visions came to him. No Man's Land. Gunfire zipping past. Sprinting forward, gazing upon the dead and dying. Explosions sending body parts into the air and covering him in dirt that fell like rain. The swooshing of fire. The hiss of gas. Hands reached out for him, eyes pleading for him to save them.

"It's suffering."

He opened his eyes, focusing them on Gretchen and Mary and their absolute innocence. Their faces showed they were still laughing, but the laughter didn't reach him, only the screaming. He stared at them, demanding his brain to make the connection and match the sight with the correct sound. And it finally did. He felt as if he was surfacing from underwater. He did his best not to gasp out loud but failed.

"Are you alright, Johnny?" Lorraine asked, hovering between the living room and the kitchen, a towel on her shoulder.

"I'm fine," Johnny said.

"Do you want some water?"

"No, I'm good, thanks."

Yes, I'm dying for some.

He breathed in through his nose and exhaled through his mouth, and seconds later, for an unknown reason, the spell had passed.

Tomato helped clean up the cards that had been kicked all over the living room and then, he, Hotsy, and Johnny grabbed their fedoras and headed to the door.

"We'll see you later, girls. You be good. Listen to your mother. Unless she talks bad about me. What do we do then?" Tomato asked.

"We ignore her," his daughters answered.

"And what do we actually do?" Lorraine asked.

"Agree with mother," both answered.

Tomato kissed both of his daughters on the forehead, and risking it all, planted a kiss on Lorraine's lips.

"Got one for me too, Lorraine?" Hotsy asked.

"If Tomato doesn't come home tonight, I will," Lorraine said.

"Very funny, Lorraine," Tomato said.

"Do you see a smile?" she asked.

"No, that's why the girls are taking you outside later, so that face of yours melts," Tomato said.

"I think you better cut your losses, Tomato," Hotsy warned.

"Tomato knows if he gets in a battle of wits with me, I'll turn him into Heinz ketchup," Lorraine said.

Johnny smirked and whispered to Tomato, "better than turkey."

"See you, cheater," Mary called out to Hotsy.

"You're a sore loser like your old man. He cried yesterday when he lost in cribbage. I mean big, fat baby tears," Hotsy said.

"I will run you over with the car," Tomato said.

"I know. Imagine what he could do if he knew how to drive," Hotsy countered.

"Thanks for lunch, Lorraine," Johnny said.

"Anytime. You and Hotsy are always welcome. Tomasso… well, that's a different story," Lorraine said.

"You're just full of knee slappers today," Tomato said.

"You don't come home tonight, and I'll have food and water out in a bowl like I would for any other stray," Lorraine said.

Tomato smiled. Lorraine allowed herself only a faint smirk.

"I will see you later tonight!" Tomato called out as he left the apartment.

They had killed time and set picking up a list of supplies as their next task.

The Green Mill, located on North Broadway, was known equally as a jazz club that sold booze and a speakeasy that played jazz. Despite being in rival gang territory, it was partly owned by a fellow South Sider and the best machine gunner in the West. Born Vincenzo Gibaldi, he had changed his name to Jack McGurn to help himself get better billings in his boxing bouts. To the press and to the greater Chicago area, he was known as Machine Gun Jack McGurn.

McGurn had a deep hatred for the North Side. They had murdered his stepfather, Angelo DeMory. So it didn't take much convincing for McGurn to give Johnny, Tomato, and Hotsy two sticks of dynamite so they could blow up a distillery owned by the Irish North Side. Tomato kept them out of Hotsy's hands, not trusting him with something that could level a building. They stayed for three or four rounds of drinks, listening to the band, bullshitting with McGurn, and waiting as the clock made circles. They ate a supper of Salisbury steaks and baked potatoes. As the strong heat of the afternoon gave way to cooler, late-evening temperatures, they left The Green Mill and drove toward the distillery, parking a block away. In silence, they smoked and watched the distillery. The waiting was awful.

"Not all of us can doze off or we'll die in here," Hotsy said.

It was a joke with more truth to it than he knew. It was damn hot inside that Cadillac.

Hotsy fell asleep first. Both Tomato and Johnny knew he couldn't be counted on to scout. He just didn't have the attention span for it.

"You had one before… back at the house, didn't you?" Tomato asked.

Johnny nodded but kept his eyes trained forward.

"What caused it?" Tomato asked.

Johnny shrugged. "I don't know. They just come on and… there's nothing I can do to stop it."

"No, nothing you can do."

"I can't stop thinking about those godman coffins at Al's neither. That doesn't help."

"Nothing to be embarrassed about."

Johnny scoffed. "I looked like I was drowning on your couch, Tomato. Your girls are probably scared of me."

"You're an uncle to those girls. I sleep with the light on, Johnny. You think anyone in my house would judge you for losing your breath for a few seconds?"

"I'm thirsty," Hotsy complained from the back seat.

Both Johnny and Tomato turned to look at him. Hotsy hadn't even taken the effort to open his eyes.

"Act alive. Sit up," Tomato ordered.

Hotsy groaned but obeyed.

"We should see maybe one or two guards inside," Tomato said.

"We don't go in there intending to kill, got it? We let them walk," Johnny said.

"Let them walk? Straight to Diamond?" Hotsy said, leaning forward from the back seat.

"These are men trying to support their families," Johnny said.

67

Tomato looked at Johnny. It was impossible to decipher if he agreed. But he nodded in assent. "Johnny's right. No one deserves to die at work."

Hotsy threw up his hands and leaned back. "Which building is it?"

"The same one Johnny and I have been scouting for the last hour," Tomato said.

"Ah, yes," Hotsy said confidently. "Which one is that?"

"The white brick one," Johnny answered.

In Chicago, there was never total darkness. Natural sunlight only gave way to artificial electric light. When the latter took over, Tomato spoke.

"Make sure you're loaded," he said.

Hotsy pumped his Remington Model 17, a huge smile on his face. There were few sounds more terrifying than the pumping of a shotgun. It was like a lion's roar—a warning that sheer carnage was about to be unleashed.

"Leave your fedora in the car," Johnny said.

"Why?" Hotsy asked.

"Because they'll recognize the gray," Tomato said.

"I lead," Johnny said.

Tomato and Hotsy followed Johnny across the street at a brisk pace.

Johnny paused before he opened the distillery door.

Do not let it happen again. If it does, we're all dead.

Both Hotsy and Tomato nodded that they were ready. Johnny paused further, ensuring an attack wasn't on its way, then opened the door and rushed inside.

"Hands up! Nobody move!" he yelled.

"Up against the wall!" Tomato ordered.

A guard reached for his gun in his shoulder holster. Hotsy smacked the butt of his shotgun into his nose, breaking the bridge of it, and sending blood flowing from both nostrils like water rushing out of a destroyed dam.

Johnny let his disapproval be known with a stern look aimed at Hotsy.

"What? He was reaching for something," Hotsy said.

The eight men inside lined up facing the wall, hands spread high and wide above their heads.

68

There were two types of men lined up along the wall. Those who were there to work, to simply earn money. They came willingly—looking dejected, but willingly. The others were there out of loyalty. It was more than a day job. Those who fell into the latter category wanted to reach for their weapons. Both Tomato and Hotsy recognized which category each man belonged to and aimed their weapons at them.

"Hey, hey, hey! Don't be a tough guy," Tomato warned.

"Stay against the wall! No sudden movements!" Johnny said.

"We done nothing wrong here," a man said, in a thick Irish accent.

"Really? Smells like booze to me, mick," Hotsy said.

"You know whose distillery this is?" the man with the broken nose asked.

It went unanswered.

Diamond's distillery didn't produce high-quality whiskey. It was quantity he was after. Before prohibition, three years was the standard time for which whiskey had to be barreled. Diamond waited three or four months at most. The factory was expansive, containing washbacks and stills that spanned three levels. The washbacks were over twelve feet across, twenty feet deep and contained a sugary water mixture known as wort. The copper stills looked like massive beakers found in science classrooms with pipes that traveled across the ceiling, branching off in half a dozen directions. Like so many buildings from the 19th century, the distillery had a brick veneer, but much of the interior was made of timber.

Johnny and Tomato searched the men for firearms. Only three had them. They removed the weapons and flung them across the room.

"Now get out of here!" Johnny yelled.

The men looked at one another, confused. Hotsy fired a shotgun blast to the ceiling that shattered the overhead light and echoed about the room. The fixture swung down, holding on by a single chain.

"Get out of here!" he yelled.

Five of the men scurried out of the building. The three men who had been armed stayed behind.

"You lose a few cards or were you born with a missing deck? Get outta here!" Hotsy said.

"If Mickey Diamond finds out we been running, what he'll do to us is far worse than anything you can do," the man with the broken nose said.

He was the ugliest and largest of the three, with a face that had seen its fair share of knuckles. He let the blood flow into his mouth instead of trying to spit it out.

"You stay, we arrest you," Tomato said.

The man chuckled. "You're an agent?"

Even if he had believed Tomato's threat, incarceration was a temporary thing—weeks, months, maybe a few years. Death, on the other hand, was permanent.

"Tell me something, *agent*. Mr. Diamond pays good money for this place to not be harassed like this, so what the hell are you doing here?" the broken-nosed man retorted.

Tomato thrust out his arm. "Back up against the wall, and keep your mouth shut!"

"Can I see your badge, *agent*?"

"You want to see my badge?"

"I'm dying to. What does it look like?"

"It's silver, rounded, about an inch and a quarter long and comes to a hollow point, and since you're dying to see it, I'll show you."

He fired a bullet into the man's chest, the sound echoing before being swallowed up by the washbacks and stills. The man slid down the wall, the faded gray concrete splattered and smeared with blood.

"Get out of here!" Johnny yelled, a command and a plea to the remaining men.

If they stayed any longer, they would be gunned down. That would be unnecessary but inevitable. Johnny fired a shot above their heads. It was enough to scare them into action, and the two men took off in a sprint.

"We don't got much time," Johnny said.

Tomato removed the two sticks of dynamite from his belt line and handed them to Johnny. He dashed to the base of the stills and lit the fuse. They blazed like a sparkler.

"Go! Go! Go!" Johnny shouted.

"Burn, baby, burn!" Hotsy yelled.

They sprinted across the street, trying to outrun the deafening sound that would come in seconds. And it came like thunder. The windows shattered. Sections of brick shot out into the street. Flames erupted with a swooshing roar. The timber acted like kindling and the alcohol an accelerant. The upper floors caved in, burying the factory in rubble. Black smoke billowed, wafting up to the Chicago skyscrapers for the whole city to see.

Melted Ice Cream

Sometimes, the secret to getting away with a crime is not running from the scene but walking. And that's just what Johnny, Tomato, and Hotsy did. They walked back to Tomato's Cadillac and drove away, showing the same interest in the flames as every other passerby. Tomato dropped Johnny and Hotsy off at The Moonlight, and then he returned home to his wife and daughters as promised.

The following day, they stopped for lunch at a place they often frequented. It was "cleverly" named "The Diner." It had once been "Al's Diner," "Will's Diner," "Kate's Diner," and so on, but with each reopening, the diner saw less customers, something that was only normal. Frequent closures forced customers to wonder why it had closed in the first place. Had they been selling expired food? Rat meat? Business would pick up again as the rumors faded, only for a repeat of the same process. Then, one owner had the presence of mind to drop the name and simply let the place be called The Diner. Now, nobody knew when the diner changed ownership. There was no flux in the number of customers. And the food didn't change, at least not enough to be of note.

Johnny hadn't cared for the place under any owner, but it was the favorite place of a friend and mentor. Jack Salvatory was seated at a booth, the morning paper neatly folded beside his plate of broasted chicken. His hair was in desperate need of combing, but seeing that he was approaching his late-fifties, worrying about his appearance for the sake of the opposite sex was two decades in the past. He might not look it now, but Jack Salvatory was one of the toughest men in not only Chicago, but the entire world. He had survived events most men would have died from. He'd been shot, stabbed, beaten, even thrown from a three-story window. Surviving all this had earned him the nickname The Immortal. In Johnny's opinion, it was the most deserved moniker any man had ever received.

"Good morning," The Immortal said well before he should have been able to see Johnny, Tomato, and Hotsy.

Tomato and Hotsy exchanged perplexed looks, as if they had just seen a magic trick.

"I can see your reflection in the window," Salvatory said, pointing to the window ahead of him.

No doubt that helped. But you didn't get stabbed, shot, and beaten without acquiring some inexplicable spatial awareness. The Immortal knew how many people were in the diner, how many of them were children, women, and men, and how many of those men were comfortable handling a gun.

Out of respect for The Immortal, all three squeezed into the booth across from him.

"You heard about Two Shits?" Johnny asked.

Salvatory frowned. "I did. Makes me wonder what Valcoro is going to do."

Johnny and Tomato exchanged what they thought was a discrete glance, but of course, Salvatory caught it. He smiled, not out of joy or humor, and Johnny guessed that he knew something had already been done. If he hadn't, then Johnny and Tomato's demeanor confirmed as much.

"What did he have you do?" he asked.

Hotsy smirked. "Start a barbecue."

"Diamond's place?"

Johnny nodded. The Immortal leaned back in his booth and chuckled, but not from humor.

"What Valcoro doesn't understand is that this whole thing… it's a circle. No beginning, no end. Just… constant revolutions, constant retaliations," The Immortal said.

"He's taking it personal," Tomato said.

"If Johnny or Hotsy were in a casket right now, wouldn't you?" The Immortal asked.

A rhetorical question. They all knew the answer. Every one of them would go down in a blizzard of bullets trying to exact revenge.

"You watch yourselves," The Immortal said.

"Those that had a problem still ain't been dug out of the rubble," Hotsy said.

Hotsy was aware that the Immortal had once been in the life, but he failed to recognize the experience and wisdom older people had. Someday, like Johnny and Tomato, Hotsy would fully realize just how significant a gift The Immortal's mentoring had been. Of the three, Johnny was the most drawn to him. Jack was a Heinz 22 in terms of ethnicity—some Irish, some English, some German, and some Italian. But he was respected by everyone—the Polish, Jews, Irish, and Italians.

"Mickey Diamond will find witnesses," The Immortal said. "The men working at the distillery, the priest at Holy Name, nosy, old women looking down from their windows… wherever they might be, he'll find them and get your names. He'll get enough details on the three of you to paint a picture he'll post all over Chicago…"

He had said all he would. After confirming the conversation was over, Tomato and Hotsy moseyed down to the counter to order lunch.

"Can I ask you something personal?" Johnny asked.

74

The Immortal smiled. "I never understood that. *Can I ask you something personal?* I don't know how personal you're planning on getting. Go ahead and ask me, Johnny, and I'll let you know."

"Why'd you get out?" Johnny asked.

Chicago had been home to vice long before prohibition. The Immortal had made good money before, but he could have made tenfold under prohibition. But he had denied something most mortal men fall victim to—greed.

The Immortal leaned back in the booth and took a deep breath. "The game changed," he said before pausing. "Three years ago, there was money for everyone—Torrio and Capone, O'Banion and Weiss, the Genna brothers, the South Side O'Donnells, Saltis, and McErlane. Everybody. Chicago is a pizza. Instead of cutting it equally, they cut it into squares. And nobody wanted the corner pieces. People got greedy—constantly craved more and more. And while all the gluttonous pricks dined like kings, us rats feasted on crumbs… killed each other for crumbs."

"How'd you do it? How'd you get out of the life?" Johnny asked.

"I survived everyone. Anyone whose secrets I could have spilled died or disappeared. Most of the young faces in the game don't even know who I am. Things were different. When my gang folded into Capone's, I just left… I knew it was then or never. Capone… he doesn't take leaving well."

Johnny considered his words. He was thirty-two years old—a young man by many standards. But many of the biggest names of both the North and South Side were in their twenties. The prospect of outliving them all was doubtful. And like The Immortal said, Al Capone didn't let you walk away.

"I haven't told anyone this, and if you choose to repeat it, I understand, but I'd prefer to keep it quiet. I'm leaving Chicago," The Immortal said.

"Leaving?" Johnny repeated.

"There's nothing for me here. Every corner I go down, I've got a memory I'd like to forget. Most of my friends are in the same spot—Mount Carmel Cemetery. And God only knows I cannot handle another winter."

"When?"

"A couple of weeks."

"You'll let me know before you leave?"

"You got it."

Johnny pulled a wad of cash from his pocket to cover the Immortal's meal.

"That's not necessary," The Immortal said, waving his hand to refuse the offer.

Johnny ignored the gesture. "We'll talk soon."

Salvatory and Johnny headed to the counter. Johnny sat while The Immortal headed to the door, saying goodbye to Hotsy and Tomato with a flick of his wrist.

That night, Hotsy talked Tomato and Johnny into visiting Al's shop. Johnny could have done without seeing more coffins and caskets but agreed to go. In the darkness, with the faint streetlight illuminating them, they looked even more eerie. It was like being in a cemetery with the moonlight creeping through the clouds. Johnny forced Tomato and Hotsy to walk quicker to the basement door.

Please just get through this. Breathe. Breathe. Breathe.

"Yeah, yeah, I'm moving..." Hotsy said.

He knocked on the door.

"Sorry, we're closed," a voice said from behind it.

"I was told I could see a man here about a horse," Hotsy said.

Judging by the sound, the person behind the door had unlocked and unbolted a half-dozen locks. The door opened, revealing a man slightly older than Hotsy standing at the foot of the steps. He nodded respectfully and let the three men through the door and down the steps. The sound of music drifted around the walls. With each step, the volume of the music increased. Laughter erupted. When they reached the room downstairs, Hotsy took in the atmosphere and beamed. It reeked of sweat, booze, and smoke—all aphrodisiacs to him.

Al waddled over to them, a welcoming, albeit anxious, smile plastered across his face. The shop had been reverted to its original pristine condition as promised, but the sight of the three men no doubt put a nervous knot in his already bloated stomach.

"I hope it's pleasure that brings you here," Al said like it was prayer.

"Sorry, Al, it's business," Hotsy said.

Al's eyes lit up like a camera flash, and he looked like he would break into tears any moment.

"My business is booze and women, and I'll need you to supply both," Hotsy said.

Al nearly pissed himself from the relief Hotsy's words brought. Tomato pulled a wad of cash from his pocket, fanned out the notes and held out enough to buy fifty beers.

"I told you it was only business, Al," Tomato said.

Al graciously took the money and barked for his bartender to fill three pints of beer for them.

"Now, listen, Al. What you did, involving your daughter, I can't respect that. You need to be a different man here than you are at home. The man you are at home stays at home, and the family stays there too. You understand?" Tomato asked.

Al nodded, looking ashamed for having used his daughter as a scapegoat earlier.

"There won't be a second warning. You involve your family again…"

Tomato didn't need to finish. Al's face told them that the message had been received.

Hotsy barely had a beer in one hand when a curly haired blonde grabbed the other. As she dragged him to the dance floor, he gulped down his pint so as to not spill it.

"There's men who will be here for hours and not have one woman approach them like that. He's here for thirty seconds, and the women are already at him like hyenas on a fresh carcass," Tomato said.

"I see a few glancing your way," Johnny said.

"They're looking at you, and if they aren't, I don't want to know. I plan on leaving here sober and alone. I'm laying low with Lorraine and the girls the next couple of days. I'd like to sleep in my bed, not the hallway," Tomato said.

"I'm not staying long either," Johnny said.

The band finished their song to a round of courteous applause.

"You should stay. Unwind. Relax, save one of these dames from Hotsy," Tomato said.

"Not in this place," Johnny said.

"Too hot?"

"It's too hot everywhere."

Tomato's demeanor shifted. "The caskets?"

"Yeah, and it doesn't help that we're buried underground right now either."

"Those damn coffins… takes you right back there, doesn't it?"

"Right back there."

Fortunately for Johnny, both of them realized that the two men talking next to them had just described a man who was "an arrogant son of a bitch who thinks he owns the place." There could be only one man they were talking about—Hotsy.

Johnny and Tomato glared at them, but it was Tomato who spoke first.

"You have an issue with someone?" he asked.

The two men, both with hair styled in a wide part, turned to Tomato and Johnny.

"I came with the doll he's dancing with," the shorter of the two said.

"You two handcuffed?" Tomato asked.

"What?" the man asked.

"Is she your wife?"

"What? No—"

"Then he's doing nothing wrong."

"I came with her, and I don't think any man here would disagree with me that what he's doing is crass."

"You came here with her. You're not leaving with her. If you're thinking of doing something stupid, let me tell you that I don't have to look far for a coffin."

Tomato's patience with Hotsy was hair thin, but God have mercy on anyone else who took offense at him.

78

"No, nothing like that," the man said.

"Why don't you and your friend take off? Your date is well-taken care of. I don't know if I'm comfortable with you two here. Booze… it makes people react impulsively. Foolishly. Violently."

"You don't have to worry about that with us," the man's friend said, clearly wanting no trouble.

"I wasn't worried about you," Tomato said.

The message was clear. If the men stayed, their fortune would take a severe turn for the worse. They set down their unfinished drinks and headed upstairs like the place had been raided by agents.

Tomato was true to his word, only staying a couple of hours before leaving. Johnny hung by the bar, the dampness of the humid air weighing his clothes down. Al's whiskey had gone down smooth. Too smooth.

A woman in a tight black dress tapped Johnny on the shoulder. "I've got a bone to pick with you."

Her hair was Hollywood blonde, cropped with short bangs, her lipstick blood red. The hairstyle was a fad that had swept through the country like the Spanish flu and generally elicited the same reaction. It was a horror. Johnny agreed for the most part. Some could pull it off, but on most, it looked like a wig had been pasted on, and for the most unfortunate, it looked like the hair dresser had slapped a bowl atop their head and cut any exposed hair. She was a flapper through and through.

"Yeah, and why's that?" Johnny asked, keeping his eyes on the saxophonist and not the road kill on her head.

"I've been carrying a torch for you all night, and you've just stood over here like a statue, all stoic and mysterious," she said.

"Sorry, I'm not much of a dancer," Johnny said, signaling at the bartender for another refill of his Old Fashioned.

"I'm not in the mood to dance."

"Looks like we came to the wrong place."

She rubbed his wrist, laughing disingenuously at his comment. Her eyes reflected her desire for Johnny to see the inside of her bedroom.

Hotsy dashed over, dragging along the curly haired blonde and a fiery red-headed dame.

"I see you met Margaret," he said.

Johnny nodded politely to her.

"Did you ask him?" Hotsy asked Margaret.

"Not yet," she said.

A normal person would have asked what they wanted to ask him, but Johnny was miles away from being a normal conversationalist.

"There's a petting party at an apartment a couple blocks away," Hotsy said.

A petting party was a father's worst nightmare, and his son's wildest dream come true. It was a gathering of people with the sole purpose of kissing and fondling multiple partners—or what Hotsy called a normal Tuesday night.

Johnny hadn't really paid much attention to the band all night, only turning to watch when a good solo was performed. But for the first time, it had his undivided attention. He watched as the drummer pounded on his drums, sweat rolling down his portly chin.

And then it happened again. The banging of the drums morphed into artillery fire. The breath was sucked out of his lungs.

No... no... no. Not here. Not in front of these dames.

He leaned on the bar, a cold sweat breaking on his neck. He grabbed his Old Fashioned and chugged it, ignoring the confused look on Margaret's face. She was rightfully offended that the idea of kissing her made him down his alcohol. But her indignation was short-lived. She was the only one who noticed him gasping for breath. For Hotsy and the two women clinging to him, the petting party had already commenced.

"Are you alright?" Margaret asked.

Johnny nodded. "I'm fine. I have to go."

Sure, her haircut was far from something he considered attractive, but there was something about an easy and free lay and the few seconds of pure clarity afterward that enticed him. But the attacks came too often. And besides, she probably thought he was a merman who had been granted a Cinderella-type escape, and that at midnight, instead of a carriage turning into a pumpkin, Johnny's lungs were transforming back into gills.

"Johnny, what gives?" Hotsy shouted after him.

Al's was packed full of people, all of them sweating in the sweltering heat. The wisps of breath he was allotted were disgustingly hot and tasted of salty sweat, offering no relief. He pushed past the dancers and chit-chatting groups, using his shoulders to force them out of his path. Everyone in Al's was in awe of the musical crescendo, but to Johnny, the drummer's rattling solo was machine gun fire, the cymbals were explosions, the trombone an artillery barrage, and the trumpet a terrifying trench whistle.

Johnny was drowning, feeling the same panic of only having a few seconds of air left. The stairs led to the surface, and he bounded them three at time.

"Let me through," he ordered the man guarding the door.

The man opened the door and stood back, like a matador side-stepping a charging bull.

Those goddamn coffins and caskets did nothing to help his breathing. The music was far in the distance now. He pushed through the glass door, the bell atop ringing, and stepped out into the street.

And then it passed like a fast-moving storm.

He removed a cigarette and puffed on it, comforted by the tobacco. The only plan he had was creating as much distance between himself and those damn claustrophobia-inducing coffins and caskets as possible.

The fire at the distillery seemed to have increased the temperature the next couple of days. Johnny's father used to say, "You can always put on more layers, you can only take off so many." Even if Johnny was inclined to stroll Chicago in the nude, he would still be wearing too many layers. He'd take the frigid negative-twenties chill of winter than slowly burn alive in this fire.

While Tomato stayed at home with his wife and daughters, celebrating the fourth of July, Johnny and Hotsy escaped to the one place that offered the best chance at defeating the heat—Lake Michigan.

Most of the women at the beach followed the rules of the required swimsuit length, six inches above the knee, but Hotsy quickly discovered those who didn't mind breaking it. Lake Michigan offered as much relief as a reasonable person could ask for. Johnny was not reasonable, and therefore, disappointed. While his legs and waist were offered relief, the water only magnified the sun and caused sunburn on his shoulders and scalp. Johnny didn't have wool-thick hair like Tomato, his was wavy and thin, and the sun burnt any exposed scalp. While Johnny's combination of pasty-German and olive-Italian skin burned to a lobster red, Hotsy only went from dark to darker.

Lake Michigan stretched 307 miles but it seemed as if all of Chicago had decided to swim in the same hundred-meter section as Johnny. It was impossible to swim without catching an inadvertent slap from a swimming stroke or an elbow from a frolicking child.

Children on the beach waved American flags, celebrating the hundred and fifty years since America broke free from England's tyranny. The city was flooded with thousands of tourists over the weekend. Later that night, fireworks would be launched down at Municipal Pier, but for now, all of Chicago was content lying on the beach or splashing around in the water.

Custard's Last Stand was a solid back-up plan to beat the heat, but the line made Johnny and Hotsy wonder if they would have enough custard left by the time they made it to the front. Johnny downright despised lines. Patience wasn't one of his prized traits. His suit dried unwelcomingly fast, and the wool made him feel as if he had put on a winter jacket inside with the furnace cranked.

Hotsy was like a dog playing fetch, and the stick was the women of Chicago. The sunbathing beauties didn't need to worry about sharks in Lake Michigan, just Hotsy. From time to time, he would return to tell Johnny of a busty blonde or long-legged brunette.

All lines, no matter where, moved at the same pace. Someone would find a person they knew in line and cut in. People who had been reading the menu for over twenty minutes would step up and have no damn idea what they wanted to order. They had to read the whole menu like it was scripture or ask the worker to name everything off only to order the first item listed. It was custard. Chocolate, vanilla, Neapolitan. It should not be the most complex choice a person made in a day. Further adding to his annoyance, some children were whining ahead of him. The youngest cried while the older ones continually asked their parents, "How much longer?" Their parents' answer was not acceptable, and so, they asked again and again and again. One child screamed at such a high-pitched tone that it sounded like a combination of a high-powered dog whistle and an angry rooster. Of course that kid's parents were oblivious to the ear-bleeding noise.

"I didn't know they served half-breeds."

The opening in line revealed Paris, in a Kelly green two-piece bathing suit that not even the sun could blind him from seeing. Her skin was smooth, burnished with a healthy glow from the sun.

"I guess you'll find out first," Johnny said.

Paris was with three other women of The Moonlight, one of whom Johnny had slept with. An arrogant man would have thought that the fact she showed no signs of recognizing him was her following The Moonlight's code of secrecy. But Johnny was a realist. The woman had slept with too many men to remember their one-night embrace months earlier when there had still been snow on the ground, and the lake shore had been a sheet of ice. That had been a different time, and in this heat, seemed like an entirely different world.

"You swim?" Paris asked, her eyes falling on Johnny's muscular arms.

"I like to call it failing at drowning," Johnny said.

"Well, you can't be good at everything."

Johnny smirked.

"No fedora? It would have complimented your suit quite nicely," Paris teased.

"You better be careful with your bathing suit. Police will hit you with a fine for ten clams," Johnny said, nodding at how much of her thighs were showing.

Her swimsuit hovered the line of beach appropriate. The beach was littered with men who would pay to see the rest.

"Look who's looking at my thighs," Paris said.

"Just trying to keep the beach family friendly and change in your pocket."

"If I get caught, I guess I'll have to charge you extra for our next conversation then."

Her eyes went from his arms to the scar on his chest, trying to decipher what had caused it. He pulled on his suit discretely in an effort to conceal it.

"Are you here alone?" Paris asked.

"My friend Quintu is around here somewhere chasing women."

"But not you? Not in a chasing mood?"

"Nah, I tire too easy."

Paris flashed an enchanting smile. "You don't look too worse for the wear."

Her eyes twinkled in the sun, wiping Johnny's mind blank, and it took everything in his power to not look at her creamed chocolate skin glistening like it had flakes of gold in it.

"What about you? Is Mr. Finger roaming around somewhere?" Johnny asked.

"No, I haven't seen him since," Paris answered.

"I guess he's looking for a longer finger."

"Or maybe one of greater girth."

"Well I hope he finds that perfect finger."

"No, I'm bitter. That's missing pay for me."

"Sorry about that."

"I'm only teasing," she said reassuringly, putting her hand on his arm.

Somehow her fingertips were cool, causing goosebumps to erupt on his arm. A complete anomaly considering the sweltering heat.

The line crept at a glacier pace, the sun hanging mere feet above their heads. The sweat dripped down Johnny's forehead and the sweat on his back caused his suit to stick to his skin like it had been glued. He could only hope that Paris thought he was still wet from his dip in the lake and not sweating like a whore in church.

"I haven't seen you at the hotel," Paris said.

"No, I have been hanging low. Trying to avoid the heat," Johnny said.

"Heat from the sun or the fire on Wabash?"

"I don't know what you're talking about."

But lying had never been in his skill set. Every sign of a lie—fidgeting, avoiding eye contact, voice cracking—he showed them all.

"Vencini gave us the whole story last night," Paris said.

A dozen questions were ready to spew from his mouth, but Johnny settled on asking what Valcoro had said.

That dumb shit had bragged about destroying the distillery in a room full of nearly a hundred people. To police, councilmen, congressmen, and prohibition agents. Valcoro had given vital information that Diamond would pay big kale to get. Valcoro took credit for everything—beer deliveries, payment pickups, victorious fist-fights, scaring away rivals in a gunfight. Part of the reason Valcoro only wanted full-Italians working for him was he thought they'd be more loyal. "It's too hard to trust mutts," he would say. All that and the dumb shit had leaked the story himself to a hotel full of guests, no doubt trying to impress women he hoped to take upstairs. How pathetic that his money wasn't enough.

"I couldn't hear everything. But it was the talk of the night," Paris said.

She bit down on a frown—a gesture Johnny translated as an apology. He only shrugged. She had nothing to apologize for.

Custard's Last Stand was a small wooden shack with barely enough space for three workers and the frozen custard inside. The four corners of the building were shaped like plastic ice cream cones of vanilla, chocolate, strawberry, and Neapolitan. They baked in the hot sun, and it seemed entirely possible that they would melt like the real thing.

"What are you having?" Johnny asked.

"Vanilla," Paris answered.

"Should I read into that?"

Paris flashed a smile, one that could evaporate his breath like one of those attacks.

Johnny ordered two vanilla cones and one chocolate, then removed a handful of dimes and nickels, sorted through them for the necessary amount, and tossed it on the counter. At the beach was one of the few times he carried change. Coins could get wet, dollar bills couldn't. He gave one of the vanilla cones to Paris and gave his chocolate a lick around the cone to stop it from collapsing.

"Chocolate. Should I be reading into that?" she asked.

Johnny smirked. "I would have gotten a twist."

Hotsy, who had been keeping an eye on Johnny's place in line, jogged over once he saw the two cones in Johnny's hands.

"Better eat it fast. Melting all over the place," Johnny told him.

Hotsy took the cone and licked it around the base to stop it from dripping all over his hand. But his eyes fell on Paris, and he diverted his gaze, causing his nose to graze against the cone.

Hotsy had done much to be compared to a dog. He had played "fetch" with the women on the beach, he had splashed around the shore, he had come running when he saw a treat, he was currently licking his cone like a dog drinking water from a dish, and if Paris didn't put a quick stop to it, he would be humping her leg soon.

"Who's this?" he asked.

"Paris," Johnny answered.

"Paris," Hotsy said approvingly, already in love with the name. "Can I gaze upon your Eiffel Tower under that suit?"

"You better marvel from afar," Paris said.

"Rude Europeans. Don't you know you're supposed to share culture?" Hotsy said.

"What culture were you sharing with the other women down here at the beach?" Paris asked.

"I was helping with their breast stroke," Hotsy replied.

"I think he means stroking their breasts," Johnny said.

Paris laughed. "Well, Giovanni, I have to be going. Thanks for the cone."

Her friends had drifted away and were waiting for her, but their expressions showed that they wouldn't wait much longer. Johnny only nodded, wishing he had some clever farewell line.

Paris strutted away, apparently immune to Hotsy's venom. With her lips wrapped around the melting custard, she left both men weak and flushed.

"Suddenly, I'm in the mood for chocolate," Hotsy said.

"Would you settle for a napkin?"

That night at The Moonlight, the heat threatened to knock Johnny out. Only by continuously sipping his Old Fashioned was Johnny able to fend it off. The muddled orange and cherry satisfied his taste buds, the whiskey stifled the permanent annoyance brought on by the heat and haunting images of caskets and coffins, and the iced soda pop cooled him as it traveled down his throat. But the hotel lobby, packed elbow to elbow, was a furnace. Each person was a space heater. The sweating dancers sent a foul odor wafting through the lobby that not even the stench of cigarette could mask.

Hotsy was like a male lion surrounded by a pride of lionesses. Male lions attracted females with their thick, full manes. Rarely did they look for a mate. Instead, the females approached the males of their choosing. Hotsy was the same. He let his oily black hair droop over his eyes. He'd shake his head to flip it back over, causing the women around him to go weak in the knees. He used enough pomade to lube a squeaky wheel, but somehow his hair always had free reign to fall over his eyes.

Tomato sulked at the end of the bar, enjoying another French 75, while the girl he planned on taking upstairs danced the night away. Judging by the guilt on his face, it would have to be one hell of a lay to be worth it. But it was a lay he had committed to when he had moved his wedding band to the other hand.

The band played patriotic tunes like *The Star Spangled Banner, God Bless America,* and *America the Beautiful.* The crowd sang along boisterously, arm in arm and applauding emphatically after each song.

"Torch?" Johnny offered.

When he had worked in his father's shop, cigarettes had been called Torches of Freedom. Though the slang may have died out, Johnny liked the nickname and continued to use it.

Tomato pulled a cigarette from the pack of Chesterfields. Johnny lit his and Tomato's cigarette with his lighter, then took a relaxing puff.

"Sometimes it's easier to fight with her," Tomato said.

He looked ill at the prospect of what he would do. *Would*, not could. He knew he would break his vow of fidelity. An internal battle raged, but the faint voice that pleaded he remain faithful was overpowered by man's greatest weakness—lust. The Moonlight was where a man could embrace his inner beast. And for Tomato, it was always a full moon. He could never resist his urges, no more than a man could stop transforming into a beast during a full moon.

Johnny pulled two one-dollar bills from his pocket and slid them beside Tomato's drink.

"What's that for?" Tomato asked.

"It's up to you. You can buy yourself a couple rounds. You can get a taxi and go home. Or you can take that girl upstairs..." Johnny said.

Tomato would mouth off to any man but Valcoro and Al Capone. But Tomato's wife could put him in his place. He genuinely feared the pain her true words caused and the collateral damage that came with them. Maybe a better friend would have tried to stop him. But to Johnny, that was too much of a "holier-than-thou" attitude. And feeling holier than anybody was something Johnny had never experienced. People have demons. They are different for each person in how they manifest, but their effect is the same. How one either exorcises or succumbs to those demons is for each person to decide and no one else. Johnny hadn't managed to overcome his. How could he judge anyone else?

"She knows," Tomato said. "She knows where I am every night. Knows what I'm doing. And I know it... I know it..." He cleared his throat and finished his drink, the gin burning away the emotion coagulating in his throat.

Johnny had considered using the two dollars for his own vices, but it was too unfathomably hot. He could have put it on black at the roulette table, but that would require traversing the crowded lobby and squeezing into a spot at a table. Those tables were for suckers too. Nobody won big at The Moonlight and left. They either re-gambled it, believing they could get lucky a second time or there was a high likelihood of a beating and a mugging after they left. So, if you won a grand, it was wise to drop two hundred back on the table to appease The Moonlight Gods.

But Johnny's thoughts were eviscerated in an instant when the band started their next song. It was a song that had dominated the airwaves in 1917 and 1918. A call of patriotism for the young American men on their way to France.

"Over There, Over There
Send the word, send the word over there
That the Yanks are coming, the Yanks are coming…"

Johnny and Tomato shared looks, neither acknowledging how much the song affected them. How it devastated them. They sat in silence, the words of the song bringing it all back. Johnny had always held reverence for music. It could entice dancing, cause smiles and laugher, cause sadness and tears. It was powerful magic.

And then it happened again. That damn suffocating, drowning feeling.

Now, he was on the USS Lapland, going from New York to Bordeaux, and feeling the rocking of the waves. Staring up at the two smoke stacks, blowing clouds of black smoke into the crisp Atlantic air. He closed his eyes, counting in his head and slowly letting out deep, exaggerated breaths. The ship ride there had been filled with joy, even glee, with each soldier vowing to personally punch the Kaiser in the face. The ride home had been silent, somber, and filled with pain.

And then the song was over, snapping Johnny back into the lobby. Breath flooded through his nostrils, inflating his lungs with life.

When the applause ended, Tomato spoke again.

"Hard to imagine if we'd lost... none of this would be here," he said, gesturing at the tiny American flags lined everywhere, the chanting of patriotic songs showcasing the glory of America, and a room full of people celebrating the birth of the greatest nation in the world.

Johnny raised his glass. "Happy birthday, America."

Tomato raised his. "150 years old... you good-looking son of a bitch."

"You keep getting better with age."

They drank to their country, a country they had fought for, bled for, nearly died for.

Should have died for.

"You heading out?" Tomato asked.

"I think so. I plan on sleeping under water tonight," Johnny replied.

"Well if you run into Mickey Diamond, I'm sure he can help with that," Tomato said.

Johnny grinned. "Yeah, I'm sure he'd be more than willing."

Tomato raised his empty glass and shook it so that the ice clanged, signaling the bartender for a refill. Alcohol helped numb the guilt of cheating on his wife, but it also numbed his reason, decision making, and senses. And in essence, loosen the restraints of his inner beast. A few more drinks, and he wouldn't have to worry about cheating on Lorraine. He wouldn't be able to. But Tomato lost that battle too—he was always able to stop one short.

"I'll see you tomorrow," Johnny said.

Tomato rested his head on his right hand but managed a wave with his left. Johnny gave his torch a final puff, tossed it into his empty glass, and left.

The naïve fool in him had hoped that the minute he stepped outside, he would be attacked by a cool gust of wind. But the wind was a rotting corpse that had died weeks earlier. He groaned—it would be another night of nothing but micro-naps of fifteen to twenty minutes.

Fireworks exploded in the nighttime sky, their awe-inspiring sight completely blocked by the surrounding skyscrapers. Johnny lit another torch and followed the exploding fireworks toward Municipal Pier. The firework finale commenced and was an unrelenting blast of *Bang! Bang! Bang! Bang!*

And then it happened again.

Or was it the same attack? Had everything in between been just a brief respite? Surfacing for a gulp of air, before falling back under?

He leaned against the stone building, sucking on his torch, flashes of those 75 mm guns kicking back and firing sixteen-pound shells poisoning his vision. It took the whole torch for the attack to pass and his breathing to return to normal. He verified the attack had truly passed, standing there and breathing rhythmically for a minute before continuing on his way.

During the day, Chicago belonged to millions of people. But at night, it belonged to a single person. Johnny never loved Chicago more than he did at night. It was just the two of them, Chicago offering itself to him and he to it. A time when he could reveal his thoughts, and the city would listen without judgement.

During the bustling days, it was easy to lose track of why and how he had fallen in love with the city in the first place. It was over-crowded, lines everywhere, traffic jams clogging the streets, and there was a person on every block with the potential to piss him off. But, at night, it was like seeing an old flame, thinking you were over her, only to fall in love with her all over again.

After abandoning his plan to head toward Municipal Pier and the fireworks (he didn't need a third attack), he had no conscious goal or destination in mind, but an evolutionary instinct for survival brought him block-by-block closer to the lake and the cool sanctuary it provided. The massive skyscrapers blocked the breeze each step of the way, and Johnny felt like the dove flying from Noah's Ark, looking for land.

Johnny removed his fedora and wiped his sweat. The Chesterfield dangling in his mouth threatened to wilt and break off. He strolled from empty street to empty street. There was not a soul around until he passed a pudgy man leaning against a brick building, puffing away on his cigarette. Another poor bastard who had fallen victim to the heat and didn't even attempt to sleep. Johnny nodded at him, silently communicating that he was equally miserable, and then left the man behind. But when Johnny crossed the street, the chubby figure stepped out from the shadows and followed.

The Hit

Johnny had taken the man trailing him to be harmless. He followed too closely to be a threat. There was skill in shadowing someone, and the man behind him had none. They just so happened to be traveling in the same direction. Johnny crossed the street. The man followed, staying in the crosswalk. But with each turn and intersection crossed, the odds they were going to the same destination went from decent to coincidental to highly unlikely and, ultimately, to astronomical. After all, Johnny had no destination in mind. He was simply wandering through Chicago.

The man had a nervous energy about him. He scampered more like a mouse than he walked like a man. Even his shadow was peculiar. Where Johnny's was an elongated giant, the man's was shorter and fatter than he actually was.

Was he lost and too embarrassed to ask for directions? Had he celebrated the fourth a bit too much and lost his buddies? Or was he also miserable in the heat and had decided to walk the night away?

When Johnny cut across another street, a second figure, a block away, stepped out. The figure lit a cigarette, his face cast in the light of the struck match.

Johnny stopped and pulled a fresh torch from his pack of Chesterfields, turning his head so the pudgy figure behind him was in his peripheral. He had stopped, awkwardly trying to avoid Johnny's gaze, his eyes widening from fear. It was clear that the man was definitely following him. Now, it was only a question of whether he was a rival or a badge. He seemed too fresh to be a man sent to do a hit, but he was also too fat to be a street cop. At that weight, he couldn't even catch a cold, let alone a perpetrator. Maybe he was a prohee, but would he follow Johnny for blocks in the hope that he was selling? His near-panting told Johnny he wouldn't. The man was an anomaly, someone whose attributes and physiology didn't match any of the three occupations.

Johnny continued on. The lanky man ahead and the fat man behind hesitated a few intentional seconds before closing the distance. Johnny had kept his pace lazy and slow, but when he came to the next intersection, he rounded the corner and stormed ahead to the next alley, creating distance between himself and the two stalking figures. He hid in the alley, waiting. The streetlight betrayed the stalker, casting his fat, dwarfish shadow across the concrete. The shadow paused, tilting its head to scan the street and sidewalk.

Johnny charged out. The shocked look on the man's doughy, thin-mustached face was laughable until he raised a shimmer of black, a blur in the darkness—a beretta. Johnny and his stalker wrestled over control of the gun, both fighting to keep the barrel pointing away from themselves. The man slammed Johnny against the glass storefront. The glass cracked. Johnny countered, driving his fist into the man, finding its way past the fat to the jaw bone. Fireworks erupted in the distance with thunderous booms.

Johnny slammed the attacker's hand against the hard, unforgiving stone of the alley way. The gun fell from his grip, skidding across the sidewalk and coming to a stop in the street. His attacker froze, uncertain of his next move.

The lanky man across the street looked even more undecided, checking with frenzied paranoia for traffic or pedestrians. Johnny used their indecisiveness to his advantage, drawing his M1911 from his shoulder holster. The sight of it was enough to cause the man to flee down the street in a pathetic scamper in which he nearly tripped over his own feet.

Johnny raised his pistol, undecided if he would wound or kill the fleeing man. But a sharp pain ripped through his side, causing him to hunch over. He brought his hand to the source of his pain, coating his fingers in sweat. But they were far too saturated for it to be sweat. He held them out into the street light. They were coated crimson.

It was blood.

His surging adrenaline had protected him from the bullet's pain. But, now that the attack was over, his adrenaline pool had run dry. He demanded his body react to his command, that his arm lift the gun to shoulder level. His attackers were gone, temporarily at least, but he fired three shots into the air to keep them sprinting.

He stumbled into the lamp post, the light revealing dangerous amounts of blood flooding from his wound. The hot blood was indistinguishable from the sweat coating his body. Seeing the blood spreading through his gray vest finally caused his brain to make the connection. His legs got weak. His heart raced. His side throbbed.

He made it to the next streetlight before he had to stop and hold the lamppost for support. The street sign read Dearborn and 20th. He only knew one person close by. But would he get there before his legs quit on him? He had been in this situation before. A situation that was purely animalistic. Survival mode kicked in. He was a wounded animal fleeing for its life. Nothing more.

He grunted, trudging forward, his wound stretching and tearing, leaving a trail of dripping blood.

The princess blend tan brick apartment building was a dwarf in comparison to the skyscraper giants surrounding it, but standing in front of it, bleeding and grimacing with pain, the building was the beanstalk Jack had climbed. The building had as many rooms as Hydra had heads, and as his vision blurred, the rooms multiplied. He had no idea which room was hers or if she was even home. He hadn't seen her in the lobby, but she could be in one of The Moonlight's many rooms, blocks away. If she wasn't home, he would bleed out on the steps of a strange apartment building. He smashed the glass panel of the front door with his pistol and dug his hand inside to unlock the door.

She had said that she had a great view, and it was doubtful she had been referring to sidewalks. Johnny's eyes went to the stairs. Injured and bleeding out, they looked like they led all the way to heaven, and with the amount of blood he had lost, he could only hope that was his destination. He used the railing to pull himself up each step, leaving a trace of blood on the wood, and dulling its polished sheen. His father's complexion faded, his skin taking on his mother's tone. He no longer had legs of flesh, bone, and blood. In their place were two slabs of ice connected to his torso.

He yelled her name successfully only once. The second time was a faint whisper. Each step was exponentially harder than the last. The stairs on the ninth floor pushed him back down with a cruel, invisible hand.

Johnny tried to shout, to scream out, but the words barely left his lips. His vision clouded then warped, sweat ran down his forehead and into his eyes, further hindering his sight. His toes and fingers fell numb, and like a colony of ants, the numbness crawled up his legs and arms.

On the fourteenth floor, his legs gave out. He slid down three carpeted steps, his face bouncing off. But they were as soft and soothing as a bed. Only the light reflecting off the golden chandelier, each reflection like a twinkling star, caught his eye. But then, there was nothing. And it was morbidly relieving. Freeing. Merciful.

"It's suffering, Giovanni," came a distant voice.

It dwelled in the center of the maze where his deepest, most profound memories were imprisoned. But this time, the memory was palpable. A country road. A truck speeding along, the trees nothing but blurs. A shape lying in the

96

road ahead. But this wasn't an attack. The memory didn't cause panic, worry or fear. The memory was a truth.

But something brought him back from that desolate country road to the carpeted steps of an apartment building in Chicago. His eyes opened. Only shapes came to him. The smooth skin and cold fingers lifting him up told him who had come.

"Paris…" he called.

"You need to help me, Giovanni," she said in a soothing voice.

He forced his legs to support his weight the last few steps. Paris pushed open her apartment door and guided Johnny to her couch, and he collapsed onto it.

"I have to go call an ambulance," Paris said.

"No. You can't… they'll…. call… police," Johnny said, grimacing with each word.

"Giovanni," Paris said in a way that made it clear she disagreed.

Johnny grabbed her hand. "No cops."

Her hand was coated in his blood. Her eyes went to his wound, dumbfounded at what to do. But the blank stare vanished, and she snapped into action. She dashed into her bathroom and came back out with a pair of scissors and ran them the length of his shirt.

"Check… for… exit wound," Johnny said.

She helped him on his side. He groaned from the pain it caused.

"I see one… you're really bleeding…" Her voice was grave now.

He had expected her face to be ghost white, but she handled the sight like a fellow veteran of combat.

"Thanks for noticing," Johnny said with a weak smile.

It was meant to lighten the situation for her benefit, but Paris didn't need it. She had taken those few moments of paralysis to process what needed to be done. She dashed to her kitchen and grabbed a dark bottle from below the sink.

"I'm going to clean the wound," Paris said.

"What is that?" he asked.

She twisted open the cap. "Industrial alcohol."

"Smells like… the same piss… you served me."

"This is probably the main ingredient."

The fume was gasoline, snapping him wide awake for a brief second before drugging him into a stupor.

Paris poured it over his wound. It was nothing short of acid. His skin sizzled like a flank steak on a frying pan.

She covered the wound with a towel and placed Johnny's hands atop it. "Put pressure on it."

She dashed off again, this time to the bathroom, and came out carrying a tin medical kit. Sitting on the edge of the couch beside Johnny, she disinfected the needle with the industrial alcohol, held it over Johnny's ignited lighter, and then, with the proficiency of a seasoned seamstress, sewed the wound shut.

"You know what… you're doing," Johnny said.

"No other choice, you won't let me call anyone," Paris said.

"I didn't mean it as a question."

Sewing flesh was not an easy feat, both skill wise and mentally. But Paris had a sure hand with well-spaced stitches. Most importantly, she was calm, silently instilling the belief he had suffered nothing more than a scraped knee.

"Done this before?" he asked.

"Some men get off by smashing their fists against a woman. Turn over," she said.

Johnny turned onto his side, biting his lip so the pain could spread to more than one place.

Paris wiped the blood away with the towel before sewing the exit wound. Johnny had enough experience with gunshots to know the bullet had been a full-metal jacket. The wound was too clean to be a hollow point, adding to his belief the attacker was green as grass. Most shooters used hollow point bullets. It caused more of a mess inside the body. More chances of bits of bullet piercing organs and arteries. The full-metal jacket bullet had gone cleanly through and saved his life. But the amount of blood on the couch did little to show that. It was also fortunate he had been shot on his left side. The right side was home to the liver. If the bullet had pierced it, Johnny would have died on the street.

When the wound had been sealed and re-sterilized, Paris went to the record player near the window. She brought the needle to it, sending music floating throughout the apartment. Johnny knew nothing about music. But it was the kind of music that told a story without needing words. What that story was, he didn't know. It was different for everyone. And it was clear it meant something to Paris.

"Is that... supposed to... relax me?" Johnny asked.

"It relaxes me. Helps calm me down when a man I hardly know screams my name and is bleeding out on the stairs of my apartment building," Paris said.

She had a wit more powerful than the bullet that had ripped through him.

"Sorry... you were... the only one..." Johnny slurred.

The room spun violently. A cold sweat ran down his body.

"What's happening? You're getting paler..." Paris said.

Johnny tried fighting the blackness, but like with the attacks, he was powerless, and the room faded to black.

"*It's suffering... It'd be cruel to let it suffer.*" The distant voice returned.

Words he had tried to bury, forget, hide, deny, and refuse. But they always came back to him. Words he couldn't hide from. Words he couldn't outrun.

"*It's suffering, Giovanni... We have to finish it off... It'd be cruel to let if suffer.*"

A country road stretched out before him. Then the blur of the forest. The rumble of the truck engine. An indecipherable mass in the road ahead. Speeding toward it.

"*Giovanni... Giovanni...* Giovanni," the voice saying his name morphed from masculine to feminine.

Johnny's eyes snapped open, his reflection staring back at him through Paris' piercing brown eyes.

"You scared the bejesus out of me," she said, sounding both relieved and annoyed. For a second, it looked as if she would hit him.

"Sorry. How long was I out?" Johnny asked.

"Oh, only close to an hour," she said sarcastically before her tone shifted. "Your breathing stopped just now."

The pain had been temporarily confused. It had shut off during his dream. But pain was never duped permanently. It always came back with a vengeance. Now was no exception. The pain returned with bared fangs, biting and tearing.

"Are you going to tell me what happened? Or do I have to wait for Vencini to tell the whole lobby?" Paris asked.

She sat on the window sill, glancing interchangeably at the city and Johnny.

"Someone put out a hit on me," Johnny said.

"Because of the distillery?" Paris asked.

"I think so... Can I trust you?"

She could lie. He liked to think he could tell if she was. In a world where people weren't always what they seemed, she appeared to be real. She had little tolerance for bullshit. Judging by her face, she was refraining from giving another sarcastic response.

She rose from the window sill and sat beside him. "You can trust me."

He pushed himself further up on the couch and grimaced from the pain. "I need you to do something..."

"Okay..." she said, holding the word.

Johnny fought the urge to pass out again. The bullet wound had its own heartbeat, and it *thumped* and *thumped*.

"Can you call The Moonlight and ask for Tomasso? Tell him that he and Hotsy need to stay inside and be careful. They may have to search the rooms for them. Tell them I'll contact them tomorrow," Johnny said.

Paris rose from the couch and grabbed a handful of change. "There's a payphone in the lobby."

"Take this," Johnny said.

He held his gun as far and high as he could, which was mere inches.

For only the second time that night, Paris didn't know how to respond. She looked at the gun with the respect and fear it deserved.

"I'm just being paranoid," Johnny said.

100

She grabbed the gun by the barrel and placed it in her purse. "I'll be back," she said and then left the apartment.

Every second she was gone felt like an hour. He was too sore to get up from the couch and look down the steps to see if she was on her way up. He had every intention of staying awake, but a traumatized body demanded sleep in order to heal.

The shutting door served as an alarm clock. When he woke, Johnny expected the clock on the wall to read 4 p.m., and the sun to be pouring through the window. But there was only artificial light surrounded by darkness outside the window, and the clock showed only fourteen minutes had passed. A duration that seemed impossible.

Paris set her purse and the pistol on the table. "I got a hold of him. They're okay."

"Thank you," Johnny said, exhaling the worry bottled up inside.

"Your buddy Tomasso sounded pretty zozzled," Paris said.

He was already drunk when Johnny had left The Moonlight.

Paris grabbed a glass from her cupboard and filled it with water. Then she refilled her own glass and finished it in one long, continuous drink. She returned to the couch and gave Johnny the water, but soon she was back on her feet, moving about the kitchen and then down the hallway to her bedroom. Her restlessness made him restless.

"You alright?" Johnny asked.

"Yes, just having a relaxing night off," Paris called back from her bedroom.

Paris returned with a cigarette in her hand, lighting it on her way to the edge of the couch.

But the moment it was lit, and the smoke wafted about the stale air, it became obvious that it wasn't tobacco in the rolling paper. He could pick out a brand of cigarette by the smell and not just when the person had a torch in their mouth. Cigarette smoke did not get carried away with the breeze; it clung to every fiber of clothing, every pore of skin. The smell emitting from Paris' cigarette was not a foreign aroma; most of the Jazz musicians at The Moonlight smelled like it. To the uninitiated, it reeked like skunk, but to those in the know, it was the distinct, musky smell of cannabis.

"You smoke reefer?" Johnny asked, his tone filled with judgement.

"Take a puff," Paris ordered, holding out the joint.

"I'm good."

"*You're good?* You're shaking from pain from a gunshot wound."

"It's not that bad."

"Ok. Then get off my couch and walk down those fourteen flights of stairs and then walk the whole mile back to The Moonlight."

A short-lived staring contest broke out.

"Alright, it's more than a scratch," Johnny conceded.

"Take a puff," Paris ordered.

"Why are you set on me smoking that?"

"It will diminish your pain and mellow you out."

"I'm fine."

"Listen, you're in my home."

"I can handle the pain."

"Well, I want you mellow. You're hard to handle."

She thrust out the joint.

"Won't you let me be in pain in peace?"

"You said you weren't in pain."

"You're causing pain."

Paris dangled it in front of his face. "Take it."

Johnny shook his head at her persistence. "You're pushy, you know that?"

"I'll drag you back down those steps."

Johnny reluctantly took the joint, trying to appease her childlike persistence. He brought it to his nose. His lips puckered. It was like sniffing a skunk's ass.

"Take a long, smooth drag. Now with that same breath, breathe in air," she said.

Johnny followed her instructions. Paris took the joint and did the same. When she exhaled, he exhaled.

"Now what?" Johnny said, trying to control his cough.

"Just relax," Paris answered.

Her voice was soothing, calming. With each passing minute, the couch grew softer, hugging and massaging his back, butt, and shoulders. His pain lessened, not only where he had been shot, but the chronic pain in his shoulder. All in the span of a few minutes.

"Better?" she asked.

"Better," Johnny agreed.

"We'll do this again. Maybe next Thursday you can get stabbed instead?"

Johnny smirked. He loved her sass.

"So, you don't drink, but you smoke reefer," Johnny said.

"You're the one breaking the law," Paris shot back.

Till then, cannabis had been used predominantly by two groups of people in the United States—Mexican immigrants migrating into Texas during the Mexican Revolution of 1910 and the Negros of Louisiana. From there, the drug had spread from city to city like the Spanish flu. In 1913, California was the first state to ban cannabis, followed by Maine, Wyoming, and Indiana. Other states joined the ban over the next few years. But Illinois was not among them… not yet.

"How long have you smoked it?" Johnny asked.

"About twelve years. Before bed, after I wake up. I have trouble relaxing. My mind… it doesn't shut off easily. Silence releases thoughts and memories… if that makes any sense."

It made perfect sense. If she only knew the haunting horrors that lurked in the center of his maze.

"And this works?" Johnny asked.

"Not always, but it's the best I can do," Paris said.

Johnny took a sip of his water. His throat was scratchy, reminding him of a bad cold he had gotten when he was eleven, after he had stayed outside too long sledding.

"That's normal," she assured him, knowing what he was experiencing without him having to say it.

Johnny finished half the glass, clearing his throat in an attempt to alleviate the dryness.

"So… Hotsy. He's called that because the girls swoon over him. Tomasso have a nickname?" she asked.

"Tomato," Johnny answered.

"Tomato? Big fan of spaghetti?"

Johnny chuckled, that was true but not the reason. "Tomato likes to wear white and he's got a temper. You ever drop a tomato?"

"Yes…"

"See how it explodes?"

Paris nodded.

"Same thing, only it isn't tomato juice spraying out."

"Well…" was all she could say. It was a much darker reason than she had expected.

Johnny smirked again, his eyes struggling to stay open. The trauma of the gunshot and the relaxing high combined to form a sedative he couldn't overpower, and once again, his eyes closed, and sleep took hold.

And then, the sun was pouring through the window and it was blinding enough to wake him. He shielded his eyes with his forearm. The pain in his side had diminished, but his stomach growled from hunger. His shirt was damp with sweat from the stifling heat. But a more pressing need than his growling stomach and damp shirt was his bursting bladder. He forced his feet to the wooden floor and sat up. The stitches in his stomach pulled but held together. He stood— albeit hunched over, but it was far better than falling flat on his back—and lumbered down the hall.

Paris was asleep on her bed, a sheet covering thigh to chest. A gust of wind blew through the open bedroom window, causing a ripple in the sheet. The beast in Johnny pounded on its fragile cage. He diverted his gaze from her and turned into the bathroom. Even urinating threatened to tear the stitches open. He grunted like he was passing a kidney stone.

After, he cupped his hands under the cold water. He splashed his face and neck, and then scrubbed the dried blood from his hands with a bar of soap. He dipped his face under the faucet and guzzled down the stream of water. His throat was dry, both from hours of fasting and scratchy from the reefer he had smoked. He drank until his mouth was capable of producing saliva again.

He examined his wound in the mirror and was even more impressed with her work. Like a hunchback returning to his cathedral tower, he went back to the couch and sighed as he sat down. It was a grueling hard day's work completed in less than seven minutes.

"Good morning," Paris said.

In the span of those seven minutes, she had gone from being dead asleep on her bed to frying eggs over her stovetop. The heat the oven brought was an intruder, but the smell of toast was a long-lost friend.

"Morning," he said.

Johnny was halfway through a Chesterfield when Paris placed a plate of over-easy eggs and white toast on the coffee table in front of him.

"I'll eat and be on my way," Johnny said.

"I saw you walking to the couch. You're not making it down the steps on your feet. And I'm not dragging you back up again," Paris said.

She squeezed into the corner of the couch and put her feet up on the coffee table.

"That wasn't your first time getting shot, was it?" she asked, after swallowing a bite of toast.

"No," Johnny said curtly.

"No... I think I may have earned more than a one-word reply," Paris said.

She most certainly had.

"I fought in the war."

"*The* war?"

Johnny nodded.

"I pegged you for a doughboy." She took a sip of her water. "I'll never understand war."

"Against it?"

"Against millions of men being unnecessarily slaughtered? Yes."

"You know it was against the law to talk like that?"

"You know it's against the law to sell alcohol like that?"

Johnny grinned, nodding his surrender.

"And that act was repealed over five years ago. I'm free to speak my mind," Paris said.

The Sedition Act of 1918 had forbidden the use of "disloyal, profane, scurrilous, or abusive language" about the United States government, its flag, or its armed forces or language that caused others to view the American government or its institutions with contempt. If convicted, the guilty party could face five to twenty years in prison. There were plenty of poor souls wilting away in a cell for a joke or comment taken out of context. President Wilson had used the War as the reasoning for the bill, but he had been pushing for it before the War had even started. He was ridiculously insecure and couldn't handle criticism.

"Fair enough," Johnny said.

"You were in France?" Paris asked.

Johnny nodded. "Northwest of Verdun."

"Saw a lot of action?"

"Action?" Johnny scoffed at the word. "Yeah… I saw a lot of action."

"I'm sorry for the word choice. I just didn't know how to ask."

"Everything's Jake. Most people don't know how to ask, and most of us don't know how to answer."

A confused expression formed on her face. "What do you mean?"

"Truthfully, no one wants details, any more than I want to give them."

"I can't begin to imagine."

"Don't you dare try."

"That bad?"

"You either find God or you lose him."

106

Paris pondered the severity of that statement.

"And you? Did you find him or lose him?"

"I left God in France."

Paris nodded, acknowledging without words that it was a personal matter. It was the kind of intuition some people lacked.

"Must have been hard on your mother. Worrying about you every day," Paris said.

"Both my parents died from the flu in '18. I didn't get home until a few months after."

Something that made the Spanish Flu so terrifying was that, unlike most flus where the virus was hardest on the young or old, the Spanish Flu was hardest on healthy adults. The flu had been an exterminator, killing in terrifying numbers.

"So you came home and found out your parents had died?" Paris asked.

"Somehow, my grandmother made it. But she was senile at that point. I don't know if she even recognized me anymore. She died a few months later. That was mercy though, you know? To see her go that way, so slow, each day a piece of her dying…"

Paris was genuine in her apology, it showed in her eyes and her frowning lips, but with a death toll conservatively listed at 50 million (100 million was possible), death had not been prejudiced in its attack. The War had claimed over 37 million casualties. Imagine being some lucky man who had survived storming machine gun nests, charging out of trenches, artillery barrages, and storms of bullets only to catch the flu once he was back home.

"It's just you? No brothers or sisters?" Paris asked.

"Just me."

"I'm going to stereotype and say your parents were Catholic? Your father at least."

"Grandmother and father. My mother was Lutheran, but only when my grandmother wasn't around."

"That's uncommon… to be an only child then. Don't Catholics breed like rabbits?"

Johnny laughed. "It's not a commandment or anything."

"Not a verse of scripture? *'Go forth and reproduce'*?"

"They would use 'procreate', wouldn't tell you how though. Plenty of Catholic virgins flipping through the Bible for help."

Paris giggled. "I know lots of Catholics, and none of the families are small."

"My mother had a few miscarriages, so the priest forgave them for at least trying."

Paris' smile disappeared. "Terrible thing for a mother."

"Not as terrible as getting a knock on your door and being told your son was blown up in France. That his face is gone, but the dog tags say it's him. That his body is in a pit with a thousand others, rotting next to the same men he had tried to kill."

"No… I guess not."

He could tell she looked at him differently than she had moments earlier. It was that feeling of being next to someone who had seen something atrocious.

"What about you? All alone?" Johnny asked.

"A step-sister and a step-brother, handful of nieces and nephews," Paris rambled off like it was a list of ingredients to unleavened bread.

"You don't see them?"

The cold way she had mentioned it insinuated there was distance between them.

"No. They didn't get along with my mother and didn't hide it."

"Some anger in your voice."

"Plenty. They never visited her when she was sick."

"She get better?"

Paris shook her head.

"Was it the flu?"

"Cancer. It was… hard to watch. Like with your grandmother. Watching this invisible killer murder your mother piece by piece, day by day."

"I'm not sorry I missed my parents' death. I know that's cowardly, but—"

"No, I get it."

"You keep in touch with your step-father?"

"No."

She hadn't pressed him about his faith, and he would repay her by not continuing the conversation about her family.

"You're a flower with no roots. There's nothing here for you, so why don't you leave?" Johnny asked.

"Every flower comes with weeds," Paris said. "You just don't walk away. And besides, I live better here than I would otherwise. How would I support myself? You may see me as a light-skinned Negro, but to the rest of the country, I'm just Negro. A Negro woman. There's no work for me. I know what I do won't last forever. I pray to God it doesn't. I'm trying to make as much as I can as quickly as I can."

Johnny had spent his whole life feeling like an outsider—because he was. He knew he would never be accepted by Valcoro. But it was more than that. Not belonging was engraved in his psyche. It was a constant feeling, a ball of doubt roiling in his gut.

But there was so much available to him that wasn't to Paris. He was a man. A man born in America. But Johnny was a part of the life, and you just didn't walk away.

"Listen, I've got some errands to run. Are you going to be okay when I'm gone? I don't really want to come home and find you dead on my floor," Paris said.

"You don't have to worry about me dying on the floor. I don't plan on leaving the couch," Johnny replied, forcing a smile.

Paris couldn't help but return it. She shook her head, grabbed her purse, and left.

Johnny reached for the bottle of aspirin she had left on the coffee table and shook out six. He finished off his glass of lukewarm water, then lay back down. When he woke, the clock on the wall showed ten after twelve. He struggled to his feet and into the bathroom. The eight-ounce glass of water had somehow transformed into two gallons of urine, and the instant it left his body, he was left with a mouth as dry as the Sahara.

He filled his glass at the kitchen sink, downed it in three gulps, and refilled it. Then he hobbled to the window, testing his stitches, but not at the cost of ripping them open. The window was ajar, and he hoped a gust of wind would straight up attack him like a rabid animal. But the heat that gushed in made him question the fundamental tenet of almost every religion. How could Hell be below him when the window in front of him was its gate?

At one in the afternoon, he cleaned and redressed his wound, glancing at the clock often. Paris had said she had errands to run. But given how long she had been gone, the appropriate phrase would have been *errands to crawl.* As boredom threatened to cause more damage than the bullet, he went into the kitchen and looked for something to cook. Her refrigerator and cupboards were almost empty. He loaded the counter with everything he could use—garlic cloves, a box of long-strand pasta, eggs, lemons, and an onion. He chopped, cut, diced, boiled, and cooked.

When Paris did return, the apartment smelt of minced garlic and lemon zest with a complimentary haze of smoke rising from the stove top.

"Make yourself at home," Paris said thick with sarcasm.

"Just trying not to die as instructed," Johnny said.

"Thank you for the effort. What are you making?"

"Bucatini with lemony carbonara."

Paris hung her purse on a kitchen chair and then grabbed two plates from her cupboard.

"Did you do my laundry too?" she asked.

She twirled the pasta onto the fork and took a bite. Judging by her reaction, she had not expected to like it.

"This is fantastic," she said.

"Not like I made it up, just following a recipe," Johnny said, brushing off the compliment.

110

"Whose?"

"My grandmother. She cooked for friends and family every Friday when I was young."

"You helped her cook?"

"As a kid I thought so. Looking back, I'm sure all I did was annoy the hell out of her."

"Your grandmother and I would have gotten along so well."

Johnny smirked again.

"She come over with your father?" Paris asked.

"About a year later, after my father had some real estate and a paycheck," Johnny answered.

"And a grandson."

"My grandfather had died some years back before I was born, but she left a lot of family and friends behind. I don't think she ever truly considered New York home."

Paris had no wine, so instead they drank milk between bites of their pasta. Liquor was such a huge part of the culture. They drank wine and beer at dinner, at parties, at birthdays and weddings. Johnny had eaten that meal hundreds of times, and not once had it been unaccompanied by wine. For Johnny, not sipping Pino Grigio or Gavi with this food was more criminal than breaking the Volstead Act.

Johnny ate with his head down and kept his eyes on his plate. But Paris' stare was strong, impossible to ignore. He looked up from his plate to meet it. A gaze that somehow intimidated yet emboldened him, weakened him yet instilled strength—a gaze he didn't how to read.

"What?" he asked.

"I don't get you," Paris said. "You come home from the War a hero. How do you get involved in this life? I mean selling booze is one thing. Burning down distilleries and getting shot at is something else entirely."

"Kind of personal, isn't it?"

"Bleeding all over my couch is kind of personal, isn't it?"

Johnny nodded, a smirk on his face. Their conversations were like chess matches, and she didn't even surrender a pawn. She had a fearlessness about her that was intoxicating.

"I don't know," Johnny said.

Paris rolled her eyes and rose from the table, grabbing her empty plate.

"Growing up, all I ever heard was that I could do or be anything," Johnny said.

The only thing he could do was talk and hope that she found worth in some of what he said.

Paris stood still.

"America is where dreams come true. I never had any. Growing up, I helped my father at his store. He sold fruit, vegetables, canned goods, the homemade pies my mother and grandmother made, stuff like that. I'd watch people shoplift or say they'd be right back with the money they owed. My father let it slide. The worst offenders were the cops. He had to give them a cut of what he earned. Sometimes twenty percent, sometimes forty. There was protection tax, delivery tax, stocking tax, holiday tax, processing tax, you name it. They used fancy words to defend what they did, but they robbed him. Plain and simple. They did that to every immigrant. Everyone but Carlisle Salconie. They never took his money."

"Why?" Paris asked.

"Because they knew what happened to the swine that crossed him. Salconie sold Italian meats—pepperoni, salami, pastrami. Rumor was he once made a sausage out of a corrupt pig—"

"Pig?"

"Police officer."

Paris looked sick.

"Rumor said he sent it to the other officers. I don't know if that's true. Makes for a good story... Anyway, I'd pick up deli meats from his place. He was always nice to me. We had hour-long conversations during Friday afternoons for years. Then Uncle Sam told me I had to go fight. When I came back, I struggled. For over a year, my job was violence, existing in this dog-eat-dog world. And then I was just supposed to assimilate back into civilized society. My father's shop closed after my parents died. Then my grandmother passed. I had nothing. I couldn't find work, and when I did I couldn't hold it. Then one day, Salconie set me down at a table and gave me a free pastrami sandwich on rye bread and a lime Miller soda pop. We talked for hours. He told me about the Wets and the Drys and the Temperance Movement, and that the country would be alcohol free soon. But people would still want it. He said there would be money in it, but more importantly, it was a service. Men who worked fourteen-hour days wanted to unwind with a beer. Women gathering together wanted to sip wine. The rich had stockpiled enough liquor to last years. The loophole in the law allowed a person to keep whatever they had before Prohibition went into effect. It was another law only the poor felt. I guarded booze from the same criminals who had stolen my family's money, and now claimed to be upholding the law. Hotsy was in New York on business May of '21. He ran a job with me. Things went south, I put a pig down. Salconie told me I needed to hang low and leave New York. He told me his friend Jack Salvatory could get me set up in Chicago. Hotsy told me it was the place to be. I boarded a train and never looked back... the violence, the life, it's all I've known."

"Don't you want to know something else?"

It was a question he had asked himself a thousand times. A question buried in the center of the maze surrounded by other questions, answers and truths, some of which he accepted and some that he denied. Paris' question was one that stayed on his mind. It had for years.

Retaliation

That Friday, after eighteen new dressings, and four more servings of bucatini with lemony carbonara, Johnny was able to leave Paris' apartment. She had been gracious enough to pick up his black Chevy FB-50 touring and drive it back to her apartment and field daily calls from Tomato and Hotsy, assuring both that Johnny was recovering well. Both were dying to see him, but there was a family in Cicero running low on money, and that took precedence.

The drive was what he had hoped for. Though it made his wound tight, it was meditative but too short lived.

Johnny pulled alongside the curb across the apartment building and killed the engine. He dug into his pocket and pulled out the wad of folded cash he had had on him the night he was shot. Because of the blood stains on them, every president on the bills looked as though they had been assassinated. He separated those, not wanting to give Cilly literal blood money.

The small stoop to the apartment entrance had never once been intimidating until now. He felt indebted to the Gods that they lived on the first floor. The street, usually filled with playing children, was empty. It was more than likely they had been called inside to clean up for dinner.

He struggled up the stoop, grimacing and releasing a four-letter curse. The front door stuck, then jerked open, hitting Johnny's injured side. He let out another curse word, this one far more colorful.

Would knocking on the door release another curse word? Before he had to figure that out, Wally opened the door.

"Evening Johnny. I saw you crossing the street. You moved like a turtle. Lucky no cars were coming by or I'd be scraping you up with a shovel," he said.

Johnny smirked.

"Wally!" his mother exclaimed from inside, "what kind of way is that to talk to someone! What an awful thing to say!"

Wally smiled, knowing he had gotten a rise out of his mother.

"We're just getting dinner ready. We can set another plate," Wally said.

He opened the door fully. But Johnny waited for Cilly's invite. As hospitable as Wally was, it wasn't for him to invite him in.

"Of course we can," Cilly said.

Johnny waved his hand, politely refusing the dinner invite. "It's okay."

The food she had prepared would scarcely have been enough for the three of them, and now she was willing to reduce their portions to feed Johnny. You can't measure the goodness in people until they are down and out. The Nettesheims were far down and way out. And they were good to the very bone. It was the kind of goodness that made most people question their intelligence. Self-preservation should have kicked in by now. Instead, the Nettesheims had a selflessness few possessed and even fewer understood.

During the War, Herbert Hoover, the head of the Food and Drug administration, had called for "Meatless Tuesdays" and "Wheatless Wednesdays" in an attempt to save food for the troops fighting over in Europe. What those rich Washington politicians had failed to realize was there already were "Meatless" Thursdays and Saturdays and "Wheatless" Sundays and Fridays. Hell, entire weeks were "meatless" and "wheatless." Poverty wasn't something you simply announced as being over.

Wally grabbed Johnny's hand and half-escorted half-dragged him to the kitchen.

Cilly dished potatoes with cheese onto each plate. Five Idaho potatoes total. They must have had some baby red in their lineage because none were of impressive size.

Clarence was at the table, his arms dangling lifelessly at his sides, a blank expression on his face and drool ready to slobber onto the floor. But Cilly had it timed perfectly, keeping an internal clock, and was always there with a rag to wipe his mouth before the slobber dropped to the floor.

"Looks good, mom," Wally complimented.

"Can't go wrong with cheese," Johnny agreed.

He would be able to get a nice fattening meal at The Moonlight in a couple of hours. The Nettesheims would have to wait until morning for a couple of eggs and a piece of dry toast, the butter dish empty after being used for dinner.

Wally helped his father, cutting his potato into pieces.

"Here you go, dad," Wally said.

He piled the potato on the fork and brought it to his father's mouth. Clarence opened wide, his eyes never blinking, chewing the forkful of potato with as much fervor as a goat chewing grass.

It was a quick meal. You could only eat a medium-sized potato so slowly before it was obviously intentional. It did nothing but tease Johnny's stomach that a true meal was on its way.

"What do you say we get some ice cream? Try to knock out this heat?" Johnny asked Wally.

"I would like nothing more. Can I go mom?" Wally asked.

"Yes, you may," Cilly replied.

116

"I tell you what though, we got to do these dishes first. Let your mom help your dad change out of his day clothes and into something more comfortable," Johnny said.

"There's always a catch," Wally said.

Johnny and Wally were on dishwashing duty while Cilly helped Clarence into the bathroom. Wally had one thing on his mind while he washed—speed. Johnny had to point out bits of potato starch and melted cheese clinging to the plates.

"You wash your face this well?" Johnny teased.

"It adds character," Wally said.

The wit on the kid.

He even insisted on skipping the drying, saying that air drying wouldn't leave lint on the plates. The weasel just wanted out of drying, so he could get his ice cream sooner.

After the dishes were dried (by towel) and put away, Wally moved with a frenzy only seen when sweets were involved. In ten years, it would be girls who made him dance with such giddiness.

Wally hopped down from the stoop without taking a step, landing on the hopscotch square and completing the corresponding sequence written in chalk.

"Your turn," he said.

"Rain check, bud," Johnny said.

Walking was challenging enough.

"How'd you like dinner?" Wally asked on their hike to the ice cream parlor.

"It was excellent," Johnny answered.

"Yeah, mom knows how to make a good potato. She does well with what she's got. She loves cooking big meals like Thanksgiving. I wish we had the money for her to do it. It really brings her joy," Wally said.

The line at the ice cream parlor, Commodore's, was longer than either Wally or Johnny had hoped. They were also stuck in the worst spot in line. The sun attacked there more than any other spot. Commodore's couldn't have loved it more. They wanted their customers thirsty and hot. It not only opened their sweat pores, but their wallets too.

"Boy, that damn sun sure has a hatred for us, huh?" Wally mentioned.

"You know my grandmother used to make me suck on a bar of soap when I cursed," Johnny said.

"Fresh breath is a courtesy," Wally said with a sneer.

Johnny shook his head and pulled the door open. They stepped inside, finally getting some shade from the stifling sun. Wally studied the menu with more dedication than he put into any of his school subjects, and within minutes, he had every item memorized.

"What are you leaning toward?" Wally asked.

"Dreamland Sundae sounds good," Johnny said.

"I thought you would have picked the Brooklyn Bridge on account of being from New York."

"I thought about it. But the mixture of orange and mint syrup doesn't sound appealing to me. What are you thinking?"

"Well I think the Commodore Perry is appealing. But it's eighteen cents. I want to make sure I can get my mom and dad something. The single scoop is only ten cents."

The kid had practically floated to the ice cream parlor. His eyes had lit up like it was Christmas morning, yet here he was, getting the blandest item on the menu to make sure his mom and dad could have dessert too.

Good to the last bone.

"Don't worry about it. Get what you want. We'll make sure we get your parents something good too," Johnny said.

Wally nodded and smiled sincerely. "Thanks, Johnny."

The line started moving, and with so many options, it didn't feel like they had been reading the menu for ten minutes when the middle-aged man wearing a soda jerk hat greeted them enthusiastically.

"Hi, can we get one Commodore Perry and two Bull Mooses—" Wally turned to Johnny. "Moose or mooses?"

Johnny shrugged. "I don't know."

Wally nodded politely, dismissing its importance. "And there'll be one more order from my pal, Johnny."

He stepped aside, granting Johnny the stage.

"Make it two Commodore Perrys," Johnny said.

"Excellent choices! Sixty-six cents please," the worker said.

Johnny removed a dollar from his pocket, making sure it wasn't stained with blood, and handed it to the man.

Johnny held the change out for Wally to take. "Here. For graciously doing the dishes."

"Oh, you don't have to pay me for that, Johnny," Wally said.

"You hold onto it. Help chip in for some groceries."

"I'll make sure to get something for my mom. She's earned it."

He took the change, placed it in his pocket, and they stepped off to the side, allowing the next people in line to order.

"Bull Moose?" Johnny asked.

"My mom likes wafers. It comes with two of them to look like the antlers of a moose," Wally explained.

Johnny grabbed a handful of napkins and stashed them in his pocket.

The four sundaes were set on the counter, each containing a glorious amount of ice cream, and more importantly, each a weapon against the heat. The Commodore Perry had a scoop of strawberry, vanilla, and French vanilla ice cream, drizzled with crushed strawberries, crushed pineapple, and grape juice, all topped off with a dollop of whipped cream and red cherries.

"Let's take a quick bite before we have to get these back to your parents," Johnny said.

"We're going to have haul some serious ass to get home before it melts," Wally said.

Johnny looked for the grin that usually spread on Wally's face after he swore. But it wasn't there. He wasn't even aware he had sworn.

Wally clinked his spoon against Johnny's. "What are you going for first?"

119

"I need to try this grape juice part," Johnny said.

"I'm right behind you."

They dug their spoons into the ice cream and shoveled it into their mouths. The grape juice was refreshing and sweet, and the ice cream brought a sugary chill. Taste buds fired and demanded another bite. Johnny had been victim to many vices Wally hadn't experienced. But with sugar, there was an addiction all its own.

Wally beamed. "Well, did I lead you astray?"

"Definitely not. This is amazing," Johnny said.

"It sure is. Let's get back home."

They each grabbed two of the sundaes and were tormented on the walk back watching them melt. The temperature had cooled, and the sun didn't follow them like a stalker, granting them more time before the ice creams were nothing but milk and crushed fruit.

When they stepped up the stoop, both realized they had no hands to open the door.

"Mom!" Wally yelled, the word echoing down the street.

It was a yell a mother felt in her soul. The door opened in mere seconds. Cilly's terrified face morphed into view, relief washing over her now that none of the hundreds of horrifying possibilities going through her mind had come to pass.

"No hands," Wally said in defense of his yelling.

Cilly ushered them in and closed the door behind them.

Clarence was in his favorite chair, dressed in a clean pair of slacks and white t-shirt. He took no notice of his son and Johnny when they stepped inside, and was unfazed by his son's scream. Instead his gaze was fixated at the open window and what lay beyond.

"Clarence, Wally and Johnny got us some ice cream," Cilly said.

She pulled a kitchen chair next to him, and Wally set the two Bull Mooses (moose?) on the windowsill ledge.

Cilly alternated between eating her own ice cream and feeding Clarence. But each mouthful Clarence consumed required his mouth to be wiped. By the time Cilly could concentrate on her own, it would be nothing but milk. But it didn't bother her in the slightest. She thanked Johnny at least three times.

"Wally picked them out," Johnny said.

Wally finished his sundae the quickest. He used his spoon to get into every crevice and corner of the dish. In the military, the phrase "Leave No Man Behind" was a mantra. Wally held the same belief toward ice cream.

"Flavors worked well together," Wally said.

"Sure did," Johnny agreed.

He checked the time. He had stayed later than anticipated. Tomato and Hotsy must be waiting to see him.

"I have to get going," Johnny said, rising from the couch.

"Thanks for the ice cream, Johnny," Wally said.

"Anytime. Thanks for supper, Cilly," Johnny said.

"Of course. I'm sorry it wasn't more," Cilly replied, blushing.

She wasn't dumb or naïve. She knew a medium-sized potato, and kindly called medium, was not enough to fill a grown man's stomach. But it had been a week of delinquent payments. Every dime they had in the place—apart from Wally's jar of change (which Cilly would never take from him)—had been used to keep the collectors at bay. Johnny wanted to hate them. Cilly had enough to worry about without having collectors hang around outside the apartment building waiting for her. But how could he judge them? They either sent letters in the mail or incessantly knocked on the door. Johnny destroyed property or broke bones.

He removed a wad of cash from his pocket and set it in the dish next to the door. Cilly could have used it all, even the ones with the blood-stained assassinated presidents. Cilly knew his business was booze, but she didn't know about the bullets and the blood. The red-stained bills would paint a clear picture. There was a chance he wouldn't be welcome anymore. They needed the money, and Johnny needed them.

"Johnny—" Cilly said, looking at the money, but Johnny wouldn't let her finish.

"You eat somewhere, you pay."

"Had you eaten someplace else, you would have gotten more food."

"But worse company."

Cilly appreciated the comment, but the blushing didn't fade. She was a proud woman, not in a hubristic way, but a woman raised on the pillars of hard work and never accepting handouts. It was one of the many reasons Johnny never hesitated to help her out. She had offered a free meal, a cup of coffee and conversation long before he had first given her money.

"Tell you what, I'll stop by tomorrow night and make an Italian dinner if it's alright with your mom," Johnny said.

"That'd be nice," Cilly said.

A smile spread on Wally's face, his eyes twinkling. "Will there be cheese?"

"There's always cheese," Johnny said.

"Thank you, Johnny... again," Cilly said.

Johnny only nodded in response. "See you later, Clarence."

Clarence only stared out of the window. Each time he failed to acknowledge being spoken to killed Wally and Cilly a bit more. There was a small glimmer of hope in their eyes that sparkled like a star, but like a dying star, it faded away. There had been ten thousand moments to reiterate the inevitable. But love is blind, forgiving, and hopeful.

Cicero was a city controlled by vices, but it was impossible to tell at that moment. At that moment, it was as peaceful as a sunset over the horizon in the Old West. Somehow during potatoes and ice cream, Johnny had forgotten about being shot. The drive back to Chicago was quiet, the traffic increasing the closer he got. Suburbanites rushed into the city to get zozzled, gamble their paychecks away or score a fresh lay. Johnny parked across The Moonlight, directly behind Tomato's Cadillac Town Sedan. He pulled a torch from his pack of Chesterfields and lit it, delaying before he would have to address the shooting and the repercussions it would bring.

The cold ice cream had helped lower his body temperature, dulling his pain. But the ice cream's effect was long gone now, allowing the pain and the great annoyance brought on by the heat to return uninhibited.

When Johnny stepped inside The Moonlight, Hotsy and Tomato rushed at him like two bullets. They yanked him into a hug, inadvertently hitting his stitches and causing Johnny to grimace.

"Thank Christ," Tomato said.

His eyes were bloodshot. It was obvious he had spent a large portion of the last week crying and just a small portion sleeping.

"What I said before... about Diamond helping you... I..." Tomato said. He looked sick about his last words the night Johnny had been shot.

Johnny shook his head, dismissing Tomato's comment before he could even finish it. It had been a joke, and he didn't believe in jinxes.

"Johnny... I'm sorry," Hotsy said.

Hotsy looked even worse than Tomato. Guilt was something Johnny had never seen him wear. All the times he had slept with married women, stolen or destroyed property, he had never given it a second thought.

"This isn't on either of you," Johnny said.

"No, I should of known we'd have heat on us," Hotsy said. "I was too worried about getting tail—"

Tomato cut him off. "It's on me. I never would of forgiven myself if you had been killed. I can't take back what happened. But I can promise you we're going to find the man who shot you. And when we do, I'm going to put him in the ground."

Tomato may not have upheld the vow of fidelity, but the words he spoke were an oath. He would search all of Chicago, all of the Midwest, the whole world to find the man who had shot Johnny.

"The Cardinal wants to see us. But first, a drink," Tomato said, guiding Johnny to the bar.

A tall whiskey Old-Fashioned was waiting for him. Its orange-red mix was as sexy as a long-legged dame. But it was the drink to the right of the Old Fashioned

123

that caught Johnny's attention—a cranberry vodka. There was only one occasion that Tomato drank it—a hit.

"Don't make a scene here," Tomato said when he caught Johnny's look.

He raised the glass to his lips and gulped down the blood-red liquid.

Johnny looked to Hotsy. He had a fierce, almost maniacal, expression.

"Tonight, he sees his last sunset," Hotsy said.

He grabbed his own drink—the Southside Fizz, a combination of gin, lemon juice, club soda, mint and simple syrup. The same drink Al Capone bought them any time he visited the hotel. It wasn't the best tasting drink, but Hotsy knew what to drink for what he wanted to do. If he wanted to play catch up, it was Panther Piss (whiskey) on the rocks. Most often, he drank the Gin Rickey. But the Southside Fizz was the drink he went to before dealing South Side business.

Not even the weight of imminent murder could dim the satisfaction of drinking the Old Fashioned. The whiskey numbed Johnny's aching abdomen. It was like reuniting with a former lover—the one who got away.

The dinner crowd would soon rush in, and the women of the hotel strutted out to offer dessert first. Paris was among them, looking radiant in a svelte silver dress. But it wasn't her low-cut dress that had caught his attention. It was her eyes. Those sultry eyes.

Tomato always had an intimidating presence, but now his cold, threatening stare chilled the liquor on the bar shelf. Hotsy, who would usually cast winks and devious smiles at the women while undressing them with his eyes, only stared at the shelf of liquor, his back to the women.

Johnny had killed men—both planned and as a random reaction. In war, reaction was everything. Sometimes, survival was gifted to those who reacted the quickest. There was no time to think when you charged out of a trench. You ran against instinct, against reason, against sanity. You just ran and hoped the hail of steel and brass missed you.

But war in Chicago meant planning. Killing someone was discussed, contemplated, and thought through. Johnny preferred the randomness of Europe. To sit and wait for a time or place, knowing you were going to end a life was a heavy burden. The same questions went through your head as in Europe. But in Europe, you didn't know the poor bloke you had killed. Sure, you wondered if he had family. You pictured his sobbing mother standing over one of those God-awful bland caskets. Did he have a young bride at home? A high-school sweetheart or a woman he had met some random, yet fated night? Did he have children? Had Johnny sentenced a son to grow up without a father? Had he forsaken a daughter to never know a father's unconditional love? But those men in war had always been unknowns. Not here. Not in Chicago. Here you knew the man you planned on killing. You knew his name, his nickname, his friends, his family. And if you didn't, the *Tribune* enlightened you in the obituaries. It was a courtesy to kill in a way that allowed for an open casket. Like that mattered. It didn't diminish the amount of tears shed. Murder was murder, open casket or closed casket. And once again, caskets and coffins broke through to the surface of his thoughts.

Don't let it happen again. Just breathe. Sip and breathe.

They imbibed their drinks, pretending to pay attention to the Negro jazz band on stage, but Johnny's eyes stayed on Paris mingling with the rich guests. It had been mere hours since he had last seen her, only blocks away. But that was impossible. That was decades ago, and a world away.

Tomato finished his drink, and Johnny and Hotsy knew to do the same. Whether she felt his stare or had been scanning the room for him, Johnny didn't know, but Paris ignored the men lobbying for her attention and cast that knee-weakening, bulldozer smile at Johnny. But he couldn't return it. Her smile vanished, replaced by the same look she had worn when Johnny had been bleeding out on her couch. Their stare remained unbroken the entire distance from the lobby bar to the conference room.

Inside, The Cardinal was standing as still as a statue.

"Johnny, I'm glad to see you on your feet," he said, hugging him much more appropriately for a man recovering from a gunshot wound.

Johnny nodded his thanks. It was awkward being congratulated for having survived being shot.

"Vencini okayed retaliation," Tomato said, not wasting any time on small talk.

"Against who?" Johnny asked.

Tomato had promised to exact revenge. Johnny believed he wanted to, but against whom? No doubt, it was Mickey Diamond who had ordered the hit. But he had dozens of men working for him, and not just bootleggers and gunman, but police too. Both Tomato and Hotsy had grilled Johnny (via Paris) over the phone for descriptions of the perpetrator. The only details he could definitively give was that it was not Mickey Diamond nor his right hand man, Sean O'Malley, and that the man who had shot him was overweight with a thin mustache and looked horrified at what he had done. Someone Hotsy had referred to as a "trigger virgin."

The Cardinal reached into his breast pocket and pulled out a two-by-four photograph.

"Is this the man who shot you?" he asked.

The man in the picture was overweight with a chubby face and a pathetic mustache. The only thing missing was the shocked expression when he had lost control of the gun.

"That's him," Johnny said.

It was strange to see a photograph of a man who had tried to kill you, and Johnny couldn't help but be in awe of The Cardinal. He had found the man who'd shot him based on the most basic of descriptions.

"That man is Earl Kowalski. Apart from his name and address, I don't know anything about him. It is my recommendation we hold off until we know more," The Cardinal said.

Tomato scoffed at the suggestion. "Hold off?"

"Don't go in blind," The Cardinal warned.

"This man put a bullet in Johnny! I don't care who he is! It demands retaliation!" Tomato yelled, loudly enough that it was unlikely that even the band had drowned it out.

"For if you forgive other people when they sin against you, your heavenly Father will also forgive you," The Cardinal quoted. *"But if you do not forgive others their sins, your Father will not forgive your sins."*

"What the hell does that mean? Are you saying we should forgive this guy?" Hotsy asked. He hadn't been raised a Catholic nor did he practice it now as an adult. Churches were nothing to him but the site of weddings and funerals.

"What I'm saying is this was not a personal hit. It was retaliation for the distillery. I'm just saying, you don't know who this man is. He could be a prohibition agent or a police officer," The Cardinal explained patiently.

"If he is a cop, then he is a crooked son of a bitch and deserves to be put down like the rabid animal he is. Vencini okayed the hit," Hotsy said.

"He okayed it because he wants revenge for Two Shits, blind revenge. God gave me eyes to use them," The Cardinal said, his voice remaining calm.

"You want to quote scripture?" Tomato asked. "You like the New Testament. I've never been a fan of that turn-the-other-cheek bullshit. I prefer the Old Testament. Wrath. Anger. Pain. Vengeance. Zephaniah chapter 1, verse 18. *'Neither their silver nor their gold will be able to deliver them on the day of the Lord's wrath; and all the earth will be devoured in the fire of his jealousy, For He will make a complete end, indeed a terrifying one, Of all the inhabitants of the earth.'"* He pointed to the picture of Kowalski in The Cardinal's hand. "I'm going to deliver the Lord's wrath on that man."

The Cardinal shrugged, his hands folded in front of him. He had given his advice, but he wouldn't fight to have it heeded. Johnny's face could only show half an apology. The Cardinal was great because he knew booze was a business. He wanted it to be like any other business—lower costs, more proficient ways of producing, and more attractive advertising to outsell the competition. But contracts in booze were signed not by pens, but bullets, and not with ink, but blood. But Johnny couldn't condemn the level of loyalty Hotsy and Tomato were showing either.

Hotsy and Tomato stormed out of the conference room. Johnny lingered behind for a moment. The Cardinal wore the look of a parent who knew their child was making a mistake.

Even the buzzed strangers knew Tomato was in a hot mood and kept their distance from him. Paris was at the bar, not fully engaged in the conversation she was currently caught in. Her gaze fixed on Johnny once more. He met her eyes for only a moment—a courtesy. She had an ability to read eyes, and he wouldn't let her read his. He wouldn't give her any idea where he was headed.

They stepped outside into the fresh, muggy nighttime air, crossed the street, and took their designated positions inside Tomato's car.

"Listen, I appreciate what you're willing to do for me but—"

Tomato rounded on Johnny. "Listen to me. You're my brother. Someone takes a shot at you, that doesn't go unanswered. If I had been with you like I should have been, he'd already be dead, and you wouldn't have a hole in your side."

Johnny fell silent. Tomato had his mind made up, and Hotsy, who always went for rash thinking, was adamant in his stance too. It was the kind of loyalty only dogs possessed. The Moonlight, hell the whole world, was full of fake friends. Friends who gossiped behind a friend's back. Friends who were only friends when it profited them. Friends who would cower at the first sign of trouble. Anyone would be so lucky to have friends as loyal as Tomato and Hotsy.

The speed at which Tomato drove deserved a ticket, but the police of the North Side suburbs better hope they didn't try pulling him over. Not tonight. And they didn't. They were too busy looking for reasons to arrest the poor. If being rich protected you from war and prohibition, it protected you from minor traffic violations.

The address The Cardinal had provided led to an extravagant apartment complex.

"Look at this," Hotsy said, gawking at the ritzy residence.

How some could live so large while others lived so small was infuriating. A caliber of wealth where people had a laundrist, a chambermaid, a parlor maid, and a mother maid to ensure every possible need and want was met and met promptly.

"Gate probably costs more than my apartment building," Tomato said.

The gate, a rich black in color and polished to a high sheen, had two spiral lion heads forged into it.

"Shall we depreciate the value then?" Hotsy asked, holding up a crow bar.

He opened the car door and jogged to the gate. Johnny and Tomato leaned out of the windows to better see any potential threats, while Hotsy snapped off the lock and pushed the gate open. It was so well-kept that it didn't even creak.

Tomato put the car in drive, turned off the headlights, and crept forward through the gate at a speed that allowed Hotsy to hop into the backseat without the car having to stop. Tomato parked the car a hundred yards away from the front entrance of the apartment complex. They watched the windows like ravens scouting for twitching worms. The only movement outlined in any of the sixty windows—ten on each floor—was an old woman rocking in her chair, crocheting a blanket, and two little children dashing in and out of frame in a game of tag. Johnny checked his watch—8:57. The sun had descended enough to conceal the car, but the complex had lamp posts every fifteen feet. God forbid the poor aristocrats had to go out in the scary dark. The parking lot was clear, so it was only a question of if there would be any surprises when they were inside.

"Should we go?" Tomato asked.

"If we wait a bit longer that old lady may have that blanket done," Hotsy said.

Tomato raised his hand to strike Hotsy but settled for shaking his head. "You'll end up sleeping with her."

"Come on Tomato, don't tempt me," Hotsy said.

They tiptoed out of car, closing the doors as quietly as they could, so the surrounding silence didn't betray them with an echoing, resounding clang. The nice thing about the rich was they loved glass. While the poor and middle class had doors of pine and oak—which would require a shotgun blast to break—the rich had frosted or stained glass.

Tomato broke the glass with his revolver.

"You think to check if it's unlocked?" Hotsy asked.

Tomato scowled.

Hotsy shrugged. "I'm just saying."

"Yes, I checked," Tomato said.

"Good. You woulda told me the same thing, that's all I'm saying."

Their argument grew louder with each rebuttal.

"That blanket's about done," Johnny said.

Hotsy had gotten the last word, and Tomato literally bit his tongue to keep quiet. He inserted his hand through the opening and unlocked the door. *Click*.

Of course, the building had an elevator. Hiking up a stairwell was an absurd, barbaric concept to the tenants. But Johnny, Tomato, and Hotsy always avoided elevators. You never knew who would be waiting outside when the doors opened or if the damn thing would get stuck.

"What floor?" Johnny asked.

"Sixth," Tomato answered.

The steps pulled Johnny's stitches but walking up them—and not crawling, like last time—was a nice change of pace.

"Why can't these guys ever live on the first floor?" Hotsy asked, glancing up at the mountain of stairs above him.

"Same reason you can't keep your mouth shut—it's a cruel world," Tomato said.

"Yeah, yeah. You keep singing me to sleep, Tomato."

After ascending the three remaining flights, Tomato spoke. "This is it."

They stood outside room 609. Johnny removed his M1911, Tomato his Colt Police Positive revolver, and Hotsy, dejected that he had not been allowed to bring his shotgun, settled for a Smith and Wesson revolver.

They exchanged a series of nods, confirming they were ready.

Tomato kicked the door in. One by one, they barreled inside.

"Don't move!" Tomato yelled.

Earl Kowalski was seated at his kitchen table, a plate of half-eaten brownie squares in front of him.

But he wasn't alone.

Tomato Splat

When it came to a hit, planning was the most important task. Scouting was a slow, sometimes mind-numbing, process. It was like going on a diet and ignoring the temptations. But scouting was the reason you could charge into a room and know who was inside. When you rushed in without due diligence—like Johnny, Tomato, and Hotsy had—surprising unknowns greeted you behind the door.

Seated around Earl Kowalski was his family—a woman in her mid-thirties with auburn hair and two young girls, no more than six and nine. Each of the four had been doing different things: Kowalski was reading the morning news and polishing off the remaining brownies, his wife was completing a crossword puzzle, the older girl was coloring, and the younger one was rocking her doll to sleep.

Johnny, Tomato, and Hotsy glanced at each other. None of them had expected Kowalski to be surrounded by a wife and children. But it was foolish to be surprised. They had known nothing about the man except his address and his face.

Johnny stepped forward. A maternal instinct seemed to take over all three women. Kowalski's wife shielded her daughters, the older girl squeezed her little sister's hand, and the younger girl whispered to her doll that she was safe.

Johnny desperately hoped they had gone to the wrong address or, at the very least, the wrong apartment number. But when Kowalski's eyes lit up with fear, the same as the night he had put a bullet in Johnny, there was no mistaking they had the right man.

Kowalski's terror-filled eyes darted about the kitchen, probably calculating if he had enough time to reach one of his pistols stashed about. Hotsy shook his head—a warning that if he lifted his ass from his chair, he'd be shot dead in his own kitchen, even if his kids had to see it.

"We're here for a word. We need to step outside," Tomato said, keeping his pistol pointed down.

He wouldn't risk accidentally harming one of the young girls. Nor would he cause them any more fear than what was currently surging through their bodies. Any decent human being would have been conflicted in this position. But for Tomato, he was a stranger breaking into his own home and gazing upon his own family.

Kowalski didn't move. For a man who had shot someone, he acted too sheepish to be capable of it. Johnny half-expected him to use his children as a shield.

"Be a man. Get up. Walk out," Tomato said.

"Don't go! Please don't leave!" the woman begged her husband when he stood, grabbing his shirt like she was clinging from a ledge. When that didn't work, she pleaded with Tomato. "Just leave, I beg you! You don't have to do this! Please! Why are you doing this? Please God, just go!" Thick tears ran down her cheeks.

Johnny often pictured the surviving family members of the men he had killed. A wife and child looking down at their dearly departed. His viewpoint was always the man in the casket. The faces gazing down at him had always been vague. A woman with brown hair but a featureless face, tiny children sobbing hysterically. But that anonymity wouldn't be granted to him now. A woman with curly dark brown hair that matched her eyes, a long, pointy nose and high cheekbones. The two young girls who were clones of their mother. There would be no obscurity in the faces that haunted him now. A photograph of this moment would etch itself on to his mind forever.

You didn't fight over there and not imagine your mother or wife getting the knock on the door from a soldier telling her that you'd been killed. How would the news be broken? How would it be received? With instant devastation or delayed shock? Now, Johnny knew what went through their minds. How do you convey calmness and passivity when you were going to end the life of a husband and father? How do you look into teary eyes like those of the two young girls? Upon family portraits lined along the walls and a hamper full of clothes that would never be worn again?

Tomato opened his mouth to speak again but to his surprise, Kowalski did so first.

"It'll be okay, Ellie. We're just going to talk. Girls, help your mother with the dishes. I want those washed and dried by the time I get home," Kowalski said.

He kissed his two daughters, breathing in their scent, whispering his unending love for them. He broke free from his wife's vise-like grip. He kissed her, stroking her hair one final time. He followed Tomato outside the apartment, artificially smiling to assure his family all was well. Tomato dug his revolver into Kowalski's shoulder blade, forcing him to continue.

Every thought and voice in Johnny's head told him to not look at Kowalski's family. No good could come from seeing the terror, shock, and utter devastation in their faces or the sense of palpable dread that hung in the kitchen.

Don't do it. Don't you do it.

He had pleaded the same in France. It hadn't worked then, and it didn't work now. His vision was crisp, his mind journaling every detail about the kitchen—

the sink of unwashed dishes, the unfolded laundry, the uneaten brownies, the unfinished coloring book, and the doll with half its hair brushed.

Hotsy back pedaled out of the room last, making sure Kowalski's wife didn't make a dash for a concealed weapon.

"Please. It was just business," Kowalski said.

"Shut your mouth. You talk again, your teeth will be scattering across the pavement like marbles," Tomato said, digging the barrel of his gun into the man's spine.

When they reached the car, Hotsy opened the back door, and Tomato and Johnny pushed Kowalski inside. Hotsy stomped on Kowalski's hand to stop him from reaching for the door frame. To prevent him from trying anything further, Hotsy forced the barrel of the gun into Kowalski's mouth past his teeth and into the back of his throat. His finger rested precariously against the trigger.

"You better pray we don't hit as much as a bump," Hotsy said.

There was no doubt that Kowalski's wife had alerted the police. As Tomato floored the gas pedal, and the car stormed through the open gate, they passed the speeding police cars hurrying to the apartment complex, their sirens wailing. But Tomato had kept his speed under the limit, and soon, the police and the North Side suburbs disappeared into the rear-view mirror. They drove until the extravagant homes and spacious lawns turned to maple-leafed forests and corn fields. When there was nothing man-made within sight, Tomato pulled over to the side of the road and killed the ignition.

The silence was only disrupted by the rhythmic chirping of crickets and occasional hooting of owls. It didn't matter how old you were, there was something about a dark, desolate cornfield that was always frightening. But Earl Kowalski had so much more to fear.

Johnny and Hotsy exited the car on opposite sides, both checking for oncoming headlights. There were none. Tomato leaned into the car and dragged Kowalski out. He plopped to the ground like a bag of flour, curling into the fetal position and sobbing into his hands.

"Be a man… get up," Tomato said.

Kowalski continued sobbing.

"Come on!" Tomato yelled.

But Kowalski still didn't move.

Tomato bent down to pick him up. "Get up—"

In a flash, Kowalski heaved all of his weight into a vicious haymaker, striking Tomato in the face and knocking him onto his back. He growled a curse word.

Kowalski bolted, glancing back nervously every second or so.

Hotsy gave chase, his gun raised, ready to shoot.

"No bullets!" Tomato shouted.

All three, even Johnny with his injury, were faster than Kowalski, not that that was a noteworthy achievement. Hotsy was the quickest and grabbed Kowalski by his suspenders. He spun him around, shoved him to the ground with a Confederate rebel yell, and pinned him down with his foot on his chest. His Smith and Wesson hovered a measly foot from Kowalski's forehead, ready to deliver death like a threatened cobra.

Johnny and Tomato joined him, one on each side, all of them looking like scarecrows in fedoras.

"You see this man?" Tomato asked.

He tapped Kowalski's ribs with his foot to get his attention. Kowalski groaned. Tomato nodded at Johnny. "That's family to me. You tried to kill him."

"It was business!" Kowalski yelled, hoping someone would hear him and answer. Something did, but it was only owls hooting their annoyance at his yells.

"Then you know the price of the game. Die like a man. Stand up," Tomato ordered.

Kowalski grabbed handfuls of Johnny's pant leg, tears trickling down his cheeks. "Please, I'm sorry! I'm sorry! I have a wife! Children! You saw them! You lived! I didn't kill you! I failed! You're fine!"

Seeing a grown man beg was embarrassing. Perhaps, Mickey Diamond had put such a large price on their heads that everyone had thought it was worth the gamble. There was money in booze. But there were bullets in it too. The Yin and the Yang.

But Kowalski ruined any chance of mercy when he drove his fist into Johnny's groin. Johnny was well-versed with pain. His side had been in a constant state of pain and was still trembling from the gunshot wound. The bullet lodged in his chest since France ached every day, his shoulder grinded in and out of place. A bullet and a blade hurt like hell, but nothing matched the pain of getting hit downstairs. For a brief moment Johnny thought Kowalski was off target, for no pain came. But it was only delayed. Johnny hunched over, the pain setting in like an avalanche gaining speed. Then Kowalski drove his fist into Johnny's injured side, rupturing at least two of his stitches.

Kowalski spun toward Hotsy and delivered a rising uppercut, knocking Hotsy onto his ass. But Tomato wasn't going to get sucker punched again. He whipped his revolver across Kowalski's forehead. A gash split open. Blood ran out. Kowalski fell onto the road, no doubt seeing a thousand more stars than there were.

Tomato went to the car and returned with a tire iron in his hand. He stood over the dazed, bleeding Kowalski. Tomato's kicks were no longer light taps meant to gain his attention; they were meant to pulverize bones. His kicks alternated between Kowalski's ribs and face depending on which parts he didn't defend. Then Tomato swung the tire iron across Kowalski's face. His teeth flew out like home runs at Wrigley. The blood splattered on Tomato's pants and the white spats covering his black shoes. Bits of Kowalski's flesh would provide a morning meal for crows.

Tomato raised the tire iron again.

"Not like this," Johnny said.

Any more damage to Kowalski's face, and it would be a closed casket.

"This is the man who shot you," Tomato said, pointing his tire iron at Kowalski.

"And I'll be the one to end it," Johnny said.

Tomato stepped aside. Johnny removed his gun and stepped over Kowalski.

A strange, indescribable entity crept through the cornfield. Invisible to everyone else. Powerless to everyone else. A predator with eyes only for Johnny.

Not now.

That invisible parasite leapt from the darkness. He waited for that drowning feeling to come. But this parasite didn't go for the air in his lungs, it went to his mind—eroding it, tormenting it.

Kowalski was barely conscious, only groaning incoherently. He looked desperate to say something, but his jaw was broken and wouldn't form the necessary sounds. Would his words have formed another plea for mercy or were they a goodbye message to his family?

And then Kowalski fell silent. It was worse than when he had been sobbing. Eyes speak a language, a mouth words. A mouth can lie. But not eyes. There is an exposed truth in them. Eyes reveal emotion in their purest form, untainted by exposition. Earl Kowalski was speaking to Johnny. Caskets and coffins flooded Johnny's thoughts. The parasitic serpent uncoiled inside him, bludgeoning his brain, constricting his chest, tightening his throat.

Kowalski would be laid to rest in one of those intricately designed coffins. But in the end, it was still just a wooden box.

The power to take a life was a rush, a thrill some loved. But not for Johnny. His breathing raced, his mind transporting him back to France. The night sky was like it had been during those precious bits of respite between battles. But France's fields weren't filled with corn. The blackened earth had been littered with corpses.

"It's suffering."

The sweat running down his brow was cool and clammy. The faces of Germans he had killed flashed before him, each man screaming for mercy, holding out their hands. *"Nein! Bitte!"* they would shout. "No! Please!"

And then the battle field was covered in the dead and dying Americans. Those clinging to life, pleading and screaming in unforgettable cacophony. Hands reaching for him, eyes filled with terror.

Calm your breathing.

Johnny had no idea how long he had been standing over Kowalski. Seconds? Minutes? He wasn't in Illinois, he was back in France. And Earl Kowalski followed him there, his near-black eyes imploring him.

Johnny stared into them, at the reflection of himself. Internally, his mind was at war. But physically, his body responded like a well-trained machine. Muscle memory took control. Even when all hell was going off inside, the gun was sturdy in his hand. It never shook, never moved.

He squeezed the trigger. Four rounds in all. Each centered at Kowalski's chest. The shots echoed. The crickets fell silent.

The gun fell limp to his side; air he hadn't had for the last thirty seconds—or what felt like hours—flooded out in an exhale.

Hotsy patted his gashed chin, coating his fingertips in blood. It was the first kink in a flawless face. Tomato stepped away, trying to kick the blood and bits of flesh off his shoes. Then he lit a cigarette and took a long drag.

Johnny stared at Kowalski's lifeless body. Moments ago, his eyes had been speaking to him. Pleading with him. Now, there was nothing. They lay open but unseeing, emptied of emotion. Eyes that had fallen in love with his wife, witnessed his children's first steps. Johnny had dragged Kowalski out of his home, and he would never return to it.

"I thought his fists would of been made of butter," Hotsy said.

Johnny stepped away and felt his stitches. His shirt was stained with a small pool of blood.

"Help me toss him into the field," Hotsy said.

"No, leave him here. We call it in," Johnny said.

Hotsy's mouth slacked and his eyes went from Johnny to Tomato. "Call it in? We should bury him in the field."

Tomato caught Johnny's look and knew what it meant to him.

"Johnny's right. Let him be blessed and buried. Every man deserves that," Tomato said.

Johnny was grateful he wouldn't have to argue. Hotsy clearly opposed but didn't protest. He hadn't been in France. He hadn't witnessed the horror of mountains of bodies bulldozed into a mass grave. Johnny had seen too many unmarked graves, too many bland wooden coffins. He couldn't see a single one more.

"Let's get out of here before a car drives by," Hotsy said.

He crawled into the back seat and spread his arms across the back. Tomato tossed his cigarette to the ground and put it out with his heel.

He put his hand on Johnny's shoulder. "You alright?"

Johnny broke his gaze from Kowalski. He only patted Tomato on the shoulder, a gesture to show he appreciated him asking, but a gesture that told Tomato he was far from alright.

Frequently, his mind brought him back to the places in the center of the maze. The questions, answers, and truths imprisoned there sometimes escaped, wafting through the hedges and dead ends. Aided by memories and thoughts, they manifested themselves in his attacks, and like a poisonous gas, sucked the air from his lungs.

Johnny helped Tomato drag Kowalski to the side of the road. In the end, he was laid out with his feet on the road and his head covered by the five-foot corn stalks. The lavender-colored wildflowers and snowflake-shaped queen anne's lace growing along the road's edge made for a somber, yet peaceful background.

And, once again, Johnny looked down at a man who had left the world decades before he should have. And, once again, it was Johnny who had caused it.

He filled his lungs with the country air and sat in the passenger seat. The headlights flashed on, flooding the road and Kowalski's body in light. The crickets chirped, the engine purred. They drove in silence, only the space in front of the headlights free of darkness. And like the road, his own life was nothing but darkness save for a few precious patches of light. Out in the shadows were the unspeakable sins he'd committed. Earl Kowalski was just one of them, his body well-accompanied by cursed specters of other men. With each passing day, the darkness further encroached the light.

Back in that apartment building, a mother consoled two young girls who had lost their father, because he had been part of a war that padded the pockets of richer men. Or maybe she held out hope that he was still alive. One phone call would end all of that. How many mothers and wives had received calls or visits notifying them that their beloved husband or son was dead? Johnny continued to add to that number. Paris had asked him if he had found or lost God. He had left God in France, but he had brought the War home.

Had Earl Kowalski served in the war? Had he stormed out of a trench and survived the hail of steel? Had he survived the deadliest pandemic since the Black Death only to have Johnny end his life on a desolate road in rural Illinois over some minor beer war?

The thoughts were tumultuous, but like the car, Johnny could do nothing but stay in the light, no matter how faint it may be.

Saturday Night Dinner

Johnny had never been one to read the paper. Anything worth reading was gossiped about. Thousands of years ago, it was at a watering hole. In Roman times, it was at the market. During the American Revolution, it was in town halls. In the 1800s, it was in general stores. Now, it was in the lobby of The Moonlight. Any story worth hearing about would be discussed there.

The newspaper ink would have an almost magnetic attraction over the next few days. Kowalski's obituary would appear in the *Tribune, The Daily News, Chicago Journal,* and the smaller papers in the neighboring suburbs. But no matter how much the paper called to him, Johnny couldn't bear to read the list of names of the surviving loved ones. Kowalski's wife and daughters' faces would forever be engrained in his memory. He didn't need names to further torment him.

"You coming to Al's tonight? Margaret is carrying a torch for you," Hotsy asked.

They had finished a game of Cribbage at the bar. It was minutes before four, and soon, the lobby would be packed full.

"No, I'm stopping over by the Nettesheims," Johnny said.

Hotsy sighed his disapproval.

"How's Clarence?" Tomato asked.

"The same," Johnny replied.

Tomato nodded solemnly. "Things will get better."

"Yeah…"

But neither of them were certain they would.

"You catching a bite here or there?" Tomato asked.

"There," Johnny answered.

"Okay, otherwise Lorraine's making dinner."

"What's she making?" Hotsy asked.

"I don't know," Tomato answered.

"*Mhmmm.* That sounds good. I usually take seconds of *I don't know.* How about you, Johnny?"

"Like it matters. You've never turned down a free meal in your life. Now, finish your drink. We gotta go," Tomato said, waving his hand to rush Hotsy.

"Where's the fire?" Hotsy asked, leaning against the bar to further annoy Tomato.

"The fire's name is Lorraine. And it'll burn us both if we're late for dinner. Let's go! Move your ass!" Tomato ordered.

Hotsy finished his drink and rose from the bar stool at a snail's pace.

"See you later, Johnny," Hotsy said.

"See you," Johnny said.

"This kid…" Tomato shook his head, deciding his sentence wasn't even worth finishing. "Talk to you later. No late night walks, you hear?"

Johnny nodded. "Say hi to the family for me."

"Will do."

Tomato and Hotsy disappeared into the fresh air outside. Johnny had half of his Old Fashioned left, and even though he wanted to sip it to enjoy every drop, he had no self-control and drank it all in one continuous gulp.

"Half breed," a voice called from behind.

143

Paris took the stool previously occupied by Tomato. She looked marvelous, wearing a gold dress that looked like it had been carved from a chandelier. A dress that belonged on a Greek goddess, though it seemed doubtful they had a body like Paris' to pull it off.

"Can I get you a drink?" Johnny asked.

"Sure. A cranberry juice. Thank you," Paris said.

"Just… cranberry juice?" Johnny asked.

"Ice too." Paris smirked, knowing it wasn't what he meant.

Johnny waved the bartender over. "A cranberry juice for the lady… with ice." The bartender nodded and scooped ice into a glass.

"I saw Hotsy and Tomato take off," Paris mentioned.

The bartender set the tall glass of cranberry juice on a coaster in front of her. Paris thanked him. Johnny nodded to his pile of cash for the bartender to take from.

"They're going to Tomato's for supper," Johnny said.

She took a sip. "Not you?"

"I'm going to Cicero tonight," Johnny said.

"They're okay with you doing business alone?" Paris asked, a hint of worry in her voice.

"Not business," Johnny said.

"What, the girls here aren't good enough?" Paris teased.

"Not for girls. Not for gambling or for drinks either if that's what you were going to ask next." He suppressed a smirk.

"Is it a secret?" Paris asked, overemphasizing the intrigue by arching her eyebrows.

"You know, the way you ask questions, you could be a spy."

"I most certainly could be. The FBI is very willing to hire women, especially ones of color."

Johnny tipped his glass to his mouth and smacked the bottom of it, causing the muddled cherries to fall.

"Are you working tonight?" he asked.

"I'm here," Paris said in an "isn't-it-obvious" sort of way.

"You want to go to Cicero?"

"Seeing as I don't know what's going on..."

"I'll give you five clams if you stop asking questions and just come with. I assure you no crimes will be committed unless it's the food."

Paris thought on it, looking to the elevators. Johnny had no idea who would be watching her to see if she left.

"What the hell. Take me to Cicero, Giovanni," Paris said.

She took another drink of her juice, leaving over half in her glass. Johnny judged her for it and finished it. His lips puckered from the overpowering tartness. Why would anyone drink that?

"After you," he said.

He followed Paris out of The Moonlight, onto the street, and to his Chevy FB-50 touring. Paris was silent on the drive, watching the buildings and trees pass by with a preoccupied air.

"Can't talk?" Johnny asked.

"I can't ask questions. I'm getting that five clams, half breed," Paris said.

Johnny chuckled. "Yeah? We'll see about that."

Paris rolled her eyes.

"So, no alcohol for you? You part of a temperance movement? Blaming men and alcohol for all your problems?" Johnny asked.

Paris blew out an exasperated puff of air. "Wow... No, I'm not part of any temperance movement. I think they have a problem with prostitution, though I could be mistaken." Her sarcasm was as thick as peanut butter.

"So you never drink?"

"I don't believe in absolutes, but I've seen what booze does to people."

"What it does to people? It relieves stress. Makes people dance. Laugh. Have fun. Forget."

"Funny, I've never seen you do any of those things... It may do those things for some, but not for everyone."

"But reefer..."

"You're judging."

"No, I'm not judging. Just curious."

"It's something different for everyone, I guess."

"It helps mellow you out?"

"On good days. I'm not going to lie to you, we all have demons that get free from time to time. Nothing can keep them caged forever."

Johnny nodded. His demons ran rampant.

"You have some?" he asked.

"Demons?"

"No, the other stuff."

"Did you drive me to Cicero to buy a joint?"

Johnny laughed. "No, and that was definitely a question."

"Bite me. I'll add the joint to your bill." Paris removed a joint from her purse and lit it. "Just a puff or two," she reminded.

Paris took the first puff, then held it out for Johnny. He took it and inhaled, following the same steps as the first time he had tried it.

"I'll give you a pass on that question," Johnny said.

"Gee, thanks."

They were both silent the rest of the ride, letting the relaxation wash over them like a hot bath. When he parked across the Nettesheims' apartment, it had been enough time for the thoughts of the previous night to fade. Even though he knew this respite was artificial—and temporary—it was a tremendous relief to shut off the constant worry and anxiety that bounced around inside his mind like a wrecking ball. So often, he would be having a fine time only to have one of the thoughts, questions and answers of the maze break free. And each was a wrecking ball—swinging from on high and pulverizing everything good he had built.

"Is this it?" Paris asked.

"Five clams stays in my pocket," Johnny said, stepping out of the car.

"Oh please, cheapskate. That does not count," Paris said, following him across the street.

146

"Sounded an awful lot like that sentence ended with a question mark," Johnny said.

"I put those stitches in, I'll take them out," Paris said.

Johnny pulled open the front door. It stuck once again, but this time he was ready and blocked his side from getting smacked.

"How is it?" Paris asked, noticing his deliberate protection of the wound.

"Tight, but healing okay. Thanks to you," Johnny answered.

He gestured for her to enter first. Johnny knocked. The lock turned, and the door opened.

"Johnny," Cilly called out with a smile.

She opened the door wider. Her eyes fell on Paris.

"Cilly, this is Paris. I owe her a dinner. Is it okay if we come in?" Johnny asked.

"Of course," Cilly said.

Paris followed him inside. "Hello."

The fact she bit her bottom lip told Johnny she was uncomfortable.

"Cilly, Paris is from Wisconsin too," Johnny mentioned.

"I'm sorry, Silly?" Paris asked.

"C-i-l-l-y. A nickname for Cecilia," Cilly explained.

"Oh, I get it. I'm starting to think I'm the only person in the greater Chicago area without a nickname," Paris said.

Cilly smiled, both hospitably and genuinely. "What city are you from?"

"Milwaukee. And you?" Paris answered.

"Brookfield."

In the span of two seconds, the two women seemed to have bonded as if they had known each other for years. No wonder, since both were from Wisconsin, a state whose residents prided themselves on honesty and hard work. They were more leery of outsiders—not rude by any means—but quick to the point and not ones to fall for bullshit.

"Where's Wally?" Johnny asked.

"Helping his father in the bathroom," Cilly said.

"The grocery is open, right?" Johnny asked.

"Yes, but it closes at six."

"I have to get supplies, and I'm afraid I'll have to take over your kitchen."

"I'm sure he'll want to go with you… if you don't mind."

"Of course not."

Cilly hesitated before speaking again. "I hate to have to mention this, but I'm not sure if Paris will be welcome. She certainly is here, but…"

Both Johnny and Paris knew what she was getting at—the Ku Klux Klan.

The Klan had been revived in 1915 by a man named William Joseph Simmons after he had seen the film *Birth of a Nation*. But now, it was not only colored people they targeted. It was Jews, Roman Catholics and foreigners. Their numbers had surged to 4,000,000, the members selling themselves on their ability to enforce the Volstead Act. And these numbers were not limited to the South. They were in the North too. Hiding under white sheets, burning crosses and businesses, terrorizing the defenseless. Racism, like alcohol, was available at every corner, including a grocery store in Cicero.

"Nothing's going to happen," Johnny assured both.

If any white sheet–wearing coward wanted to have a word, Johnny would introduce him to his black M1911 and stain those cotton white sheets a deep crimson.

"Johnny!"

He turned.

Wally had been helping his father from the kitchen to the living room, but had temporarily abandoned that task before realizing his error.

"And you must be Mr. Nettesheim?" Paris asked, stepping toward Clarence.

Clarence neither made a motion to face Paris nor showed any sign that he was aware he was being spoken to.

"That is Mr. Nettesheim, my husband, Clarence. He doesn't speak," Cilly said.

Wally's face blushed. Cilly was nothing but proud of her husband, but enlightening new guests to his condition was a difficult task.

"Oh, I'm sorry," Paris said.

"It's fine," Cilly said, dismissing the unneeded apology.

Johnny had expected Paris to be casting daggers with her stare for not having been told about Clarence, but she showed nothing but compassion.

"Wally, we have to pick up some food for supper. Care to take us?" Johnny asked.

"Sure, let me get my cap," he answered.

Wally dashed into his room, returning seconds later with a tweed wool newsboy cap on his head.

"Who is this?" Wally asked.

Paris held out her hand. "I'm Paris."

Wally placed his small hand in hers and shook it. "Walramus. I'm named after an uncle. But it sounds like walrus, so I prefer to go by Wally."

"Then Wally it is," Paris said, unable to suppress her smile.

"Mom, we'll be back in a bit. Why don't you take the time to relax? Johnny and I will handle the kitchen," Wally said.

Cilly beamed at her young gentleman. "That's very sweet of you, honey."

Wally led Johnny and Paris out into the fresh, summer air and toward the grocery store.

"You play ball today?" Johnny asked.

"Yeah, we played a double-header. Well more like one-and-a-half games. Mrs. Finkmeyer was annoyed that she almost got hit with a pop up, so we couldn't finish," Wally said.

Mrs. Finkmeyer lived in the apartment complex down the street. She was an ornery widow who liked to suck the joy out of anyone she met.

"Get any hits?" Johnny asked.

"One. No round-bagger though," Wally said, his eyes on the pavement, shoulders sunken.

"Can't always be at our best, but we—"

"Can always give our best."

149

Paris smiled at Johnny. It was a glimpse of him she had never seen and never expected to.

"So, Miss Paris…" Wally said.

"Just Paris, Wally," she insisted.

"Paris, how do you know Johnny?"

"We see each other at 'The Moonlight'," Paris said.

"I see. Johnny and I go way back, don't we, Johnny?"

"We do," Johnny agreed.

"He robbed me of a homerun first time we met," Wally said.

Paris tilted her head, confused.

"We do a lot of drop offs here. We were crossing the street, and I took a baseball to the chest," Johnny said.

"I crushed that ball, Paris. I mean you know when you listen to the games on the radio, and you hear that *pop*? I had that! And he just walks right into it!" Wally said, arching his head back to emphasize what could have been his greatest moment as an amateur baseball player, a moment that would have made him a legend in the neighborhood.

"So he comes rushing over, apologizing profusely. After he knows I'm okay, he says in a solemn voice, 'You know you just screwed me'," Johnny said.

"So, that's how you two became friends," Paris said.

"Pals ever since," Wally said.

The Piggly Wiggly grocery store was rather empty considering it was nearing dinner time. Whether Paris looked passably white with a heck of a tan or the few people inside ignored her was hard to tell. Johnny didn't care which one it was, only that they kept their mouths shut.

"What are we getting, master chef?" Paris asked.

"Eggs—" Johnny said, and before he could finish, Wally was off to procure them.

"Sorry I didn't tell you about Clarence ahead of time. I just didn't want you to act differently around him," Johnny said.

"I understand," Paris said.

But it was all she could say, for Wally was back with a carton of eggs.

"Next?" he asked.

Johnny rambled off the ingredients—flour, pepper, sage, butter, and ricotta and parmesan cheeses—and Wally dashed off to get them all, tossing in a box of wafers at the end for his mother. Then he dug out a heap of change from his pockets that totaled less than twenty cents.

"I got it, pal," Johnny said.

"What about your dad? What does he like to eat?" Paris asked.

"I don't know. He just eats. You can't tell if he likes anything," Wally said.

"He liked that ice cream," Johnny reminded him.

"He did. That was good ice cream, Johnny," Wally said.

"You like chewing gum, Wally?" Paris asked.

"I'd marry it," Wally said.

"Juicy Fruit or Spearmint?" Paris asked, her hand hovering over the packs of Wrigley gum.

"Juicy Fruit. But you get what you like, Paris. I'm not picky," Wally deferred.

"Juicy Fruit it is," Paris said.

All three enjoyed a piece of chewing gum on the walk back to Wally's home. Johnny refused Wally's offer to carry the paper grocery bag.

"We better pick up the pace or my mom will have the militia looking for us," Wally said.

When they were at the stoop, Wally turned to face Paris.

"My dad doesn't respond to anything, Paris, except for the word 'artillery.' So, I'd appreciate it if you refrained from using it."

Paris instinctively looked at Johnny. "Artillery" was hardly a word that came up in an average conversation.

He turned and opened the door. Paris looked at Johnny, her expression strangely melancholic.

"I was ready to send out the militia," Cilly said when they stepped inside.

"Told ya!" Wally said, tossing his newsboy cap on the couch. Cilly grabbed it and placed it on the stand beside the door.

Clarence hadn't moved from the chair nor did he move a muscle when they stepped inside. He was still staring out of the open window with the same blank expression, completely unaware there were guests in his home.

There are over 170,000 words in the English language, and Clarence Nettesheim responded to only one. Not *love, dad, Wally* or *Cilly*. But a word that put him back in that trench, waiting for a barrage of Armageddon. Where everything else was shattered, that memory remained unbroken.

"What are you making?" Cilly asked.

"Yeah, what are you making?" Paris asked.

"It's a secret, ladies… right, Johnny?" Wally said.

"Right. It's a secret," Johnny said, playing along.

But as soon as Johnny and Wally were in the kitchen, Wally leaned close and whispered, "What are we making?"

"Cheese gnocchi," Johnny whispered back.

"That sounds like the name of Pinocchio's grandparent," Wally said.

"It's a dumpling," Johnny explained.

Paris hovered in between the kitchen and the living room.

"You want to help?" Johnny asked her.

"Sure, put me to work. My hands. Your command," Paris said.

"Wally, you want to fill a large pot with water and sprinkle some salt in it?" Johnny asked.

"You got it," Wally said then dug through the cupboard.

"Paris, we can combine the ricotta, eggs, and parmesan in a bowl. Dash of salt and pepper," Johnny instructed.

"Is this another one of your grandmother's recipes?" she asked.

Johnny nodded. "Another staple of the De Luca household."

"She was a good cook?" Wally asked.

"If I had been a fat kid, I definitely would of deserved it. But I don't promise it'll taste as good," Johnny said.

He rambled off the instructions. Wally put the half-stick of butter into a pan and, with a pained expression, watched it slowly melt. Cilly popped in every now and again, to make sure Johnny didn't need help or to graciously say, "It's starting to smell good in here."

Wally was eager to know everything, asking a hundred questions. He was flabbergasted at how long foods took to boil or cook. Johnny told him not to watch, but Wally kept peeking at the pan or holding his hand close by to ensure it was hot. When dinner was ready, Wally helped his father from his chair by the window to his chair at the kitchen table.

"Wally, will you lead us in prayer?" Cilly asked.

Cilly and Wally closed their eyes. Clarence stared blankly. Johnny bowed his head, but his eyes were open. He could feel Paris staring at him, but when Wally spoke, she closed her eyes.

"Bless us, O Lord, and these Thy gifts, which we are about to receive from Thy bounty. Through Christ, our Lord. Amen," Wally recited.

"Wally, that wasn't very heartfelt," Cilly said.

Wally exhaled. "God, thank you for another great day, thank you for my mother and father, for my pal Johnny and our new friend Paris. Thank you for the wonderful food and the Piggly Wiggly for selling it at such affordable prices."

Wally, Cilly, and Paris motioned the sign of the cross. Johnny and Clarence did not—one unable to, one by choice.

"It looks amazing," Cilly commented.

"It's gnocchi," Wally said nonchalantly.

"Do you know how to spell that?" his mother asked.

"Sure. N-o-chee," Wally said.

Cilly laughed. "Chee? What letter is that?"

"It's Italian, mom. Johnny was explaining it," Wally said.

"Oh, really?"

"Yes… Italians…" Wally shrugged.

"It actually starts with a g," his mother said.

"Oh, silent g? Like gnat?"

"Just like gnat."

"I think this turned out fairly well," Wally said after the first few bites had been taken.

"Me too," Paris said.

"Your grandmother loved to cook?" Cilly asked.

"Loved it," Johnny said. "Hated the cleanup though. That was where I came in. She drank the whole time I washed and dried. She loved her wine, so you can imagine she was stringent on the cleanliness of the dishes, making sure she had plenty of time to drink."

"She wouldn't have been a fan of prohibition," Cilly said.

"It would of taken the entire Marine Corps to take a bottle of wine from my grandmother. She'd defend it like it was the Alamo," Johnny said.

"What's the Alamo?" Wally asked.

"It was a battle in Texas against the Mexicans," Cilly explained.

"Did we win?"

"No, sweetie."

"There were over 4,000 Mexicans against less than 200 Texans. They fought knowing they'd lose," Johnny said.

"Why didn't they leave?" Wally asked.

"Sometimes a defeat leads to further victories. Sometimes a great sacrifice can give others life," Johnny said.

"Was that like the battles you and my dad fought in?"

"They won their battles," Cilly said.

The truth was neither the Americans nor Germans had won or lost. Both sides had lost an unfathomable number of men. The winner had won a stretch of muddy, barren field.

"You haven't been to Europe, have you, Paris?" Wally asked.

"No, I haven't," she answered.

"My dad wrote letters. He said the French Coast was beautiful," Wally said.

"Your dad's right," Johnny said.

"Is the rest of France beautiful?" Wally asked.

"Parts of it are," Johnny said.

"Johnny's from New York," Wally told Paris.

"That's actually one of the few things he told me," Paris said.

"Most of our family is back in Wisconsin. Mom says the doctors here are better for dad. I don't think so though," Wally said.

"Your mom's a smart lady," Johnny said.

"I know she is. But the doctors here haven't helped," Wally said.

"Your father has shown signs of improvement," Cilly said.

Johnny knew she doubted that herself, but she believed Clarence was aware of what was being said, even if he didn't show it.

He had to be.

"Are your parents still in Wisconsin?" Paris asked, changing the topic.

"No, they moved to Florida. They hate the winters. Clarence's parents still live in Brookfield though. He comes from a large family. Thirteen siblings," Cilly said.

"So, Paris…" Wally said.

"So Wally," Paris mimicked.

"Are you named after the city?"

"The one and only."

"Are you French? I mean I know you're Negro, but do you have French in you?"

"I'm not sure, to be honest."

"My dad's family came over from Germany."

"A city called Erftstadt," Cilly added.

"Dad wrote mom that he'd take her to Europe and show her Paris and the coast," Wally said.

"I feel like I've been there," Cilly said. "Wally's father is quite the writer. He wrote such fantastic letters when he was over there. He never was much of a sweet talker, too nervous, but put a pencil in his hand…"

The light caught her eyes, and the tears in them were easy to see. She was a strong woman, but every time she thought about her trials and tribulations—Clarence's condition, raising a child alone, being dirt poor with debt collectors circling like vultures—were lessening, it was only the waters receding to join the tsunami that would crash over her. A lesser person would have succumbed to all three problems. A strong, proud person would have succumbed to one of the three. Being resilient to all three was super human.

"Why don't we get these dishes cleaned for your mom?" Johnny said to Wally after everyone had finished eating.

"Oh, Johnny, I can do them. You've done more than enough. You always do more than enough," Cilly said.

"It'll be like old times for me," Johnny assured her.

"I can help," Paris said.

"No, I'll do it, Paris. You can relax. Johnny and I sort of developed a system. It's pretty efficient," Wally said.

Johnny and Wally tackled the dishes, while Cilly helped Clarence back into his chair beside the window. She and Paris chatted about Wisconsin and their experiences growing up there. The fondness for the state was fully evident and the longing to return there quite decipherable in their banter. Life had led them elsewhere, but home was always home.

"Did you like the gnocchi?" Johnny asked Wally.

"Yeah, Italians have some good food," Wally said.

"We sure do."

"I think I might enjoy a stick of after-dinner gum. Care for one?"

Johnny smirked. "I'm okay. Thanks."

"Paris?" Wally asked.

"I don't think I should have a second," she said, politely refusing as if it was another shot of alcohol.

Cilly was beguiled by her young gentleman.

Paris couldn't sit idly by, insisting on helping to at least dry the dishes. Afterward, they joined Cilly and Clarence in the living room to begin saying their goodbyes. In New York, goodbye was an instant thing. But for those from Wisconsin, it was a process. Variations of "We should get going" were uttered four times (Jesus Christ had only fallen three times carrying his cross). However rude it would be, it seemed the only way to leave was to walk out and shut the door. But Cilly and Paris eventually acknowledged the final goodbye with a mutual sigh.

"We'll see you later, Wally," Johnny said.

"For sure," Wally said.

Johnny opened the door and allowed Paris to step out first. Darkness had descended. Music carried faintly from the neighboring blocks. Johnny opened the passenger door for Paris before plopping down on the driver's seat. It didn't take the street lights illuminating Paris' face for Johnny to know that she wanted to talk. But darkness had resurrected the memory of killing Earl Kowalski from its shallow, freshly dug grave. The day had gone fast for Johnny, but for Kowalski's widow and children, it had been the longest day of their lives. Dinner with the Nettesheims had helped take his mind off Kowalski, but now, he was all Johnny could think about. The incident was too recent to cage in the center of the maze. Right now, it was behind every turn, waiting for him at every dead end—not with terror-filled, but pleading eyes. Even when he did bury the thought, it was always in a shallow grave of loose soil that Kowalski's corpse hands could easily rip through. Johnny raced through his own maze, struggling to outrun the demons hunting him.

Keep the car on the road.

He stood over Kowalski, staring down at those pleading eyes.

And then it came again.

Swooping in like a gale, sucking the air from his lungs.

Don't crash this car with her in it. Focus. Breathe. Get through this.

"Is something wrong?" Paris asked.

Johnny shook his head, but the gesture had zero conviction.

"Did I do something?" Paris asked.

"No… nothing you did," Johnny said.

"You look like something's wrong."

He held his head out of the open window like a dog panting. He breathed the rushing air in, allowing it to fill his lungs. His breathing steadied, and the attack passed.

"You got another smoke?" Johnny asked.

"Cannabis isn't a cure-all, Giovanni. At some point, you're going to have to confront what's tormenting you," Paris said.

"Some day. Not today," Johnny said.

Paris lit the joint and handed it over. Johnny took a long drag and blew the smoke out of his open window.

"You're going to want to limit that. Smoke too much, and it's not going calm you. You're going to get paranoid," Paris said.

Johnny wanted to smoke the whole damn thing, but if what Paris said was true, it would release every single buried and caged truth, question, and answer he had ever imprisoned in the maze. And if that happened, he'd never recover. He handed the joint back to Paris, hoping he had smoked the perfect amount to numb his anxiety and not give himself unrelenting paranoia. The silence that followed only lasted seconds.

"I thought at first, that you and Cilly were—" Paris said.

"Intimate?" Johnny interjected.

"Yes."

"No, nothing like that."

Paris nodded, accepting his answer. "Wally looks up to you."

He shrugged off her comment. "He's a good kid."

Paris laughed. "Talks like he's forty."

"Swears like it too."

"So, you just kept running into them?"

"Yeah, a bit more mindful for fly balls though."

"And you give them money?"

Johnny looked at her, surprised she was able to ascertain that.

"I could tell by the way she said 'You've done more than enough.' There was guilt in her voice."

"They need it. Cilly can't rake in enough kale. Not with the doctor bills breeding like rabbits. Every time one of the white coats thinks he has an answer or cure for Clarence, it ends up being a cruel joke that only costs them more money."

"Nothing's worked?"

Johnny shook his head.

"Did you serve with him?"

"No, not directly. But you feel like you did, if that makes any sense."

"It makes sense. What happened to him?" She shifted positions, so that she was nearly sitting sideways.

"Shellshock."

"War can cause that?"

Johnny nodded, showing all the solemnness such a horrible affliction deserved.

"Wally never knew his father as he was, did he?" Paris asked.

Johnny shook his head. "No, Clarence left for the War when Wally was only a year old."

"Such a terrible thing."

"He is still his father."

"Of course, but that can't be easy for a young boy to understand."

"No, it isn't. But there's hope for Clarence."

There has to be.

Paris put a hand on Johnny's. Her fingertips were cool, her touch soft. She met his gaze. "That's very admirable of you to help them out."

Paris removed her hand and shifted her gaze to the world outside. Johnny fell silent again, a feeling of guilt flooding over him. She had commended him on his generosity and kindness. If she only knew that twenty-four short hours ago, he had put four rounds in a man's chest. Thousands of tears had been shed that day because of what he had done. Kowalski's daughters' lives had permanently changed. They would be different people now, a trajectory forever altered. The compunction was overwhelming.

159

It was lucky nobody had slammed on their breaks or no pedestrian had darted across the road, because Johnny wouldn't have even noticed. The high that had set it in had helped dull his tormenting thoughts. There had been wisdom in Paris' warning—anymore and the maze would have fallen to anarchy.

Johnny pulled the car over to the curb outside The Moonlight.

"Are you coming in?" Paris asked awkwardly, avoiding looking directly at him.

Johnny looked over. "No…"

Paris nodded, confused about the whole night. And he couldn't blame her.

"Well, alright then. Good night," she said, reaching for the door handle and opening the door.

"Paris…" She turned to look at him. He held out a ten-dollar bill. "Payment."

"Keep it."

"No, take the night off if you want."

"The deal was for five."

"Five and a tip. Even though you did ask questions."

Paris hesitated but took the offered bill. Her hand brushed his. Johnny pulled it away and nodded.

"And you answered none of them," she said.

Paris stepped out of the car and watched Johnny drive away.

Art E. Lee

The following day, Johnny met Tomato and Hotsy at The Moonlight an hour before the dinner rush would strike. An Old Fashioned was waiting for him at the bar. Hotsy wasn't there but a finished game of cribbage showed he had been and that he had won the game. He was always red, and Tomato was green during their games.

"Vencini want to see us?" Johnny asked.

"The Cardinal," Tomato said, grimacing after sipping his Bloody Mary. Tomato, ironically, was not a fan of tomato juice. But he went to the drink when he was suffering from an unusual hangover caused by drinking something foreign to him.

Different boozes caused different hangovers in different people. For Tomato, beer gave him terrible headaches, liquor gave him a queasy stomach, and wine brought on Armageddon. He never won the next morning.

Hotsy strutted over from the elevators, a smile covering eighty percent of his face.

"You reek of wench," Tomato accused.

"*Wenches*," Hotsy corrected.

Tomato and Johnny smirked at each other.

"So kind of you to join us," Tomato said.

"Like a fish, I figured I'd come up for air," Hotsy said.

"Whales come up for air, moron. Not fish," Tomato said.

"A whale is just a specific type of fish."

"No, it's not."

"If it lives in the water, for all intensive purposes, it's a fish. I was like a fish, and she was a fish. Guess what type, Johnny?"

"I don't know. What?" Johnny asked.

"A blow fish," Hotsy answered, a smile curving toward the top of his ears.

"What about you?" Johnny asked Tomato. "Spend the whole night with Lorraine?"

Tomato nodded. "And the girls. I needed that."

"How'd you manage the hangover?"

"Wine… lots of wine."

"And Lorraine?"

"Feeling just peachy. You know women, they're immune to the grape poison."

Wine was dangerous. It didn't have the same strong taste of alcohol like liquor or beer. Some even tasted like grape juice. Before you knew it, you had drunk a bottle and a half in less than half an hour, and the ride was already underway.

"You should take Lorraine out for dinner. Maybe a show. I'll watch Gretch and Mary," Hotsy said.

"I wish every night could be like the one I had last night. You know when you first starting seeing a girl, there's that excitement? Everything's bliss? I haven't had a night like that in years," Tomato said.

162

It was the blissful feeling Johnny hadn't ever had. His mind wouldn't ever shut off long enough to afford him such a moment. But the look on Tomato's face made every man long for such a connection.

Johnny finished half his Old Fashioned in two gulps and sipped the rest over the course of a few minutes during which he asked about the game of cribbage the two had played. Tomato said the whole game had been neck and neck, whereas Hotsy said Tomato had blown a massive lead. The truth was somewhere in the middle. Tomato was too proud to admit a blown lead, and Hotsy embellished to get a rise out of Tomato.

After Johnny finished his drink, they met The Cardinal in the conference room. When they entered, The Cardinal was standing against the wall, his head hung low.

"And here I thought I looked like I was going to blow chow," Tomato said.

The conference room was only ever occupied to transfer funds into the pockets of the police and politicians or when men and women without rooms risked a quick, passionate embrace.

The Cardinal held out the day's *Tribune*, folded open to the Obituary section. He pointed to the desired deceased—Earl Kowalski.

"What about it?" Tomato asked, not in the mood for one of The Cardinal's non-violent sermons.

"Read it," The Cardinal said.

It wasn't an order, but the closest The Cardinal got to delivering one. That itself was unnerving.

The obituary photograph of Earl Kowalski showed neither terror nor pleading in his eyes, but a glimmer that spoke of a love of life, visible even in the grainy black and white image.

Johnny and Hotsy stood behind Tomato, so all three could read it at once.

"Skip to the 'survived by' section," The Cardinal instructed.

Tomato glared at The Cardinal out of the edge of his eye. He hated being told what to do. Only Lorraine, Al Capone, and Valcoro could do that.

Earl Kowalski is survived by his wife Elizabeth 'Ellie' Dimonkowski,
two daughters, Lenore (9) and Lacy (6), and two sisters, Samantha
(William) Hamels, and Georgia (Walton) Matthews.

"Yeah, we knew he was married with kids," Hotsy said, brushing off what he had read.

"Dimonkowski," The Cardinal said.

"Yeah, so?" Hotsy asked.

Johnny knew what it meant, and the grave look on Tomato's face told Johnny he did too.

"Kowalski was Diamond's brother-in-law," Johnny said.

The Cardinal solemnly nodded.

"What?" Hotsy asked, trying to quickly reread the paper.

"Michael Dimonkowski. He changed it to Diamond," Tomato explained.

The name change should not have come as a shock, but it was easy to feel betrayed. But in this line of business, nicknames were common. Men with warrants out for their arrest usually chose to go by a different name.

The Cardinal had warned them not to blindly deliver retaliation. He had given advice, and they had ignored it. And because of that, they had killed the husband of Diamond's sister. Mickey's younger sister, one he was assuredly very protective of. Diamond had wanted them dead for business. Now, it was personal.

Johnny had killed Kowalski, ended his life, removed him from the face of the Earth, but leaving the dead body to rot in the strong heat and be a meal for birds, critters, and worms was something he could not do. He would not bury another damn person in the dirt. He could not. Would Kowalski have been considered a missing person had they buried him in the corn field like Hotsy wanted to?

"Jesus, how were we supposed to know?" Tomato asked.

Taking The Cardinal's advice was a lot like listening to your parents when you were a teenager. You wanted to make your own decisions, and you failed to see the wisdom in their words. But that's how growth happens, how lessons are learned. Most often those were not life or death situations. Ignoring The

Cardinal's advice, on the other hand, would have tremendous, detrimental consequences.

"There's more," The Cardinal said.

More was never good.

"The police visited Mrs. Kowalski. She told them three men of Italian heritage, one with blue eyes, kidnapped her husband. Police showed her a pile of mugshots. She identified all three of you," The Cardinal said.

Of course she did. How many blue-eyed Italians were roaming Chicago and worked for Capone? His eyes were so vivid they even showed up on a monochromatic photograph.

"What do we do?" Johnny asked.

Tomato would recommend staying and shooting any stranger that approached. Hotsy, not one for planning nor truly understanding the gravity of the situation, would recommend doing something he enjoyed—taking a woman to bed, drinking to excess or dancing until his legs gave out.

The bullets and blades coming for them wouldn't be from a single man. It would be from Chicago itself. But that was part of the life. You accepted that fate. Though Mickey Diamond would be gunning for them, it was the police that prompted action. Accepting retaliation was preferable than rotting for decades in a prison cell.

"You get out of Chicago, out of Illinois if you can. For at least a week," The Cardinal said.

"A week?" Hotsy complained.

"I'll spread news that you three went east to New York or south to Miami."

"But where do we actually go?" Tomato asked.

"I may have a place," Johnny said.

"Where?" Tomato asked.

"Wisconsin," Johnny answered.

"Wisconsin?" Hotsy said, looking like he had swallowed something rotten.

"I need to call Lorraine before anything," Tomato said.

"Make it quick," The Cardinal said.

"Trust me, if I don't tell her I'm spending a week in Wisconsin, she'll crucify me, and upside down, to mock me," Tomato said.

"She certainly won't be jealous," Hotsy said.

"Give me ten minutes," Johnny said on his way out of the room.

"Now where are you going?" Hotsy yelled out.

But Johnny didn't stay to listen to questions or to explain himself. Tomato had a phone call to make, and Hotsy could go take a few mental photographs of The Moonlight's women to get him through the coming week.

Johnny went to the gold elevators, waited for that annoying *ping*, entered, and hit the button for the fifth floor. When the doors opened, he turned right and went to room 518 and knocked on its door.

"Occupied," a man's voice came from inside.

Johnny knocked again. This time harder.

"Occupied!" the man repeated louder.

Johnny pounded his fist on the door like it was a face.

"Alright asshole, you better be high-tailing it to the elevator!" the man inside shouted.

Johnny didn't care who the voice inside belonged to. Whoever it was could not be half as powerful or threatening as Mickey Diamond. Nor did Johnny have time to wait. The Chicago police were actively searching for them, and it wouldn't take long for The Moonlight to come up as a probable hideout.

A man roughly Johnny's age opened the door. The beast in Johnny clenched its claws and bared its fangs.

"Who the hell are you?" the man asked, the confidence in his voice trailing off as he took in Johnny's appearance.

Johnny had broad shoulders and thick arms, physical traits that scared off most men. But it was his permanent scowl and piercing eyes that were truly unsettling. He looked capable of becoming unhinged at any moment. Because he was.

Johnny pushed past him. Paris was at the foot of the bed, the worried look on her face vanished when she saw that it was Johnny. The thought of the man

166

touching her made his blood surge through his veins. He considered leaving the man beaten, broken, and broke. But there was no time.

"You up for a drive?" Johnny asked.

The confusion on her face was evident, but she had little time to process it before Johnny held out his hand.

"What the hell is going on?" the gangly man said, pulling his suspenders up and buttoning his pants.

Johnny rounded on the man. "Get lost or never be found."

He picked up the man's coat and flung it at him, scowling at him to show how resolute his threat was.

The man stepped aside, and Paris followed Johnny through the door and to the elevator.

"What's going on?" she asked.

Johnny had done his best to hide his worry, but Paris' gaze was too keen.

"We need to leave town for a bit," Johnny said.

"This have anything do with the repercussions of burning down Diamond's distillery?" Paris asked.

She was cunning. One of the many things he liked about her.

"Why am I coming?" she asked.

"I may need you to stitch me up," Johnny said.

Paris only stared at him.

"That was a joke," Johnny said.

"Yet, neither of us is laughing," Paris said.

The elevator offered no room to hide, and even though it could fit ten, it was as if they were crammed inside a shoebox.

"If you don't want to go—"

"Some details would be nice. You know, the who, what, where, when, why. I'd settle for just two of those."

"You, me, Tomato, and Hotsy, going to a cabin in Whitefish Bay, Wisconsin, leaving right now, because the man who shot me, I killed him Friday night. His widow ID'd us out of a pile of mugshots, and the police are after us."

167

Paris had gotten more information out of Johnny in one sentence than all of their previous conversations combined. The truth that Johnny was a murderer. The truth that he was not a good man. The truth that he wanted her at the cabin. Why, he couldn't say, but that want bordered on a need.

Paris studied his eyes. They were fierce, but there was something else there too—not fear, but an uncertainty of what would come.

"...okay," Paris said.

They hurried out of the elevator, trying to make their way through the crowd as quickly as they could. Both had to ignore friends and acquaintances who wished to share a word. At last, Johnny pushed through the revolving door and pointed to Tomato's Cadillac.

Tomato and Hotsy were waiting in the car. Tomato tossed his hands up in frustration, while Hotsy looked on in envy, because Johnny was bringing a woman along. The idea of being stuck in a cabin without feminine contact was worse than being arrested. Maybe even death.

Judging by the look on Tomato's face, his phone call had been a verbal bashing. No doubt he had landed himself in a massive crater he would have a hell of a time climbing out of. But worse than Lorraine's verbal artillery was the pain of having to go a week without seeing his daughters. Right now, that punishment manifested as anger, but at some point it would change to deep depression and an extreme self-loathing.

"You sure you're ready? Did you want to shower first? We have all the time in the world," Tomato jested.

"Hey, nobody said we could bring somebody," Hotsy said, sounding like a petulant child.

"Get up here, drugstore cowboy," Tomato ordered Hotsy.

Hotsy sighed but listened, and climbed over to the front. Tomato yelled at him for not stepping out of the car like a civilized person. After Johnny and Paris were in the backseat, and Tomato had dusted off Hotsy's footprints from the seats, he brought the car to life.

"So, where in Wisconsin are we going?" Tomato asked.

"We have to stop in Cicero first," Johnny said.

"More charity?" Hotsy asked.

"Knock it off with that charity shit," Tomato yelled at Hotsy. His eyes found the rearview mirror. "Johnny, sorry, but we don't have time."

"We're the ones in need of charity," Johnny said.

Paris at least knew who was in Cicero, and it temporarily stifled some of the questions sprouting in her mind like weeds.

With Tomato driving, it took only twenty-four minutes for them to arrive at the Nettesheims' apartment building. Kids played in the street and ran through the spray from an open fire hydrant. It was an idyllic, innocent day every child should be able to enjoy during their summers. But a day that hadn't existed for children twenty years ago. Johnny had grown up working in his father's store. Though he complained on occasion, he knew it was a better job than most of his friends. He worked ten hours stocking shelves, mopping the floor, picking up and dropping off products, and standing behind a desk. Children who were older than him by five years or more had not been protected under the law. Only in 1900 had it been made illegal for children under fourteen to work for wages. Before then, only Massachusetts and Connecticut had a law limiting the workday to ten hours for children under twelve and fourteen. It was fair game in the other states.

"You got ten minutes," Tomato said.

Johnny opened the door and stepped out. "You coming?" he asked Paris.

Paris took his offered hand. They crossed the street, keeping an eye out for playing children and foul balls.

"I take it Cilly owns the cabin we hope to be staying in?" Paris asked.

Johnny nodded as he muscled open the apartment door. They went inside, and he knocked twice on the Nettesheims' door and stepped back. The door struggled open with a screech. Wally's bored face brightened with excitement in less than a second.

"Johnny!" he squeaked.

"Hey, pal, how's it going?" Johnny asked.

"Not too bad, doing what I can in this damn heat," Wally said.

"Wally!" his mother yelled from inside, "Watch your language!"

The boy rolled his eyes, suppressing a smirk. "Good evening, Paris."

"Good evening, Wally," Paris said, smiling at the young gentleman.

Clarence was at his chair beside the window, unaware that anyone was at the door. Cilly stepped into the frame, a polite smile on her tired face.

"Hi, Johnny. Paris, it's nice to see you again," she said.

"And you too," Paris said.

"Cilly, can we stop in?" Johnny asked.

"Of course."

Cilly opened the door fully, and they stepped in.

"Listen, Cilly, we can't stay long. I came here to ask for your help," Johnny said.

"Help? Something wrong?" she asked.

"The cabin your family has in Wisconsin…"

"Yes…" Cilly answered, looking unsure.

"We need a place where we can hang low for a few days. I don't want you to think you have to say yes though."

"Please, it's the least we can do. Let me find the key."

She hurried through the kitchen and down the hallway.

"What's going on that you have to go to Wisconsin?" Wally asked.

"I thought I'd show Johnny around my neck of the woods," Paris said.

"He's going to be blown away by the trees, having grown up in Brooklyn and all," Wally said.

Before Johnny or Paris could reply, Cilly was back, holding a key in her outstretched hand.

"We haven't been up there in ages, so I apologize for the shape it's in," she said.

"Nothing to apologize for, Cilly. I appreciate it," Johnny said.

"Can I go with Johnny?" Wally asked.

170

Cilly knew whatever was taking Johnny to Wisconsin was not leisure. Her maternal instinct could sense a nervousness in him.

"No honey," Cilly said.

"Why not?" Wally asked.

"Because we'd miss you too much."

Wally shrugged it off. "He wouldn't notice if I were gone."

"Of course he would."

"No he wouldn't."

"Wally, you watch your tone. Of course he would miss you. You're his son."

"No, he wouldn't! He doesn't notice a damn thing! He only knows one word! Maybe you should have named me that! Art E. Lee!"

Cilly slapped him across the face. Wally broke out in tears and sprinted into his room.

Cilly was mortified at what she'd done, and what the word "Art. E Lee" could incite. She prayed nothing came from it. But "Art E Lee" was close enough to "artillery" to unleash the trauma imprisoned in Clarence's mind. With an agility Johnny had never witnessed in him before, Clarence leapt from his chair and dove under the kitchen table. He covered his ears, screaming and mumbling incessantly.

Nobody knew what to do, each person instinctively reacting in different ways. Paris was horrified at Clarence's reaction, her mouth agape and eyes bulging. Cilly appeared as though her heart had been ripped from her chest and tossed under the table beside Clarence. For Johnny, it brought the War back to him. Wally had paused at the hallway, appalled at what he had done.

And then it happened again.

An invisible force pushed Johnny against the wall, a gasp of air erupted from his mouth. Clarence's scream was a scream Johnny knew all too well. A scream that brought back all of the horrors he had tried his damnedest to bury and cage.

Cilly dove under the table, striving to calm Clarence and coax him back to their beaten-down Cicero apartment and out of that trench.

"Dad! I'm sorry! I didn't mean it!" Wally shouted through his sobs.

171

Paris looked at Johnny pinned against the wall by invisible hands. But Clarence's shark-like thrashing brought her eyes back to him.

Cilly stroked Clarence's hair. "Honey, it's me Cilly. You're okay... you're okay."

Wally sobbed, his apologies indecipherable.

Johnny scrunched up his trembling fist, his eyes closed, hyperventilating.

Cilly rocked Clarence and gradually succeeded in calming him down. She pulled Wally close, kissing his forehead.

Paris could only look on at the heartbreaking tragedy unfolding before her in mute helplessness.

And then it passed.

Air flooded into Johnny's lungs like it had for Lazarus. The invisible force pressing him against the wall relinquished its hold on him.

Cilly helped Clarence to his feet and to his chair.

Johnny went to Wally and crouched down beside him. Wally's sobs had drenched his gray shirt.

"I didn't think that would happen. Really, Johnny," he managed to say through his sobs.

"I know you didn't."

Johnny offered his hand, but Wally shook his head.

"Come on Wally, we know you didn't mean it."

"That was a terrible thing I did. Worst thing a person can do."

If you only knew the terrible things I've done.

Wally scurried out from the table and ran down the hallway to his room.

"I'm sorry you had to see that," Cilly said.

Paris struggled to speak. "Oh, Cilly... I'm sorry."

"Let me talk to Wally. He'll want to say goodbye before you leave," Cilly said.

She hurried down the hall, looking like she had aged a decade since the conversation had started.

Johnny crept to Clarence in front of the window. His gaze was fixed on the world outside his window. He showed no signs that the last five minutes had even happened. To him, they hadn't. His memory was a broken clock, never advancing. The glass of water beside him on the window sill was empty. Johnny grabbed it, went into the kitchen, and refilled it. When he came back, Clarence opened his mouth. Johnny held the straw, and Clarence leaned forward like an egret and slurped. After drinking his fill, Clarence brought his attention back to the window and to the world outside that only he saw. Most thought he saw nothing or nothing different than anyone else and was only unable to process it. But Johnny knew. The Great War replayed outside that window. Clarence's eyes were like no one's Johnny had ever met. It wasn't the color—though eyes as black as ravens' wings are rare. Eyes revealed emotion. They showed when a person was offended, when they were sad, angry, confused or joyful. But to most, Clarence showed none of those. His eyes were black, lifeless, and forever void of emotion. But a trained eye like Johnny's could detect an eternal agony in them, a permanent poignant heartbreak caused at the pinnacle of human tribulation that set apart Clarence Nettesheim's eyes from anyone else.

Johnny put the glass down as a guilty-looking Cilly and a sulking Wally returned.

"I'm sorry for what happened. I truly am. Paris, Johnny, forgive me, please," Wally said.

He had cried too much for a person so young. Paris bit the inside of her lip, unsure of how to respond. Johnny nodded his approval at Wally's courage. He crouched down, meeting Wally's tear-filled eyes with his own.

"Every person makes mistakes. We all say things we don't mean. It takes a man to acknowledge them and apologize. We all know you didn't want that to happen."

Wally nodded, trying his hardest to stifle the second round of sobs.

"I have to go. I will stop back by soon though. I promise," Johnny said.

Wally held out his hand. Johnny shook it, smiling at the formality.

"We'll make another meal soon," Johnny promised.

He removed a wad of cash and held it out to Cilly.

"Rent for the cabin," Johnny said.

"Johnny... you just gave us money last night," Cilly said.

"Don't worry about it. It's just paper. Just make sure you take Wally and Clarence for some ice cream to help beat this heat," Johnny said.

Wally smiled appreciatively at Johnny's words and at the promise of better days double-scooped into a cake cone.

Cilly put her hand on the money but didn't take it. Johnny nodded at her more emphatically, and with great reluctance, she took it.

"Take care, Clarence. We'll see you soon," Johnny said.

"I'm sorry we have to leave so quickly," Paris added.

Cilly dismissed Paris' unneeded apology with a flick of her wrist. "Drive safe."

Paris and Johnny both knew Cilly would cry most of the night. It showed on every inch of her face.

Johnny tipped his fedora and followed Paris out.

"Wally," Johnny said.

"Yeah?" Wally answered.

"Can you name a city in Italy besides Rome?"

Wally thought on it and then shook his head. "Can you?"

"Mirabella Imbaccari."

"Is that a pasta dish?"

Johnny smiled. "It's where my father was born."

When they had gone down the stoop, Paris put a hand on Johnny's arm, turning him to face her.

"That was the most heartbreaking thing I've ever seen."

The Wisconsin Woods

The city appealed to drive, determination, and dreams. It was a place where a living was made. Soon, they had left it behind, and the lakeshore came into view, its waters sparkling like diamonds and sapphires. Steel skyscrapers could make a man feel small, but natural giants like forests, mountains, and lakes could make a man feel inconsequential.

The ride was filled with periods of silence and moments of arguing between Tomato and Hotsy. Arguments over everything—what routes to take, how fast to drive, and when to stop for the bathroom.

While the front seat had sound, the back had nothing but silence. Though they stole glances at each other, Johnny and Paris spent the time mostly looking out of the window and at the majestic lake and then at the giant pine trees.

When they reached Milwaukee, they stopped for gasoline, snacks, and a bathroom break. The two pairs swapped seats, Johnny taking the driver's seat and Paris the passenger seat. As the night plunged the world outside into darkness, Hotsy and Tomato fell asleep, filling the car with annoying snores, but it was better than the bickering.

"It's so strange being back here. It feels like ages," Paris said, staring out the window at the sights flashing past.

Johnny knew what she was feeling, what she was thinking. It was the strange feeling of being a foreigner in your own hometown. Recognizing all of the buildings but none of the faces. Having a memory on every street corner and having a rogue wave of nostalgia crashing over you.

In a way, it was the ultimate betrayal. The whole ship ride home from France, Johnny had thought home would still be there. That everything he had been through would somehow be set right in his hometown.

I was wrong.

"A few blocks from here is the house I grew up in," Paris mentioned.

"Do you want to drive by?" Johnny asked.

"No."

There was more to her refusal, but Johnny let it be. Her expression confirmed she had been betrayed by her hometown too.

"So, we're going to Whitefish Bay?" Paris asked.

Johnny nodded. "Northeast part of the state."

"Did you know that almost every single person is born with a map of Wisconsin?" she asked.

Johnny looked over, beyond confused. "I think you smoke too much reefer."

Paris slapped his arm in mock indignation, then raised her left hand, her four fingers tight together and thumb spread out.

"See?" she asked, holding her hand out toward him.

"Well, I'll be goddamned," Johnny said.

It really did look like the state of Wisconsin.

Johnny smirked. "Then we're traveling to your upper thumb."

Northeastern Wisconsin was so far removed from Chicago, it seemed impossible that they were of the same continent. One was built of stone and steel, and the other overflowed with forests and fields.

"At what point do they qualify as being in a coma?" Paris asked, stealing a glance at the back seat over her shoulder.

"The last week has been hard on them," Johnny said.

"Some of the girls were talking about when Hotsy and Tomato found out you had been shot," Paris said.

Johnny was quiet; he looked down the road or at his mirrors—anywhere but at Paris.

"Tomato cried. Right there at the bar. And Hotsy didn't blink for minutes. Looked sick from it. You've got loyal friends Giovanni," Paris said.

"I don't deserve it," Johnny said.

"What's the story behind that?"

He finally looked at her. "Story behind what?"

"*I don't deserve it.* You hold onto something that happened, this cloud that hangs over you, makes you think you're unworthy. Let it rain, Giovanni, and let the cloud pass."

"I'm that easy to figure out?"

"No, you're far from easy to understand, but I know the way you think."

"And how's that?"

"I've always considered life a car ride. We spend so much time looking at what's ahead or in the rear view mirror and what came before, that we forget to look out of the windows. Putting so much emphasis on what's coming that when we get there, it's a let-down. Only realizing the beauty of something until we see it in that mirror, and by then, it's too late. All of us will fade into history. None of us will make it out alive. At some point, we all go the way of the dodo bird. We might as well enjoy the time before we do."

She fell silent and turned her attention to the black expanse out of her window, but her message had been received.

"I guess I should apologize for interfering," Johnny said.

"You didn't force me to come. How's the wound?" Paris asked.

"Another scar."

"You have quite the collection of those. I saw the one on your chest."

177

"I knew you weren't looking at my eyes."

"How can I? You hide them all the time."

Johnny shook his head and suppressed an uncomfortable laugh. But it was far from a joke.

"Did you get that one during the War?" she asked.

"Yeah."

He slowed the car and veered onto a gravel road. Tree branches hung over the road so far, it looked as though the road would disappear into a thick forest. But just when Paris motioned to point that the road would vanish beneath the drooping willows, a clearing opened and exposed a secluded two-story wooden cabin. Johnny parked and killed the ignition. He leaned over the seat and shook Tomato's shoulder.

"We're here," Johnny said.

Tomato awoke with a curse. Hotsy only woke when Paris and Johnny slammed their car doors shut. The wooden cabin was in fair shape but showed signs of neglect. The air was still warm, but much cooler than Chicago and considerably less thick. It was also fresh, an exciting thing after a nearly six-hour drive. City air was filled with exhaust, pollution and cigar and cigarette smoke that had permeated the walls of almost every building. Outside that cabin in Wisconsin, it was the same air Indians had breathed hundreds of years earlier. The whole area had a timeless quality to it, from the air to the trees to the soil. In a word, it was calming.

Johnny removed the bronze key Cilly had given him and unlocked the cabin door. The door crack was clogged with dirt, and it took a strong shove to push it open. He had expected an overpowering smell of dust or mildew to attack his nostrils but was pleasantly surprised when it was cedar that caressed them.

Tomato dropped his suitcase off by the side of the door. "I saw a generator outside. I'll go fire it up."

The stars and the waxing crescent moon hovered just beyond the surrounding tall Silver Leaf maple trees, too far away for their light to reach the inside of the cabin. A loud vibrating rumble told them that Tomato had successfully started the generator.

Hotsy hit the light switch. The lights flickered to life. The inside had looked much cleaner in the near-blackness. Now with the room bathed in light, it was clear the cabin had had two species of occupants since Cilly's family had last set foot inside—spiders and dust bunnies.

"Any chance there's food?" Hotsy asked.

"Take a look around, bozo. Does it look like there would be food?" Tomato asked.

"What's that saying? Don't judge a book by its cover?"

"There was no power on! Do you think the cupboards are stocked?"

Their bickering continued like rounds of a boxing match. While they argued, Johnny and Paris looked around. The kitchen was to the left upon entering, with an island counter separating it from the living room. There was an ice box in the corner. A long maroon couch sat in front of a dirty, soot-ridden fireplace with bedrooms on both sides.

They strolled around, taking in the wood trim, black curtains, and hardwood floors while Hotsy tried to get a fire going. Tomato stood by, silently critiquing. The interior of the cabin had a draft of neglect, but it was far too hot for a fire. But if no one else complained, Johnny wouldn't either, not aloud at least.

"Jesus Christ, haven't you ever started a fire before?" Tomato snapped at Hotsy. He stormed to the fireplace and crouched beside him.

Johnny had hoped that, for once, Tomato could stifle his need to correct or criticize everything Hotsy did. A fire was the last thing they needed.

"I'm crumpling the paper," Hotsy said.

"You want to create surface area," Tomato said.

"Well if you're a pyromancer, be my guest," Hotsy said, stepping aside and pointing at the fireplace.

In less than two minutes, Tomato had a fire started. "God, kid, you're helpless."

"Or maybe it was my goal to dilly dally and wait for your overbearing nature to kick in, so you'd end up starting the fire. With that and the generator, when it comes to household chores, it's Tomato two, Hotsy zero," Hotsy said, a victorious smile on his face.

Tomato's face turned red, the vein in his forehead bulging.

"He'll shoot you," Johnny warned.

"Nah, from that distance?" Hotsy said, folding his arms over his head.

Tomato held a rolled piece of newspaper into the flame. As the flames crawled onto it, Tomato launched it at Hotsy. It soared through the sky like a fireball. He swatted at it, nearly falling off the couch.

"You crazy son of a…!" Hotsy yelled.

"Plenty of places to bury you out here," Tomato said.

"You can find me buried under the sheets in the master bedroom."

"The hell I will!"

Hotsy jumped off the couch and dashed toward the bedroom on the right. Tomato was slow to his feet, but closer. He grabbed Hotsy by his shirt, pulled him out of the door frame, stepped inside, and slammed the door shut.

"Rat bastard!" Hotsy cursed through the door.

"Sweet dreams!" Tomato yelled back.

Hotsy was a womanizer, and sometimes obliviously rude, but that didn't mean he didn't have manners. He granted Paris and Johnny the other bedroom. But Johnny would have preferred if now would have been one of those obliviously rude moments. The living room was a communal gathering place to laugh, eat, drink, and enjoy company. It was a room for extraversion. The bedroom insinuated so many things—private things. A room for introversion. No room was home to more pressure, excitement, revelation, and nervousness.

His eyes on anything but Paris, Johnny nodded for her to enter first. She did. The air in the room felt heavy, as if thick with anticipation, a sense of suffocation no number of open windows could alleviate. Johnny hadn't done as much as hold her hand. Paris was far from bashful nor did she normally convey her thoughts or feelings in her eyes like Johnny did. Her eyes were a fortress. But there was no way she wasn't wondering where the next several minutes would take them.

"I'll… sleep on the floor," Johnny said.

Paris only nodded.

A palpable awkwardness rose between the two as Paris lay on the soft bed while Johnny lay on the cold hard wooden floor. It wasn't the fact the floor was as comfortable as a rock, it was the thoughts swirling around in his head that kept him awake. At quarter to five, he crept out of the bedroom and walked to the lakeshore to catch the sunrise.

There is something soothing about sunrises. Something about them kept the attacks at bay. There was nothing more hopeful than a new day. There's nothing like the gentle warmth of the sunrise hugging your skin, bringing with it a promise of better. This sunrise was no different. It was a sunrise that made you believe there was something better out there, somewhere. But as he turned and walked away, it was another reminder of how much of a trickster the sun was. It was all a mirage, a dream, a lie. The fleeting glory of the rising sun only reiterated how inconsequential you were—a mere speck of dust in an infinite universe, left to fend off the darkness alone.

When he returned to the cabin, only Paris was awake. Hotsy had his face buried so deep into his pillow he risked suffocation. The fire had long died out. Thank God for that. For as cold as the woods had gotten at night, the cabin had cooked like an oven the higher the sun rose. Paris was at the kitchen island finishing off Hotsy's bag of potato crisps from the night before.

"A small fraction of me wondered if you had gone to get us some breakfast. But then I remembered chivalry isn't really your thing," she said.

"Sorry, I went for a walk to get some fresh air," Johnny said.

"I was thinking of getting out of this cabin. Maybe walk to get a newspaper and some groceries."

"Okay."

"The subtext there being that you're invited to join me…"

"Sure."

181

No one could deny Hotsy had achieved fluency in the language of women. But Paris must have thought none of his skill had rubbed off on Johnny. And, truthfully, it hadn't. Johnny kept his relationships with women to minutes at a time. When things went from casual to serious, women wanted to know more, but too much of what Johnny wanted to keep buried. Too much of what he was afraid to reveal. Any time a woman had tried to enter the inner-levels of his maze, he had ended it, and ended it quickly.

Johnny opened the door for Paris, and the two stepped out into the rural air. Thankfully, it was free of mayflies, gnats, and mosquitos that normally swarmed the lakeshore.

"It's peaceful here," Paris said.

"Yeah, it is," Johnny said.

"Look at the sun over the water. Have you seen anything like it before?"

"Once."

"Back in New York?"

Johnny shook his head, studying her face to see if she was truly interested in his reply. So often a question was asked even when a person truly didn't want an elaborate answer. But Paris' face showed she starved for a detailed answer. And he owed her that much.

"France," Johnny said. "A giant forest reaching the clouds. We set up camp in this field, waiting for the Germans. During the mornings, a fog would come. Looked like ghosts floating past. It was eerie but oddly relaxing. When the sun rose, you'd hear fifty different types of birds. But nighttime was unbelievable. More stars than I'd ever seen. More than I thought there were. Growing up in Brooklyn, I think I saw about half a dozen total. But in that field... it was like you were in space. It was just you and the stars. But then the attack began. That whole forest was destroyed. That's not exaggeration either. Every last tree was upended, every leaf and blade of grass in that field was turned to ash and dirt. The smoke was so thick that you couldn't see the sky any more. Not even the moon could burst through. By the end, that field... that sky that'd been a site of such beauty... had become an apocalyptic wasteland."

182

Paris studied his face. Behind his blue eyes, he was reliving the horrors of war. He expected the attack to come. He had opened a book of monstrosities. He had unlocked every door, opened every window. But whether it was that powerful sun or the look of compassion on Paris' face, the attack didn't come.

"There are still places in this world uncorrupted by man," Paris said. "Places that are the same now as they were hundreds of years ago. I'm drawn to places like that. I have a dream of moving to a beach house in California. Listening to the waves as I drink my morning coffee, the sunshine magnified through my tall glass windows overlooking the beach. I don't think there is any greater feeling than having the sun on your shoulder. That comfort, that warmth... Every dollar that I am able to save goes to that."

He had revealed a snippet of himself, and she had done the same.

"Why California?" Johnny asked.

"*Manifest destiny,*" Paris said with a forced smile.

"Gold rush ended seventy years ago."

"Truthfully? I wanted to be an actress."

And for the first time since Johnny had known her, Paris looked vulnerable.

"*Wanted* to?" Johnny asked, emphasizing the past tense.

"I grew up. Life doesn't ask what you want."

"No, it doesn't."

The most heartbreaking truth a person has to learn.

"Why did you want to be an actress?"

"I loved the idea of being someone else. Every day someone different."

"And now?"

"I am hoping to earn enough money to leave and get a place. Start new. Be someone new."

"Would you try to make it in Hollywood?"

"Maybe, I don't know. I'm not relying on that to work out. Besides acting is just that. All your problems don't go away with a costume. Now, I think I'd like to help people."

"What do you mean help people?"

"Help people cope with things they've experienced. Everyone has a cross to bear. I'd like to help them accept what's happened and move on. There is this stigma that we should keep our demons to ourselves, that we have to fight them alone. And we don't."

Johnny looked at her. "Is that why you're here?"

She returned his gaze. "Is that why I'm here?"

Paris would have been able to get a wolf to submit to her gaze.

The gas station was open, but there were no cars at the pumps. The door was propped open in an attempt to help circulate fresh air and reduce the temperature inside. The older man behind the desk sipped a cup of black coffee while he read the morning paper.

Johnny nodded politely at him. Paris grabbed a newspaper from the stack beside the door.

The gas station was far from a grocery store, but there was a refrigerator stacked with cola, milk, cheese, and juice and aisles stocked with potato crisps, bread, peanut butter, jams, and cans of soups and vegetables. Johnny grabbed two colas and a block of cheddar cheese from the fridge, two bags of potato crisps, a loaf of bread, a jar of peanut butter, a jar of strawberry jelly, and a few cans of vegetables—corn and green beans—from the shelf. He barely made it to the counter when the contents fell from his hands. He went to Paris and took the paper from her and set it on the counter beside the hodgepodge of food. He asked for two blocks of ice, and the attendant dug into his zinc-lined ice box and pulled out two, each weighting twenty pounds.

The attendant added the total on his cash register, bagged the items, handed Johnny his change, and wished him a good bye in the most insincere, formal way. Johnny hated coins. Hated the way they jingled in his pocket, and the way they fell out when he sat. Therefore, he normally left his change. But the attendant had cast disapproving glances at Paris standing outside his store, so Johnny kept every last penny and cast a dirty look of his own.

He closed the door behind him, trapping the thick, stagnant heat inside. In the span of the six minutes they had been inside, the temperature felt like it had risen by ten degrees.

Paris offered to carry the bag of groceries. Johnny declined, but she took it anyway.

"You always read the paper?" Johnny asked.

"I like to know what's going on," Paris replied.

Johnny scoffed at the comment.

"You agree?" Paris asked sarcastically.

"I think the average person has enough awful things to face in a day that they don't need to read about what happened to other people."

"It isn't all bad."

"There's a whole section detailing who died."

"Here, read the weather." She playfully thrust the paper into his chest. "Ninety and sunny."

"That's the most devastating news in the whole damn thing."

Paris laughed. "You're a Cola half-empty type."

"Yeah, keep it up, and I'll drink your half too."

Johnny was incapable of a fake smile, and he wasn't too well-practiced in genuine ones either, so his cheeks nearly cramped from the one on his face.

It was only half-past nine, but the beaches were already lined with children who had bugged their parents into allowing an early swim. They frolicked in the water, while their parents sat on lounge chairs in the sand. Far from shore, boats lined the horizon, fishing or cruising for pleasure.

"Let's walk in the water," Paris suggested.

"Not exactly dressed for that," Johnny said looking down at his pants and boots.

"Weren't you ever a kid? Take your shoes off and roll your pants legs up or do you have webbed feet you're trying to hide?"

Johnny rolled his eyes and dropped the two blocks of ice. He leaned over, untied and yanked off his black-capped boots and socks. They strolled through the water, its cooling refreshment stopping at their knees. Paris filled the stroll with conversations about the beaches along the Milwaukee shoreline she had visited during her childhood. Most of the best swim locations were segregated. Coloreds had their own section of beach, a place she had spent hours at. She talked about walking to school, about visiting small towns in the summer. Towns where you could walk from the start to the end in an hour. Towns where you could call things by the type of business—the gas station, the restaurant, the store, the Church—because there was only one of each.

When their toes had turned to prunes, and the blocks of ice had started to melt, they put their socks and shoes back on, and returned to the cabin. When they walked in, Hotsy was scavenging through the cupboards.

"If you missed food the first twelve times, you're the world's biggest moron," Tomato said.

"I'm being thorough," Hotsy shot back.

Paris set the bag of groceries on the counter, and Tomato and Hotsy flocked to it like hyenas to a fresh carcass. After all four had enjoyed a peanut butter and jelly sandwich—apart from Hotsy who only had peanut butter (he didn't care for jelly (it was a consistency thing)—and several slices of cheese, they played cards, ranging from poker, sheepshead, Hearts, and the most popular amongst the four—cribbage.

At twelve thirty, the four walked to a local restaurant called Good Eats that specialized in German food. Johnny and Paris didn't mind the walk. It was preferable to being canned in a car like sardines. The fresh air and sun could do wonders on a person's body and mood. But Tomato loved driving and despised walking. Hotsy didn't care either way, but sided with Johnny and Paris only to tick off Tomato.

"I'd die of starvation if I was German," Tomato said, reading the menu.

"Blood sausage?" Hotsy asked, looking like he had inhaled manure.

"How do you pronounce half this shit?" Tomato asked, dropping his menu in frustration.

The menu contained foods Johnny's mother used to prepare. Chief among them was the *kartoffelpuffer*. It had been a family staple—her mother had prepared it and her mother before her had prepared it, passing it on like a family trait of dark wavy hair and blue eyes. But the menu did contain items that could be risky for the uninitiated.

Tomato and Hotsy were not going to take risks with their choices, each ordering the *spätzle*—egg noodles covered in melted cheese. It was the closest thing to pasta the restaurant had. Paris, on the other hand, was curious to know about each menu item and challenged Johnny to find a suitable comparison to something she may have tried. Both settled on a *schnitzel*—a staple of German cuisine. The *schnitzel* was a cutlet coated in breadcrumbs, with ham and cheese sandwiched inside the deep-fried coating. When the food was brought out, it was obvious that Tomato and Hotsy had banked on having to manually massage the food down their throat, but were instead pleasantly surprised at the flavor. Deciding to dive into the deep end of the pool of German cuisine, Hotsy ordered a blood sausage for all four to try. His excited smile completely vanished when the black sausage was set before him.

"Who wants to try it first?" he asked.

When no one spoke, he cut the sausage into four pieces, hoping it looked more appetizing. Lord Jesus was he wrong.

"Aren't you two a couple of wet blankets," Johnny taunted.

He dug his fork into one of the pieces and chomped down on the sausage. It was not a favorite meal, but he had eaten it before. It tasted no different than getting punched in the mouth. It was all iron.

"When in Rome," Paris said.

"You won't find that abomination in that Holy City," Tomato said.

Paris took a deep breath and ate her piece. It was an obvious struggle, but it went down and stayed down.

"Tomato?" Hotsy asked.

"I'm not eating that. I wouldn't have eaten that on the front line. That's sick. Some Dracula-type shit," Tomato said, adamant in his resolve.

"Do it for your children," Hotsy said.

Johnny and Paris laughed.

"Do it for my children? Me eating blood is for them?" Tomato asked with a dumbfounded stare.

"Isn't that the whole Jesus thing? You drink his blood?" Hotsy asked.

"That's a metaphor. We Catholics drink a nice dry red wine."

"If I eat this, I need to stand taller in your eyes."

"You won't be taller when you're hunched over the can."

Hotsy took five rapid breaths and plunged the blackened, bloodied slice into his mouth. Initially, he had hoped to swallow it whole, but it was too large, and to prevent himself from choking, he had to bite into it—the flavors swarmed his mouth. The horrors of what he tasted showed in his dark eyes. He grabbed his napkin and spewed a combination of chewed blood sausage and vomit into it.

"It wasn't that bad," he said when he finally stopped gagging.

"You lying…" Tomato said, trying not to smile.

The waitress talked them into a slice of *schwarzwälder kirschtorte* (Black Forest Cherry Torte). But only after she had confirmed it did not contain bits of tree bark or leaves. After all, Germans were apparently literal with the names of their food.

"What is the plan for tonight?" Paris asked.

"I'm about to have plans," Hotsy said, watching their young, smiling waitress return to their table.

She placed their check and four peppermint starlights on the table. Hotsy placed his hand atop hers.

"Of course," he said.

"I'm sorry?" she asked, his touch causing her cheeks to flush.

"Of course I'll take you out tonight. I'm a stranger to these parts and could use an experienced guide. I mean what if I get lost? You wouldn't want that on your conscience, would you?"

"No…" She bit her lip to stop herself from smiling.

"I knew God wouldn't give a smile like yours to someone who would."

"What did you have in mind?"

If she turned any redder, she'd be a strawberry.

"In mind? Whatever you want. On my mind? You."

She nervously ran her free hand through her curly blonde hair, giggling like she was half-seas over.

"Call your friends up, and we'll meet you back here at six."

"Okay."

The conversation was over, but her eyes were locked on Hotsy. He shook his hair from out of his eyes, transferring an invisible spark that caused her to trip on her way back to the kitchen.

"Unbelievable," Tomato said.

But he was hardly mad. Hotsy had gotten a friend for him too.

"The blood of Christ flows through me," Hotsy said nonchalantly.

"No, that's pig blood," Tomato said.

"Tomato, I am touched by God." He held up his hands as if they had performed miracles.

"Oh, yeah? Then turn your napkin into some kale and pay for this."

Dinner and a Movie

After enjoying their slice of delicious cake (something that completely changed Tomato and Hotsy's stance on German cuisine), they returned to the cabin. Hotsy agreed to play only one game of cribbage. After he and Johnny had narrowly defeated Paris and Tomato, he darted to the bathroom before Tomato could force him into a rematch. He was in the bathroom for an hour and twelve minutes, an exact duration according to Tomato's watch.

When Hotsy stepped out, his hair shined with enough Brilliantine hair product to grease a squeaky wheel. There had been a time when Hotsy could not afford the real thing and had to settle for petroleum jelly. What a mess that left. He'd run his fingers through his hair and transfer an oily smear to everything.

His black sleeves were rolled to the elbow, the top two buttons left undone to expose his tanned chest. He kept a gold-chained pocket watch in his gray vest, not because he cared about the time, but because it was stylish.

Tomato had a few choice words for him, most of which related to the ridiculous amount of time he had spent in the bathroom. It took Tomato a tenth of the time to get ready. They said goodbye to Johnny and Paris, grabbed the bottle of whiskey they had brought, and drove back to the German restaurant to meet the waitress and her friends.

"Do we have anything planned for tonight or are we spending it in awkward silence?" Paris asked.

"We were going to, but you ruined it," Johnny said.

"Sadly, I don't know if you're joking."

"I thought about going to a petting pantry. I saw the show times in the paper."

"I thought you didn't read the paper. Look at you."

"I'm growing."

"So, we're seeing a picture. Any plans for supper?" Paris asked in a way that evoked suspicion.

"Have something in mind?" Johnny asked.

Paris raised her eyebrows and kept the mystery intact. "I need to get some clothes, I can't wear this all week."

"Fair enough."

They walked to a small clothing store less than half a mile away. It was no Sears, but Paris found a few items—an emerald green summer dress, a cotton cloche hat of the same color, and a denim blue day dress. Johnny grabbed a few extra shirts, underwear and socks, and Paris selected a pair of golden brown pants and matching vest with an art deco tie, a swirling wash of beige and gold. She dug into her purse, but Johnny stopped her.

"This is on me. I didn't exactly give you time to pack."

When they were back in the cabin, Paris allowed Johnny to get ready first. He used a wash cloth to scrub his body and then shaved, insuring his face was smooth to the touch. He fell somewhere in the middle of Tomato and Hotsy's time, mostly because he couldn't pull his head out of the sink with the cold water streaming down his neck. He stepped out wearing only his pants and A-shirt—

191

the rest could wait. Paris went next. When she stepped out, an invisible fireball swept over Johnny. She was as breathtaking as the sky above that field in France had been.

Johnny's suspicion about supper was well-founded. Paris wouldn't say exactly what or, more importantly, where she had in mind for supper. The only hint she gave was that it was a "Friday Wisconsin Tradition." She may as well have spoken Chinese, because "Friday Wisconsin Tradition" meant absolutely nothing to Johnny.

Though it was muggy, Johnny would have enjoyed the march even if Paris had led him to the middle of nowhere, because the whole town was refreshing. They passed three restaurants, a candy shop, a boutique, and butcher's stop. But Paris stopped at none of them. Several times Johnny came close to asking her if she was taking him on a one-way ride (walk.) He opened his mouth to ask if she knew where she was going, but just then, a crowd of people emerged from seemingly everywhere and headed in the same direction. Paris had used her Wisconsin intuition to know where to go. Maybe it had something to do with that built-in map everyone was born with. Reading the lines in her hands like they were streets.

Searing and sizzling sounds came from behind a restaurant, followed with *ooos* and *ahhhs*. Johnny followed Paris, not to the front door but around the side and to the back. Fifteen tables stretched over an open gravel area that was around fifty-feet wide and sixty-feet long. In the center of the tables was nothing but empty space, save for a giant black cauldron of the same kind found in stories involving witches, potions, and poisons.

"You brought me to a séance?" Johnny asked, unsure if he was joking.

"No, don't be silly. This is a cult. You're the human sacrifice. They don't like half-breeds with blue eyes," Paris said.

"Well, you better hope I appease the Gods or you're next, half-breed."

Paris laughed.

The fifty people at the tables had either finished their food or were waiting for it, so it was impossible for Johnny to decipher what the menu offered. The hostess greeted them and led them to a communal table. The folks were friendly according to Paris. He insisted they were being nosy, just short of interrogating, but Paris assured him it was a Wisconsin thing. Something that soon became an annoying refrain.

"Is this restaurant going to serve food or is it still being caught?" Johnny asked.

Paris leaned into him. "Patience is a virtue."

"A virtue trumped by hunger."

Suddenly, the children beside them leaned forward on the table with excitement. Johnny and Paris turned around and faced the bubbling cauldron. Two men were standing over it. Apparently pleased with what they saw in the pot, they added a wire basket filled with over a hundred red potatoes. Minutes later, whitefish was added, followed with two pounds of salt. The flames beneath the kettle surged, licking the sides. One of the two men cautiously approached the bubbling cauldron and doused the fire in kerosene. The flames shot into the air, fifteen feet high with the terrifying roar only fire could unleash. The crowd *ahhh'd* at the sight. The relief the time of day, the blocking trees, and lake breeze had brought vanished as an invisible flame swept over Johnny. One that had nothing to do with the flaming cauldron.

No. Not here. Not now.

He closed his eyes and instantly regretted that decision. The heat vaporized the air in his lungs, drying his tongue to a block of stone. With his eyes closed, he was back in France. The flames. The explosions. The screams. He opened his eyes. He was back in Wisconsin, but the sounds playing in his head were those of war. He could feel Paris' stare. Had she spoken? The sweat ran down his forehead, spreading across his lower back and under his chest.

Breathe. Breathe damn it.

He was no different than the whitefish, twitching for one final breath.

Paris was speaking, but no sound reached him. He read her lips, which seemed to be moving in slow motion—"Are you okay?"

Other than the fact I'm going to drown on land and die in front of all these people, everything's Jake.

Johnny tried steadying his breathing without her noticing. But of course she noticed. He struggled to breathe as if he had a plastic bag over his mouth. The whole damn crowd probably noticed. Memories came to him in flashes, like rising and falling under the rapids of a strong river.

And then the attacked morphed, mutating like a deadly virus. Air flooded into his lungs, like water onto a sinking ship. He couldn't breathe it in fast enough, hyperventilating. His chest heaved up and down, his hands shook. With unbelievable fluidity, he was transported to France and back to Wisconsin for seconds at a time.

Standing at a trench ladder, eyes closed.

Staring at the boiling cauldron.

A whistle shrieking, shells exploding, climbing that ladder into Armageddon.

The small town people cheering and clapping.

The sunlight unable to penetrate the thick, gray blanket of smoke and the blackened earth below it.

The bright sun-filled day, the earth alive with vivid greens, blues, and browns.

Crawling under barbed wire coils through glue-like mud.

Sitting on that wooden bench, gravel under his boots.

Artillery launching and exploding across the night sky.

Mayflies swarming through the air in black clouds.

German machine gunners unloading without pause. Blood pouring from the dead and dying.

A frenetic bubbling, water and oil spilling over the sides.

White-faced corpses lining No Man's Land, open, unseeing eyes. Expressionless, motionless, cold and rigid.

Tanned smiling faces, excitement and happiness glimmering in their eyes. Warmed by the caress of sun, bodies contorting for a better view.

He closed his eyes again, demanding his mind retake control over his mutinous body.

Paris squeezed his hand. In an instant, he was back at that table in Northeast Wisconsin, having traveled the four thousand miles in a second. His breathing steadied, air slowly filling his lungs.

Paris removed her hand and continued as if nothing had happened.

"All the fish fat boils over," Paris explained, leaning closer to Johnny.

"How do you know so much about this?" Johnny asked.

"Friday fish fries are a tradition here. They're especially popular during Lent."

The fish and potatoes were scooped onto plates and handed out to the hungry guests. For no seasoning except salt (only added to increase the gravity of the water or so the woman at the table told them), it was surprisingly tasty, mostly aided by the melted butter drizzled over the plate.

"Now you're one of us. A true Wisconsinite," Paris said.

It seemed that in Wisconsin, if you ate a meal together, you would be lifelong friends, and it took ten minutes to say goodbye to Taylor, his wife Susan and their three children, Thomas, Peter, and Marcy. The picture was at quarter-to-eight, and the movie house a twenty-minute-walk away. With the sun low, the lake breeze went unchallenged. Johnny was almost comfortable, but Paris was chilled. The title "The Phantom of the Opera" shone in black letters on a white marquee, while the name of the movie house, The Majestic, was lit with blinding white gold bulbs surrounding the vertical golden letters. Even now, at thirty-two, the eye-catching marquee sparked a sense of wonder in him. Life had unlimited possibilities on the big screen. It offered relief. Relief from worry, from angst, from pain, and from despair. For a couple of hours, it numbed Johnny's thoughts. It hypnotized his demons, securely burying and caging them, granting him the ability to be someone else. He could be heartthrob Rudolph Valentino, the stoic physical comedian Buster Keaton, the tragedian John Barrymore or the Jack-of-all-trades Charlie Chaplin.

The movie they would see had been released last November, but it was just now making its way from the bigger cities to the more rural areas of the country. And of all the movie characters he'd seen on screen, The Phantom was the one Johnny related to most.

The line at the ticket counter stretched the length of the sidewalk, and the young man in the booth struggled to keep up. People in line talked to each other about the film, discussing how good they expected it to be or what the reviews in the paper had said. Johnny continually checked his watch. The show was minutes away from starting, and they were still outside. He grew more frustrated by the second. Paris put her hand on his wrist to prevent him from checking his watch again.

"Just relax," she said.

"I don't relax," Johnny said.

"Don't or can't?"

"Both."

Johnny was certain they wouldn't get a ticket, but when he asked for two, the overwhelmed man tore off two and took the offered money with nothing more than an "Enjoy the show." That was Johnny's kind of worker. No small talk, just getting down to business.

Gold-trimmed glass doors were held open by a door stopper, keeping the air inside fresh and allowing for an easier transference of travel. Chandeliers reflected gold and silver twinkles around the room. The steps were lined in gold. Vendors sold bags of popcorn, that holy smell of melted butter wafting through the lobby. It was a smell Johnny had never been able to resist. In an oblivious daze, he had gone from the entrance steps to the popcorn stand. He only snapped out of the daze when the vendor repeated his question about what he wanted to get.

He ordered a large popcorn and munched on it as he stood in the concession line for two soda pops and a Hershey bar. Then he and Paris followed the crowd into the dark theatre. As always, all the open seats were in the middle and getting to them required doing an awkward slide and shuffle while balancing a soda pop in one hand and an overfilled bag of popcorn in the other. Johnny apologized on his way through, popcorn falling on the laps of the people he slid past.

The white screen was massive, stretching from floor to ceiling and wall to wall. It wasn't as grand as the movie palaces in Chicago or New York, but it was impressive the little Wisconsin town even had a theater. But once the lights dimmed and the screen came to life, they were all the same—a place of magic. A place that transported you into the life of a different person.

What a blessing that was. It was only too cruel it lasted less than 120 minutes.

"Maybe I'll see you up there some day," Johnny whispered.

Paris acknowledged the comment with a smile then took a handful of popcorn. Neither were overly hungry, but the human body is designed to always save room for popcorn.

Throughout the film, there were moments when the theatre lit up. During those moments, it was impossible to miss Paris' open hand. Her palm seemed to be too upturned for it to be in a natural resting position. Was she inviting him to hold it? He stared at her hand, and when he looked up, her smoky eyes were staring at him, cruelly illuminated by the bright screen. Johnny diverted his gaze to the screen, trying to sell how vested he was in the film.

That deformed phantom on the screen had more game. But the truth was, he hadn't paid any attention to the film over the last ten minutes. He was too busy overthinking and silently cursing himself. After the last end credit had rolled down the screen, the lights powered on, and the masses headed to the exits. Johnny and Paris hurried past those unable to discuss the movie and walk at the same time.

Outside, Johnny appreciated the calming effect of the fresh air by puffing on a torch. The smoke rose into the summer air. Small talk about the film filled their walk. Away from the epicenter of the town, the streets grew increasingly barer. Paris talked about the quaint beauty of the small town. In big cities, everything was constantly changing. There were always new fashion trends, new technology, new music and new slang. The city birthed them. But in small towns, it took months, even years, for those changes to arrive. The Illinois rich were also enchanted by their charm and they vacationed in Northeastern Wisconsin, sometimes for the whole summer, or so Paris explained.

"By rich vacationers, do you mean entitled assholes?" Johnny asked.

"Maybe. I'm sure some of them are, but not all of them. You shouldn't let someone's money define them," Paris said.

"Money's a free pass."

"People with money have problems too."

"Problems can be paid off."

"Some of them."

"Most of them."

"I think Cilly and Wally would disagree with that."

"They can't afford the best doctors. If they could, maybe Clarence gets better."

Paris nodded her acceptance of her small defeat. But that was a single battle, not the war. She counted her wounded and continued the good fight.

"So what you do for a living, should I judge you for it?"

"The rich get their booze. The real stuff. Half of them are friends with congressmen, zoning commissioners, police captains, and prohibition agents. I've seen shipments of South Side booze confiscated and brought to the rich for their parties. I've dropped crates of whiskey off at the State Capitol. You walk into any Walgreens, and you'll see the rich standing in line waiting to legally purchase alcohol with the doctor prescriptions they bought. The rich prey on the poor, always have. And it doesn't look like that's going to change anytime soon. I make sure they don't got to do it sober."

The passion in his voice was evident. There was rage, maybe even hate.

"You guys are from out of town or no?" a voice said from across the street.

Johnny and Paris turned to face the source of the sound. Four men, all in their early twenties, stood by the intersection Johnny and Paris had crossed. Which of the four had spoken was impossible to decipher.

"Yes, we are," Paris answered politely.

The four men checked for traffic before crossing the street. Friendly smiles showcased an illusion of hospitality.

"Yeah, I figured as much. Old Herb at the gas station said youse two had stopped in. We were at the movie palace just now. I figured we'd take it upon ourselves to explain the rules of the town—the official and the unofficial," the apparent leader of the group said.

It was not the man Johnny had pegged as the speaker. His guess had been the burly, cinnamon brown–haired man, not the lanky blonde.

Paris held her own fake smile, but Johnny's lips were straight as an arrow—he'd heard enough already.

"You the mayor?" Johnny asked.

His friends chuckled, not because they found it funny but because he had had the nerve to say it.

"No, I'm not the mayor, but when you come to a city, it's best not to stir the pot. Not to ruffle any feathers," the self-appointed mayor said.

His blonde hair was well-kept and his smoothly shaven face was the handiwork of a skilled barber. If his appearance didn't give away his wealth, his wardrobe did.

"See, I had you pegged for poultry. You know why?" Johnny asked. "You've got this smell of chicken shit clinging to you."

The comment wiped away their phony smiles. Paris did her best to hide her own, biting her lip to suppress it.

"We won't cause any problems. We're just keeping to ourselves," Paris insisted.

They were approaching a head-on collision and running out of streets to turn off. A few more wrong words, and it would be inevitable.

"Well you aren't keeping to yourselves. See, we like to keep things the way they've been," the self-appointed mayor said.

"If it ain't broke, don't fix it," one of his friends chimed in.

Johnny's fingers instinctively twitched and bent into a fist.

"And what if I break something? You going to fix it?" Johnny asked.

The self-appointed mayor's three friends took a step forward, so that they were shoulder to shoulder with their leader.

"I'm sorry if I caused trouble," Paris said.

Johnny looked at her in disbelief, almost betrayed by her unwarranted apology.

"Just stay out of places you don't belong," the man said.

"Where she doesn't belong..." Johnny repeated, anger rushing through his veins.

"Yeah. If you wouldn't bring a dog in, don't bring a nigger in," the youngest and smallest of the three said.

He was all of five feet three inches, and in this heat, had shriveled down to a hundred thirty-five pounds. He wouldn't have been intimidating at a playground. His friendship with the other three had granted him the ability to run his mouth unpunished.

Until now.

Paris grabbed Johnny's arm by the elbow like it was the reins of a wild stallion, preventing him from charging forward.

"Giovanni, let it go. Please," she pleaded.

Johnny took off his fedora and held it in his hands, squeezing it in a futile effort to stifle his rage.

The four men laughed together, beaming with pride at having defended segregation. The alcohol on their breath was unmistakable. It was the real stuff too. Not something made in a bathtub with paint thinner, like the poor were forced to drink. No, these men had drunk straight from their daddy's liquor cabinet. Liquor stockpiled before the Volstead Act went into effect.

"Are we clear or do you need me to continue?" the self-appointed mayor taunted.

"Giovanni, let's go. I'm asking you," Paris said.

Johnny's breathing escalated but not like with his attacks. These were deep, powering breaths. He became more aware of how much the thick muggy air annoyed him, of how irritating the mosquitos buzzing around his ears were. Color and heat flooded his face.

200

With the attacks, he was powerless with absolutely no control over any aspect of his body. But in moments like these, his body was an armed force, each muscle, each nerve a soldier. Soldiers unafraid of any foe.

"Why don't you return to wherever you came from?" one of the two who had remained silent said, in a final sort of way.

"Hit the road," the self-appointed mayor commanded.

"Nah, I'll leave when I'm ready, Mr. Mayor," Johnny said.

"Enough, Giovanni. Please, let's go," Paris said.

She tugged on his arm, trying to drag him free from where he stood. But his legs were oak trees, his feet the roots holding him in place. Paris would have had as much luck moving a mountain.

"Listen to your bitch," the self-appointed mayor said.

"You need to leave," Paris warned the self-appointed mayor.

It was a warning. Johnny was immovable. Her only hope of avoiding bloodshed was to warn the four men about the danger they were in. She had seen glimpses of Johnny's rage at The Moonlight, but the real moonlight seemed to have transformed him from man to beast.

"Shut up, nigger," the self-appointed mayor said.

It was the last straw. Their last chance. Had they walked away, refrained from hurling that awful slur, he would have let them be. Not because he wanted to, but because Paris wanted him to.

"Hold my fedora," Johnny said, handing it over to Paris and breaking free from her grip.

The friends smirked. They were bullies who filled their Friday and Saturday nights with drinking and looking for weak defenseless prey to beat on. But they had been raised on lies. They weren't wolves. They were sheep dressed in expensive furs trying to mimic a wolf. And on that night, they had not come across a fellow sheep. These fools had stumbled upon a battle-tested, scarred, maimed wolf who didn't care whose territory it had infringed upon. A wolf who was willing to bleed because it loved the fight.

Their faces warranted every bruise, every cut they would receive. Johnny wasn't smiling, but a sense of elation rose in him. Rage was his lair. It was where he was comfortable. Brooklyn had made him tough. France had shown him the true horrors of war. He had charged out of trenches to face an onslaught of machine gun fire. He had placed his life in the hands of God, and whether it was fate, destiny or a higher purpose, he had overcome. For some unbeknownst reason, Johnny had survived it. The amount of fear he had experienced in that trench, waiting for the whistle to blow… he would never feel fear like that again. It wasn't possible, and these rich racists couldn't instill even a single drop of it.

The self-appointed mayor opened his mouth to speak, but only managed to get a word in before Johnny cut him off.

"We're done with words," Johnny said.

Johnny had gotten into fights since he was twelve years old. He had spent the first two years getting his ass kicked like it was tradition. The boys he fought were always three or four years older and had already reached manhood. Johnny was a scrapper and a rail-thin, little shit. But that had only taught him how to take a beating. And now, at six feet and two hundred pounds, his stick knuckles had transformed into bricks. He knew what getting punched in the face felt like. He knew what being stabbed felt like. And he knew what being shot felt like. But the most important thing about fighting was being able to take a punch. Nothing was more terrifying than getting hit in the face for the first time. Every inexperienced fighter goes for the haymakers, the blowing uppercuts or swinging hooks. But a hard punch to the gut brought every man to his knees.

"Too stupid for math? You're outnumbered," the self-appointed mayor said, but he had obviously been shaken by Johnny's threat.

Johnny shrugged. "Faced worse odds before."

The man considered what Johnny had said, and his face contorted as he tried to decipher what it meant.

Johnny didn't care to differentiate amongst the four. In a few minutes, they would all look the same—bloodied and bruised.

"I want you to think back to the last time you looked in a mirror," Johnny said. "Maybe it was after you had showered, maybe it was the rear view mirror in your car or when you washed your hands after using the rest room at the movie palace. Whenever it was... wherever it was. I want you to remember the reflection cast back at you. Because after tonight, it'll never look the same."

The color faded from their faces, but they had talked too much to back out now.

The self-appointed mayor swung for a knockout blow. Johnny ducked and drove his fist into the man's stomach. He fell to the ground, gasping for breath, the look of horror on his face clearly indicating that he had not expected such a thunderous blow. But Johnny's fists were stones launched from catapults, mercilessly striking faces and ribs. He took his fair share of hits, and the punch that connected to his injured side only enraged him further. He shoved the runt of the litter head first into the stop sign pole. The burly, cinnamon-haired man was taken out next and then the third. With the other three men out of commission, he turned his attention back to the self-appointed mayor who had continually run that stupid mouth of his. In a few, paltry moments, Johnny would ensure that no words would ever leave his lips again. He was still on the ground, clutching his side. Johnny had broken his ribs. It was most likely the first time he had been punched. His daddy's money had, up to then, saved him from such anguish. He was curled up in the fetal position—a truly pathetic, embarrassing sight.

"Stop... please!" the man pleaded, his voice cracking.

Johnny grabbed a handful of the self-appointed mayor's shirt and drove his fist into the man's face. Over and over and over. Two of his pearly white teeth clattered and rolled across the sidewalk like marbles. The whole thing sounded like someone punching a steak, and after a dozen blows, that's what the man's face looked like. He had been a good-looking guy before and with his inheritance would have acquired a good bride. But now, not even his daddy's money could buy him a wife.

Think of the last time you looked in the mirror.

The rage didn't lessen at the sight of the man's battered face. His empty threats and lack of fight only infuriated Johnny further. He pulled out his M1911 and stepped over the bloody, beaten man. If getting hit in the face for the first time was scary, staring into the barrel of a loaded gun was sheer terror. The pool of urine streaming down the man's gray pants showed he was experiencing a level of fear he had found unfathomable.

Too many times Johnny had stood over a soon-to-be dead man. Too many times he had wanted to pull that trigger. What face would be added to the maze? The handsome, devious dimpled chin and smooth jaw line? Or the bloodied, beaten pile of flesh that cowered on the sidewalk?

"Giovanni, stop!" Paris yelled.

She had been pleading the whole time, but only now did her words reach him. In his animalistic rage, words were just sounds. She tugged on his arm in a desperate attempt to pull him away. Johnny's hand pulsated from the trauma, his knuckles bruised, bloodied, and swollen. He broke free from Paris, stepped over the man, and aimed his gun at the self-appointed mayor's head. Paris only stood by in horror. She knew there was nothing she could do. The man in front of her had completely disconnected from humanity itself. Johnny was nothing but a predator now. A shark. A lion. A wolf. He was doing nothing but taking out the sick and the weak in a herd of sheep. Above all, he was a survivor. That's all war was about—those who didn't make it and those who did. He had expected another attack, like what had happened when he stood over Kowalski. But too much hate flowed through him. Kowalski had shot him, a forgivable act. These men had ridiculed Paris, and there was no forgiveness, no atonement for their sins.

Nigger. Nigger. Nigger.

That horrible word replayed over and over in his mind, each time causing his finger to twitch further on the trigger. Anymore and the bullet would fire. But Paris' horrified expression was impossible to ignore. He turned to look at her. The fear, the sadness, the shock in her eyes made him pause. Were his eyes even blue anymore? Or were they black like a shark's? Like a demon's? Forget his eyes. Did she even recognize the monster in front of her? Was he even a man anymore? Had all remnants of humanity left him?

His hand twitched. A shot rang out, echoing across the vacant streets. The man cried out, sobbing uncontrollably. Johnny had shot the pavement inches from his head, sending bits of concrete shrapnel burning and ripping into his face and more urine trickling down his leg. The bruises and swelling would go away. His nose would heal crooked, his cheekbones lopsided, and the shrapnel would leave horrifying scars. It was the best Johnny could do. The best condition he could let the man walk away in.

"We'll be staying as long as we'd like, and if I see you or your friends again, I will kill you," Johnny said.

He turned to Paris and held his hand out for his fedora. She handed it over with a trembling hand, her face twisted with a hundred emotions.

"No one's ever going to talk to you that way when I'm around. I promise you that," Johnny said.

He offered her his hand with a courage that had been absent at the movie palace. She stared at it, horrified at what'd he done but drawn to him all the same. She took his offered hand, and they left the four soft men bleeding on the hard pavement.

They walked in silence, Paris stealing glances at Johnny every ten feet or so. But by now, she knew the silence would have to be broken by her.

"No one has ever stood up for me like that. Nobody. I don't agree with how you did it... but thank you," Paris said.

Nothing was more attractive than loyalty.

Johnny remained silent. Paris knew what he was involved in, but now, she had seen it for herself. Seen that with booze came bullets and blood. Seen the person he was. If you could even call him that. Words like "murderer," "evil," and "monster" better described what he was.

Unlike in the myths, when Johnny transformed back from beast, he was well-aware of what he had done, well-aware of the sins and transgressions he had committed.

Paris examined his left hand. His mountain-hard knuckles were turning shades of blue and purple.

"Doesn't it hurt?" Paris asked.

"Not as much as his face will," Johnny said.

The adrenaline and shock would wear off, replaced with throbbing pain. It wasn't the first day after that was most painful, it was the second.

"*Faced worse odds...* You were talking about the War," she said.

Johnny nodded. Her touch was a soothing balm, and her cold hands helped dull the pain.

She released his hand and shook her head. "You're a strange man, Giovanni De Luca."

"Why?" he asked.

"I'm not quite sure what you want from me. At times, I think you're attracted to me, and other times, I think I make you nauseous."

"You don't make me nauseous."

But silence descended again after those brief words.

"Oh, good. I was hoping that would be the end of the conversation."

Johnny struggled to speak, losing the words before they could leave his mouth.

"I have a constant worry of not being wanted or good enough," Paris said. "And it helps me if you just come out and say that you don't find me attractive. It's better than wondering and tormenting myself over it."

She continued rambling until Johnny broke his own unintended vow of silence. "You're gorgeous."

"So you are attracted to me?" Paris asked.

Johnny knew he needed to speak and fast. He was a man who could go a whole day with saying less than fifty words. But if he didn't speak now, it would hurt Paris, and hurting her was the last thing he wanted to do, and that conviction overpowered his shyness and his tumultuous thoughts long enough for him to speak.

"For a long time, when I walked into the lobby of The Moonlight, I kept my eyes to the floor. I didn't want to see anyone, and I didn't want anyone to see me."

"And now?"

"Now, I look for you. And it doesn't matter how many people are packed into The Moonlight, my eyes find you. Within seconds, I find you. Every time. My eyes are drawn to you, gravitate to you. I watch you, the way you smile, your expressions, your mannerisms, the way you're there but not really there. I think that only makes sense to those of us who don't belong. I see the way you stare off—you're looking past The Moonlight and the people inside it, past Chicago. Your gaze travels miles. But then there's this moment when wherever it was that you were looking to vanishes. And the realization of what your life is shows on your face. This sadness. This emptiness. I've never seen someone convey so many small emotions the way you do. When I look at you, my body... it fails. When you smile, one second I'm stronger than I've ever been and then the next, you completely level me... When I see you, there's nothing I want more than you but..."

The word *but* was the most dreaded, worry-inducing, terrifying word in the English language.

"But what?" Paris asked.

"You scare me."

"I scare you? Why?"

Her tone was unmistakably incredulous. He had just fought four men without a trace of fear in his eyes or a tremble in his hands. Yet she scared him?

"Because you see through it all. See through everyone's bullshit. Whether it's because you're... more real somehow or you've been around it for so long... maybe both... but you see through it. And I don't want you to see me for who I really am."

"See you for who you really are? The terrible things you've done? You beat four men to a pulp right in front of me. I didn't run away."

"That's the least of the sins I've committed."

"Things you've done, things that have happened to you… it all made you the person you are. The good and the bad. Trust me, I know."

"Paris, there are things in my past that won't let go."

"The past is always going to tap us on the shoulder. It's up to us if we turn around."

"And what if it turns *you* around?"

"It only has power if we let it."

"I wish that was true."

The restaurants and shops were far behind them. It was now the lakeshore and the mighty trees that rose along the sandy shoreline.

"Those men back there," Johnny said, "I wanted to hurt them. What they said to you… But that's my choice. If you weren't beside me, I would of killed him. I like to think I wouldn't of… but I know. I've killed men. Men on the wrong side of a trench, men who stood in the way of profits, men who posed a threat. Some by choice, some by command."

Paris stared into his eyes. Hers were usually intimidating, but now, they were filled with compassion. They instilled a feeling that no matter what he said, his words were safe with her.

"If I had been shot three weeks ago, I would have allowed myself to bleed out in that alley way," Johnny said.

"What changed?" Paris asked.

"When I was over there, so many times I thought I would die. I tried to fill my head with something that would make dying easier. You know? Maybe a prayer or a poem. But every time I charged out of that trench, I didn't have anything that would bring me peace. Anything that would make dying easier. The other night, I was just wandering around when I got shot… Bleeding out, I looked up… I was on your street. Something inside brought me there. I thought I had wandered there, but maybe it was something more. I just know your face came to me, and I wanted one last look at you. I didn't care if I had to crawl up every last step. I just knew when I saw you, dying would be easier."

He turned to walk away, embarrassed, almost humiliated at what he had revealed. Paris grabbed his hand, stopping him. She stared into his cobalt blue eyes, and for the first time, Johnny didn't hide them. Her face moved closer to his. From across a room, Johnny's eyes would find Paris. But inches away, the attraction was atomic. Too close to resist. Johnny ran his fingers through her hair, squeezing the ends, cupping her face with his other hand. Their lips hovered close, each succumbing to the gravity of the other.

The tall reeds along the beach swayed in the breeze, against the soothing melody of the waves washing upon the shores. The waxing crescent moon and luminous stars were painted on the black lake.

With a sense of urgency, they fell to the sand, removing each other's clothes and leaving them scattered along the shoreline. One moment she was atop him, and the next he was atop her. His hands traveled her body, memorizing its curves. She wouldn't let him break his gaze from her eyes. Even when it was over, she held onto that gaze.

After a few minutes of uninterrupted silence and gazing at the star-speckled sky, Paris sat up. "Come on."

She grabbed his hand and dragged him into the water. The temperature was unsurprisingly and unwelcomingly warm, but the massive lake, carved by glaciers thousands of years ago, never warmed. Paris gasped from the shock of the cold water on her warm skin. Johnny smirked, because in this heat, the water felt like a lukewarm bath. They swam and danced and kissed in the water until Paris was too cold. Johnny would have been content staying until October.

He lifted Paris into his arms and carried her to the grass, the sand clinging to his feet like parasites.

"Are you carrying me so I don't get sand stuck to my feet?" Paris asked.

"And you said I wasn't the chivalrous type," Johnny said.

He set her down on the grass, and they hurried to dress, Paris out of the need to stop shivering and for the sake of decency, Johnny only the latter.

When they reached a curb, Johnny sat and swatted the sand off his feet. His socks, damp from a day of sweating, had to be tugged onto his feet. Paris elected to walk barefoot, carrying her shoes in her hands. Johnny wore only his A-shirt.

"Walking barefoot a Wisconsin thing too?" he asked.

"I love the feeling of the earth on my feet. It makes me feel like I'm a part of it," she replied.

She stared at his shoes and then at Johnny. Not a subtle hint in the slightest.

"You want me to walk barefoot too," Johnny said.

She nodded dramatically.

"Fine. I will walk barefoot if it pleases you." His sigh told her how ridiculous he thought it was.

He tugged off his shoes and socks. The pavement was cool and massaged his feet with each step. He was more aware of every step he took. At times, a pebble would painfully dig into his foot, but mostly, he felt one with the earth beneath his feet.

"And?" Paris asked.

"You Wisconsin folk have figured out the secret to life," Johnny said.

There never was true silence in the rural areas of Wisconsin. Owls hooted, grasshoppers chirped, and the trees howled from the wind whistling between their leaf-covered branches. But each sound was peaceful, cocooned in a tranquility that lulled one into a state of ease. The Windy City and its ceaseless noises instilled a need to rush through and past. But here, nature pleaded with Johnny to slow down.

But the sounds of nature were overcome with music as they got closer to the cabin. It was jazz, there was no mistaking the trumpet and saxophone. Johnny opened the door, its usual creak swallowed up by the blaring music coming from a record player, the price tag still hanging on it.

Hotsy was on the couch, underneath the waitress from the German restaurant. The music was too loud for either to hear Johnny and Paris enter. Johnny lifted the needle from the record player. The music cut out with a scratch, leaving only the waitress' giggles to fill the room. When she looked around to see why the music had cut off, she gasped in horror and crossed her arms to cover her breasts.

"What's wrong, baby?" Hotsy asked.

"Your friends are back," she said.

"Johnny, is that you?" Hotsy asked, twisting from beneath her body to look at him.

"Well, if it wasn't, you'd be dead already," Johnny said.

Hotsy simply changed positions with the woman. He was hardly bashful and didn't care if Johnny and Paris had a clear view of his backside.

"Tomato here?" Johnny asked.

"In the bedroom. Best knock," Hotsy said, his lips smashed against the woman's.

She had introduced herself at the restaurant, as all waiters and waitresses do, but there was a two percent chance Hotsy remembered her name was Lisa.

Paris and Johnny went into the kitchen, and Johnny grabbed two colas from the ice box. He put the needle back on the record player, for he had no intention of hearing the moaning coming from the couch or the other bedroom. They hurried into the vacant bedroom, and Johnny shut the door—not only for privacy, but also because Hotsy had that damn fire going again. Johnny tossed his fedora on the dresser. In bed, Johnny and Paris drank their colas and shared an end-of-the-night joint to unwind.

"I'd ask how your wound is, but I'd have to be more specific wouldn't I?" Paris asked.

"We all have our wounds," Johnny said.

"True words. Some that can't be seen… Like the attack at the fish boil."

Of course she had noticed. The whole damn restaurant had probably spent the night talking about the nut who had lost it at dinner.

"Something brings them on, and when they come… I can't stop them. Sometimes, I think I'm going to drown. I know that sounds stupid," Johnny said.

"No, it doesn't. It's sounds, smells, sights that cause them, isn't it?" Paris asked, softly running her fingernails along his arm.

Johnny nodded. "Yeah…"

"And they take you back there."

Johnny nodded again, fear swelling in his throat.

Call the devil, and he shall answer.

"I try to tell myself it isn't possible," Johnny said. "That I can't alternate from some small town in Wisconsin to that field in France in seconds. But sometimes it's so real, the taste of the thick haze of smoke on my tongue, the feeling of the mud under my boots, the stench of decay… that sometimes I wonder if I am actually in France, dreaming about making out of that trench. And if the life I'm living now is just a mirage. If I'll snap out of this day dream and find myself back in that trench, waking from a long nap."

"Have you told anyone else about the attacks?"

"Hotsy and Tomato know. It's impossible not to. Tomato understands more, I think."

"He served too?"

"Yeah."

Paris nodded, sensing, with her usual intuition, that Johnny had spoken about it as much as he wanted to.

She caressed his swollen, bruised knuckles. "Is Tomato handcuffed?"

"Yeah."

"Does his wife know about…" she nodded to the other bedroom.

"Yeah…"

"A surprising number of them do. A lot of men mention it before. Like they have a permission slip. Some are trying to eliminate the possibility of being blackmailed by being upfront about the fact that their wife knows."

Many women had schemes to find their way out of the pit they lived in by threatening to ruin the life of a rich, successful married man. Legends and myths of success stories spread and persuaded more women to try it, but the truth was that such ventures were seldom successful. And if they tried it with the wrong man, the woman disappeared. Forever.

"He loves her," Johnny said. "He'd die for her, but there's something he needs that she can't give him."

Paris sat up further, clearly taking offense at the comment. "Any woman can do what 'Miss Next Door' is doing. I hear that excuse all the time. Don't pass your unfaithfulness as some character flaw your wife has."

"Those are my words not his."

"You feel that way?"

"I don't know. I've never committed to anyone."

"Then you don't commit. Again, if she knows and accepts, I am no one to judge. But if he couldn't commit, he shouldn't have gotten married."

"Their marriage was arranged. He was only seventeen. She resented him for a while for it."

He smiled fondly, recalling the stories Tomato had told him.

"And now?"

"There's love there. Pain too. Don't be too hard on him. Tomato... there's just something missing that Lorraine can't fill. And that's not on her."

"A person can provide companionship, Giovanni. They can't fill something that isn't there. Family and friends can only do so much."

"What about yours?"

"My what?"

"Your family."

"You need to do what's best for you, and only you know what that is."

A deflection. But Johnny wouldn't let it bounce off.

"Is that why you're not close to yours?"

"I'm doing what's best for me."

But her voice was far less certain than her words.

"I don't believe you're only looking out for you. I know you said you make a good wage and all, but something drove you to do what you do."

"Prostitution. You can say the word. I won't burst into flame."

"Prostitution."

If she had expected him to drop it out of embarrassment, she was sadly mistaken. Paris knew Johnny had his secrets, and he knew she had hers.

"Well," Paris said, "maybe sex, like booze, makes people feel good, and like booze, it's been scrutinized, demonized, and stamped with legislation."

"Yeah... maybe. But I think that's bullshit."

Paris stared at Johnny. He stared back—he wouldn't force the conversation, but he wouldn't turn away from it either.

She studied his face. Was she aware when her eyes showed glimpses of weakness? They were filled with a vulnerability that only made her stronger.

"Maybe I'm missing too."

"It's suffering"

Sunlight streamed into the room through the cracks of the curtain, bathing it in morning light. The brightness broke their slumber.

Realizing that shielding her eyes would be futile, Paris rose from the bed with an exaggerated yawn and stretch. Johnny followed her out of the room, rubbing his eyes that felt like they had been glued shut. Paris went into the bathroom. Johnny sat at the kitchen island, contemplating taking a nap.

The second bedroom door opened, and Tomato stumbled out, looking like he had joined the ranks of an undead army. He didn't even dare nod to Johnny. His head was at the receiving end of an artillery barrage, and his stomach was in the middle of an aerial dogfight. He plopped down on the seat beside Johnny and held his head in his hands with the care and caution with which one holds a baby.

Minutes later, the bathroom door opened, and Paris stepped out, hair brushed and face washed.

"Tough night?" Paris asked Tomato.

"I don't know what these Wisconsin folks put in their beer, but it's Old Testament wrath I'm feeling," Tomato said.

"What happened to the whiskey?" Johnny asked.

"While Hotsy and I went to the can, she took the liberty of pouring shots for the whole place. I didn't get a drop," Tomato said.

"Where is your friend now?" Paris asked.

"In the room," Tomato said, radiating shame. "Hey, Johnny, I'm going to go for a walk, can you… tell her goodbye?"

"Yeah, sure," Johnny said.

"I've got this pounding headache. I think a walk will do me some good. I think it's easier if I'm not here, you know…" Tomato rambled on, trying to defend himself.

"Don't worry about it, Tomato," Johnny assured him.

Judging by Paris' strong glare, she did not approve of Tomato's action, deeming it downright cowardice. The Moonlight had many perks and amenities the cabin couldn't provide. Food service, live music, and housekeeping were a few. But the perk Tomato missed the most was the quick escape it provided. Had they been at The Moonlight, Tomato would have crept out into the bustling city and disappeared, avoiding any awkwardness and embarrassment.

He forced himself to stand, fought the great urge to vomit on the spot, and left. The sunlight blinded him like it was the first time he had left a dark cave in a year. Paris smirked, knowing that the blinding sun was doing little for his throbbing headache.

At five to ten, Hotsy came back to the land of the living. It seemed a hangover had finally found him, but after a two-minute piss and three glasses of water, Hotsy was in prime spirits. His date, however, was still out cold, and the woman on Tomato's bed hadn't stirred either. Hotsy wanted to wake them and tell them they should get going, but Paris broke it to him that that would have been boorish, reminding him these weren't women who had been paid for services rendered. Johnny, Paris, and Hotsy played three-handed cribbage, and Hotsy declared if he won they would wake the two women and "send them on their way." Much to Paris' dismay, Hotsy won. Johnny's twenty point shellacking did little to help the sour taste in her mouth. She went so far as to accuse him of deliberately losing. But she should have been thankful Hotsy tapped both women awake rather than roll them onto the floor. The brunette on Tomato's bed hadn't even reached a hangover yet. She was still zozzled, and Paris had to help her dress. Hotsy had expected the women to walk and find their way back into town, but Johnny objected before Paris had to.

Johnny drove, Paris was in the passenger seat, and Hotsy, Lisa and her still-to-be-named brunette friend were in the backseat. Lisa kept glancing at Hotsy, hopeful that he would find her charms as irresistible as he had the night before. But Hotsy was a horse with blinders and kept his vision straight and true, his blood pumping an antidote to her poison. They dropped the two waitresses off at the German restaurant, and Johnny explained to Tomato's still-drunk date that Tomato was sorry he couldn't say goodbye. The awkwardness Paris had expected was only lessened by the fact the woman was too drunk to remember any of it. Hotsy assured his date he would see her later, but as soon as they were out of the car, he told Johnny and Paris they would have to find something other than German cuisine for supper. Tomato was in the cabin when they returned, doing little to change Paris' opinion of him. It looked as though he had hidden in a tree or in a bush and waited for them to leave.

The rest of the day was uneventful. Tomato napped for two hours, a time Hotsy and Johnny filled by running to the grocery store. Paris insisted on staying behind, not wanting to cause any more problems. Johnny argued that she had nothing to worry about, but Paris declined, electing to sweep the floor and wash the counter and dishes from the previous night. After Johnny and Hotsy returned, the three played more card games. Hotsy referred to Tomato's nap as a "stint in the recovery room." When Tomato woke, they ate a late lunch of ham and cheese sandwiches and played more cribbage. The record player filled the room with the newest and hippest jazz. It wasn't live entertainment like at The Moonlight, but the audio quality was exceptional, providing comforting background noise.

Later, Tomato and Hotsy went to pick up some whiskey from an associate who worked the area for Al Capone. Paris gave Tomato a slip of paper but was silent on what was written on it when Johnny asked. Johnny refrained from asking Tomato because it was an opportunity for him to get out of the dog house Paris had banished him to. But he got his answer when Tomato and Hotsy returned, and Hotsy dug into a brown paper bag and pulled out oranges, maraschino cherries, and a liter of Bubble Up lemon-lime soda. As for what Johnny considered the most important ingredient, Hotsy held the small bottle of Angostura bitters in his hand like a watch salesman.

"Think I wouldn't remember bitters?" Hotsy asked.

"How'd you manage that?" Johnny asked.

"Local joint has a license to sell it as stomach tonic for medicinal purposes," Tomato said.

For someone who didn't drink, Paris sure made a great Old Fashioned. And whether Tomato genuinely agreed or he was attempting to gain back more approval points, he said it was the best cocktail he'd ever had.

Tomato and Hotsy played a game of cribbage, sipping away at their Old Fashioneds while Paris and Johnny prepared spaghetti for supper. The sounds of the boiling noodles, simmering tomato sauce, and jazz were drowned out by Tomato and Hotsy's bickering and occasional compliments at the sauce's aroma from the thyme, oregano, basil, and garlic.

Most sane people like pasta, but Tomato adored it. He had three heaping platefuls and couldn't stop commending Johnny and Paris on its taste. Paris initially thought Tomato was only trying to gain her favor, but there was no faking that level of enjoyment.

After dinner, they drove to an ice cream place called Double Scoops. It was modest in size and even more modest in choices. They all ordered chocolate, except for Johnny who ordered scoops of both chocolate and vanilla, something Paris rolled her eyes at. They strolled the lakeshore, enjoying their cones and the majesty of the lake.

When they returned to the cabin, Hotsy readied the cribbage board, Tomato shuffled the cards, Johnny got the record player going, and Paris prepared another round of Old Fashioneds. They played two games, Hotsy and Tomato winning once and Johnny and Paris the other.

"You men want to play a different game?" Paris asked.

"Choose your next words carefully or Hotsy will have his pants off," Tomato warned.

"Come on," Paris said, grabbing the empty bottle of whiskey and leaving the kitchen island.

She sat on the floor next to the crackling fire. Johnny had kept the windows open in an attempt to diminish the fire's heat. It hadn't been started for the warmth it provided, but for the relaxation it brought. The last time he was this close to a fire he had nearly drowned in front of a live audience.

Please don't happen again.

"If you say we got to kiss who the bottle ends up on, I got to say, I don't like the odds," Hotsy said.

"Person spinning asks a question. Person it lands on has to answer," Paris said.

"And if a person doesn't want to answer?" Hotsy asked.

"Then they have to drink," Paris replied.

"You don't drink," Johnny said.

"Guess I'll be answering then," Paris said.

"Anything off limits?" Hotsy asked.

He asked more questions for a game of spin the bottle than he had ever asked when it came to hits, heists, and rackets.

"Probably anything you're thinking," Johnny said.

"I'll start," Paris said. She spun the bottle, and it landed on Hotsy. "Hotsy, have you ever loved a woman?"

"You saw last night. I made her squeal with zeal," Hotsy said.

"No, have you ever been in love?" Tomato clarified, no hint of his usual impatience.

219

Hotsy thought on it, too naïve to know his contemplation was an answer in itself. "I don't think so."

Tomato was silent. He wouldn't ridicule him for that.

"Your turn," Paris told Hotsy.

Hotsy spun the bottle. It landed on Tomato.

"Let the record show, Tomasso Capuano is under oath," Hotsy said.

"Shut up," Tomato said, even though he laughed as much as Paris and Johnny.

"What is your favorite thing about me?" Hotsy asked.

"I'll drink instead," Tomato said.

"Oh, come on, be nice. There has to be something," Paris said.

"Like I said, I'll drink," Tomato said.

"Fine, but you don't get to spin," Hotsy said. He spun the bottle again, and it halted on Paris. "Paris, what is *your* favorite thing about me?"

Paris laughed. "Your friends."

"Ouch, sending some heat my way."

"That's the fire, nimrod," Tomato said.

"Hotsy, I think you're a loyal person to your friends. Women… that's a different story," Paris said.

She spun the bottle, and once again, it landed on Tomato. He groaned.

"What are your children like?" Paris asked.

It was not the question Tomato had expected.

"I have two daughters," he answered, "Mary Louise and Gretchen Marie. They both look like their mother. Something I considered a blessing, but the older they get the more grief it causes me thinking about all the boys who will chase them in ten years. They're a permanent sunny day. Every time I look at them, I miss them before I even look away… and my wife… she is the center of my world. Without her, I'd be speeding through space. I don't always stay on orbit, but her gravity keeps me straight—here and here." He tapped his heart and temple.

Johnny stared at Paris. She could feel his gaze. Tomato hadn't been asked about his wife but had brought her up anyway. Johnny knew how Tomato looked to an outsider like Paris. But Tomato was so much more than his shortcomings. And infidelity was not a sin he alone carried. The Moonlight vouched for that. Only someone who had seen Tomato at home could understand the unwavering dedication and love he had for his family. In a world filled with passing glances, sometimes you needed to stare to truly see.

The guilt flooded Tomato's stomach again, a guilt he tried to numb with a sip of his Old Fashioned. He took a deep breath to steady his emotions, grabbed the bottle, and spun it. It narrowly missed Johnny, stopping on Paris.

"Luck is on your side tonight, Giovanni," Paris remarked.

"Paris, why'd you come with us?" Tomato asked.

Paris trained her powerful, intimidating stare at Johnny. "I feel like I can read people easily. But not him. He's guarded, but I hope if I keep trying, he'll let me in."

She "spun" the bottle one turn to her right. It "landed" on Johnny. In the Old West, such an act would have gotten her shot.

"That was unexpected," she said, arching her eyebrows with dramatic effect. "What was your favorite part about Europe?"

"Besides the boat ride home?" Johnny asked, both a joke and the truth.

"And besides the forest," Paris added.

Johnny thought on it. It was like trying to find a diamond buried deep in a field of shit. The others were quiet; only the fire crackled in the background. He wasn't sure that what she was asking about even existed. It felt like minutes before he found his words.

"I was on leave for four days. I was on this bus taking soldiers to Paris. I wasn't in the mood to be with people, so when most of them went to this night club called *Les Sauvages*, I continued on, aimlessly walking those cobble-stone streets. But then this smell hit me. Freshly baked bread. I followed it like a bloodhound. It brought me to this café called *The Givre Strudel*. A woman was inside baking, but the place didn't open for an hour or so. But she opened the door and allowed me in. I ordered a strudel. She poured me coffee and let me be. It was the best pastry I ever had. I ordered a loaf of French bread, bought a bottle of Moscato from a nearby restaurant, and wandered the city. When I reached the Eiffel Tower, I sat on this bench, drinking and eating. I stayed there all night, gazing at that golden giant."

The others were silent, taking in what Johnny had said. Johnny was slow to spin the bottle. He had been struck by nostalgia. The War had given him a thousand memories that tormented him. Memories that completely dwarfed, demolished, disintegrated, and destroyed one of the few good ones from the War. It had stomped the memory into the mud, burying it beneath the soil. The memory was a gift, something he had never expected to unwrap. A memory he had forgotten years ago. He choked on the emotion in his throat. He rubbed his eyes, trying to pass it off as a scratch. Gazing upon that French landmark, he had never expected to survive another night. Contemplating death is natural. Everybody will die. But Johnny had known (or at least assumed with certainty) the time and place of his death, and knowing your death was hours away was a dark, steep decline into a pit of blackness. A pit most never get out of.

Breathe. Breathe. Breathe.

He exhaled deeply and spun the bottle. Tomato let out another disgruntled groan.

"Your worst time in Europe?" Johnny asked.

Tomato met Johnny's gaze. Apart from casually agreeing that "War is Hell," they had never gone into the specifics of their experiences over there. If you knew a man had served, as a fellow veteran you knew the horrors they had been subjected to, but there was a part that demanded you know for sure. That you knew the hell you experienced had burdened another soul.

"Hiding in a crater hole," Tomato said. "Hearing that hissing noise—like a thousand invisible snakes—coming my way. Seeing that thick, slow-moving yellow fog creeping toward me. And then the feeling of a pillow stuffed over my face. My eyes burning and then... everything going black."

His breath shortened as if that yellow fog was creeping at him once more.

"What was it?" Hotsy asked.

"Mustard gas. I was blind for two weeks. Long enough that I thought I had lost my sight for good," Tomato said.

Sweat ran down his hands and neck. His memory hadn't been a welcome, unexpected gift but a visceral nightmare.

"How terrifying," Paris said, her voice grave.

"You know, call it a blind man's senses, but everything else was heightened. I could smell the death. I upchucked more into that bucket than any speakeasy toilet sees on a Friday night. But it was my hearing that seemed amplified, more honed. I swear I could hear those poor bastards on the field at night. I don't mean to be sacrilegious, and may the Almighty not judge me, but I felt like God hearing the prayers of the damned. Hearing them plead and beg for salvation. And then, begging for it all to end. Pleading with someone to end their suffering. Men younger than Hotsy begging for death, forfeiting life because the pain was so extreme. And one by one, God granted them reprieve, and the voices fell silent."

Tomato stared into the fire with the same stare as Clarence had. A stare signifying he was in a tangible nightmare.

"Thank you for sharing that with us," Paris said.

Her words seemed to have somehow freed him. He spun the bottle once more, and it came to a rest on Johnny.

"What memory stands out the most?" Tomato asked Johnny.

Discussing the pain and hurt was not something a man did. It was weakness by all definitions. "Have a stiff drink to take the edge off" had been a doctor's recommendation. But thanks to Prohibition, that channel of alleviation was outlawed. Memories were to remain suppressed even if they were cancerous in the damage they inflicted, slowly killing from the inside.

Johnny's eyes found Paris'. There was compassion and support in her eyes, but also an indomitable strength, and she transferred that strength to Johnny. A wind beneath his wings.

"Two of them," Johnny answered.

He struggled over where to begin. Converting fluent thoughts into a foreign speech was an impossible task. Were there words for the images and scenes in his head? It is said a picture is worth a thousand words. Chaos. Mayhem. Carnage. Horror. Atrocity. Genocide. Bloodshed. He could list a thousand words. If the War was a painting, it had been painted in blood on a canvas of corpses.

"…There are duties over there that when you get assigned them, you know your luck is up. That that's it… your time is up. Going out into No Man's Land to set up the barbed wire was one of those. You never truly sleep there, but I tried to get some rest. I'm tapped on the shoulder—and even though you're not in a deep sleep, it still scares the bejesus out of you. I'm told it's my turn to set up the barbed wire. I cover my face in mud, so that when the artillery or explosions light up the sky, my face is concealed. I crawl out there into the cold mud, fingers sinking into the ground, grabbing handfuls of the dead. I lay out the barbed wire, and this ball of light explodes in the sky like fireworks. It's like I am a kid again, watching fireworks on the Fourth of July. I find myself watching the trail of light fluttering toward the ground. It lights up the German trench no more than twenty yards away. A German has his rifle aimed right at me. I look at him with this 'You got me' look on my face. It didn't even pay to flee, not with the barbed wire set up and the mud like quicksand. He just stares at me…it feels like minutes. But then he lowers his rifle and nods. I nod back… And he lets me go."

"Why?" Hotsy asked.

"Because both sides knew that job was suicide," Tomato answered.

It was a gesture the Germans hoped the Americans would remember when it was them crawling through the mud following suicidal orders.

"And the other memory?" Paris asked softly.

"Maybe another time," Johnny said.

"Let it out, Johnny," Tomato said with an encouraging nod.

The memory and the emotions it triggered overpowered him. He gasped and his hands trembled.

Here we go.

What they were asking was for him to release a memory he had tried to contain near the center of the maze. A memory caged in fragile bars away from the moonlight to prevent its transformation. But the maze was always lit by a full moon. All the memory had to do was extend its clawed hand through the cage to feel the caress of the celestial light. And when it did, the moonlight transformed the memory from the distant past into the tangible here and now. Where it was no longer a memory, but an experience all over again. And it consumed him.

The attack crept around the corners, waiting for that final sign of weakness before it struck. If he voiced the memory out loud, he would be dropping his sword and shield, leaving himself utterly defenseless.

"I don't know what month it was, but it rained and rained and rained. When I thought it couldn't possibly rain anymore, it did. I thought the Navy would have to send Noah and his Ark to pick us up. Thought that that trench was going to turn into a river. A flooded trench is horrible because if you don't keep your feet dry and clean, you get trench foot, and if it gets bad enough, they take your foot.

"We lined the trench with dead soldiers... German... American... to stand and sit on to keep ourselves out of the water. You try to find someone who was a bit heavy, more cushion. But at that point, everyone had lost weight. You also try to find someone who had just died, before the body starts decomposing. I don't know when or what day, but, finally, the sun comes out and dries the trench. It shined for days straight. We started burying the dead. They weren't needed anymore, and the sun had ripened the smell of decay. One man in my unit buried a German with his arm sticking out of the ground, his fingers curled into his palm and his thumb straight up. It became a joke in the trench to ask the German questions. Things like 'Is the weather going to improve?' 'Will the war be over soon?' 'Will Melissa Jackson marry me when I get back home?' The joke was that every time you'd ask a question, you'd get a thumbs up. We all got a kick out of that.

225

"Until one soldier, uncoordinated guy, tripped over the arm and ate a face-full of mud. We all made the joke of how fearsome the German soldier was. That even in death, they keep fighting. The guy was a bit embarrassed. He dashed off and came back with an axe and chopped off the arm. There wasn't one of us who didn't laugh. God, we screeched like hyenas. He took the arm and flung it over the trench. Someone shouted, 'How's the view?' and you just saw this upturned thumbs up sailing through the air. We laughed for ten minutes, and when it stopped, someone would think about it and start laughing again. Like kids in church. That night, it starts raining again, worse than before. Every man we'd buried rises through the mud to the surface, bobbing up and down in the water. The German with the hacked-off arm rises too. The whites of his eyes are so vivid, ghost-white… they stare right at me. His skin is pale white with blue and purple hues, his body bloated. I can't take my eyes off him. Even in death, he is pleading with me.

"I puked. Not from the sight or the smell, I had gotten used to that months back. No, I vomited because I couldn't believe how cavalier I had been about a human life. Such disregard. No empathy. No remorse. A god damn joke. I wanted to kill every last one of them… How did I get to that point? How did I become as cold as the reaper himself that I could laugh at a man's death?"

"It was war, Johnny. They did the same to us," Tomato said.

Johnny nodded, but Tomato's words were far from comforting. And judging by Tomato's face, they were words he didn't believe either.

The German soldier, one-armed, rotted, bloated, and wreaking of putrid decay, wandered the maze like it was a hallowed cemetery. Johnny tried to bury him in the mud, but he would always resurface.

Johnny brought his gaze to the fire, fully aware of Paris' stare. But he was too embarrassed, too ashamed, too regretful to meet her gaze. Had voicing the memory released the one-armed German from his cage forever? Would Johnny never be able to suppress it again? He had tried his best to trick his mind into believing that the memory was just a nightmare. It seldom worked, but saying it out loud had given it a power over him it hadn't had before. A small, weak

226

whisper instilled a hope that maybe the German could leave the maze forever now that he had been freed. But that whisper came from a naïve voice.

"Was getting shot the worst part of the war?" Hotsy asked.

The bottle hadn't been spun, and it wasn't Hotsy's turn to ask. But all eyes were on Johnny.

"No, being shot is a relief. I mean you keep thinking, 'Am I going to get hit next?' The man next to you, in front of you, behind you... you see all these men going down... when it happens, it's kind of a relief. The anticipation is worse, you know? No, my worst time was in that trench. Hearing, 'Twenty seconds!' shouted out. Your stomach drops. You take your place in line. And in that moment, you find God. There are no atheists in a trench, you may leave him after, but in there, you pray to God, to Jesus, you pray to anything and everything. You hear those explosions above and in front of you. And then the whistle blows. And it's... almost indescribable. The carnage... the chaos..."

The fire's heat sucked the air out of his lungs. His mouth fell open, his eyes widened.

Not in front of everyone. Come back when I'm alone in the bathroom. Breathe through it. Just breathe.

"To this day, if I hear a whistle I swear I'm going to piss my pants. I never thought a whistle could cause so much fear, anxiety, and... just sheer terror," Tomato said.

The faces of fallen friends, brothers-in-arms came back to Johnny in meticulous detail. Overwhelming him. Crowding him. Suffocating him.

"My favorite and worst memory of Europe was..." Hotsy said.

And then it passed.

Hotsy had broken the tension, allowing Johnny and Tomato a reprieve from reliving the horrors of war. But it was the end of the game. It had brought Johnny and Tomato to a dark place. Both stayed by the fire, staring at its mesmerizing light. A half hour later, Tomato went into his bedroom. Hotsy was fast asleep on the couch, his soft snores absorbed by the wooden walls. Paris wanted to stay a bit longer by the fire. Johnny sat beside her. The heat from the fire completely overpowered the breeze from the open window, but Paris still covered Hotsy in the plaid blanket draped over the back of the couch.

Both sat in silence, watching the flames leap in the darkness.

"You have love for fire in your eyes," Johnny said.

"It's beautiful. It dances to its own music," Paris said.

Johnny hated its heat but couldn't refute its beauty.

"Tomato left the light on. Last night too. Because of the mustard attack?" Paris asked.

Johnny nodded. "He never shuts off the light. Not since his sight came back."

Tomato was an intimidating man. Smiles looked unnatural on his face. There was little Tomasso Capuano was afraid of. The fact he feared the dark didn't diminish him in any way. It only told Paris how truly awful the mustard gas attack must have been.

"Can I talk about something I have no right to talk about?" Paris asked.

"You can ask whatever you want," Johnny said.

"Back in my apartment, you spoke of losing God. That you left him in France. But some men held onto him. Why did you go the way you did?"

Johnny stared at the fire, trying to break the trance it had cast on him. "What kind of God does that to his people?"

"God is vengeful. That gets lost sometimes. The Old Testament… the wrath of God was fully evident."

"Demanding Abraham kill his son."

"God gave his only son so that we could live."

"Jesus was one man, Paris. God needed millions of men to sacrifice their lives? For what? So maps could be redrawn? I grew up with God being merciful and compassionate. Jesus… that's all he taught. I go over there with a cross around my neck thinking I'm on some holy crusade. Guess what? The other side had crosses too. And they didn't fare any better than we did."

"I'm not saying that. I don't know why God put you in that trench, Giovanni. I don't know why millions of men had to be killed. But don't think he wasn't there with you on that battlefield."

228

"And the ones who died? He just abandoned them?"

"No, God didn't abandon those men. Jesus took the hands of every man who fell and escorted them into heaven himself."

"You believe that? You know how many men called out to God? To Jesus? I didn't see any angel's wings flying them to heaven. I saw their bodies rot in the mud, pushed into mass graves."

"There was a time I thought God had abandoned me. But maybe I only made it through because he was there."

She turned to the fire and wouldn't speak about God again. But it was clear that she had something else on her mind—it showed in her eyes.

"Can I ask you one more question?" Paris asked, shifting her weight toward Johnny. "Or do I need to get the bottle?"

"I have a strong feeling it would land on me anyway. Go ahead," Johnny answered.

"In my apartment, you said you ran a job that went south. You put a *pig* down."

"The job went fine. It was after. Hotsy and I went to this sandwich place for a bite to eat. When we walked in, there was this copper giving the owner a hard time. Wanted his cut. Hotsy, he took it as the way things were. He was studying the menu and didn't give the cop a second thought."

"And you?"

"I stared at that cop, with so much disgust for everything he stood for. He felt my gaze and met it, you know, giving me the opportunity to look away. I didn't. He ordered me to look away. I didn't. He removed his baton… and it brought me back to France, in that German trench with a Hun, a persuader in his hand—"

"Persuader?"

"A club with spikes. Most men carried that or knuckle knives," Johnny said, but caught himself using jargon again. "That's a knife with brass knuckles on the handle. In that trench, it's hand to hand, face to face. When that cop raised that baton, I took my knife and drove it into his throat."

229

"You were trained. Reaction isn't something you can stop, Giovanni," Paris said.

"I tried telling myself that. But I wanted to kill that cop the moment I walked in. In my mind, he was the same cop who had extorted money from my parents."

He fell silent and stared into the fire.

"One more question?" Paris asked.

"You know if we keep quiet, we may be able to hear the song the fire is dancing to," Johnny responded.

But Paris' eyes reiterated her persistence. Johnny turned to look at her, granting her permission.

"When you passed out, you were talking to yourself. You said, '*It's suffering.*' You were mumbling something else, but I couldn't make it out. But you kept repeating '*It's suffering, it's suffering.*' Do you remember that?"

Of course he remembered it. Those words came to him every day, whether in his dreams or during long drawn-out stares into the distance. Two days ago, he would have lied. A lie now would only hurt her, and she would see through it. But what she was asking for was at the very center of the maze. Of all the truths, memories, and answers, this one needed to be buried the deepest.

"Yeah, I remember it," Johnny said.

He gathered his thoughts, gazing at the destructive beauty of the fire. Paris only looked on patiently—no rushing, no judging, no pressure.

"When I was a kid, my father and I were walking home from church. We were staying upstate. At a place a lot like this one. I was maybe seven or eight, the only thing I don't remember clearly. In the middle of a secluded country road was a deer sprawled out. Twitching. Trembling. It had gotten hit and left for dead. My father said, 'It's suffering, Giovanni, we have to finish it off.' I pleaded with him not to. I had never seen anything or anyone die before. I thought it could live, that it could be saved. He said it'd be cruel to let it suffer. My father ran home, I chased after him. We got in the Manhattan truck my dad had borrowed and drove back. I bawled the whole time, pleading with him to try to save the deer, but he kept saying, 'It's suffering, Giovanni.' He said,

230

'Sometimes death isn't cruel. It's mercy.' I could see it, lying in the road, growing clearer the closer we got. I could hear my father press down on the gas pedal, the truck humming loudly as it picked up speed. I can still feel the skull breaking under the wheels. See the blood smearing on the road in the rear-view mirror. It never goes away, I never get it out of my mind. When I was on the battlefield, surrounded by thousands of corpses and dying men in excruciating pain, I saw that deer. I couldn't believe… wouldn't believe there was nothing that could be done for them. That the only thing I could do was stand by those scared, crying men and pray for them. I couldn't believe that, Paris. I couldn't listen to those guttural, soul-wrenching screams… I couldn't accept nothing could be done. My father's words came to me. The foolishness I'd had as a child was long gone. I knew there was no saving them. I knew there was nothing I could do for them but end it… end the cruel, unrelenting suffering…"

Paris was sickened—not by the actions he spoke of, but the situation young men had been put in. The heartbreak was reflected in her eyes.

"Ask me what I did," Johnny said.

"You don't' have to—"

"Ask me."

"What did you do?"

"I stood over them and put a bullet in their head. Up and down that field until I was out of bullets."

"I… I'm sorry that you had to do that. But it was mercy. Euthanasia."

"Doesn't silence the screams."

"No, I can't imagine it does. Thank you for sharing that with me. I know that wasn't easy, and I can't imagine the burden of making that choice and the torment you carry because of it."

With her left hand, she stroked the side of his face, and with her right, she squeezed his hand.

"Is that why you befriended the Nettesheims? Because you won't accept that he can't be saved?" she asked.

231

"There are things inside him that broke. Things that I have to believe can be repaired. They have to be."

"That's why you give them money, so he can continue seeing doctors. There's a part of you that thinks if he gets better, you get better."

Johnny didn't need to answer. Paris had found her way to a deep truth.

"Do you feel guilty about it? That he's like that? And you're not?"

"Not guilty. It worries me... scares me."

"Why?"

She stopped stroking his face, a concerned look on hers.

"Clarence was pure, you know? War... it feeds off the good in a person. It broke everything good inside him," Johnny said.

At last, he met her gaze. His blue eyes gleamed with emotion.

"And I look at myself, and I don't know if there was anything in me to break."

Party in a Barn

Dreams were often just memories for Johnny. Most often, dreams put him back in that trench, where the artillery barrage and gunfire was so vivid it had to be real. Johnny would snap awake seconds before he was killed. That morning was no different—except that when Johnny woke and took in the sunlight pouring in through the curtains, the gunshots didn't go away. For a moment, he passed it off as another attack brought on by a sight or smell. But Paris had been startled awake—she had heard the gunshots too. But to her they were a generic sound, she didn't know they were from a .32 caliber.

Johnny dashed to the window and peeked through the curtains. He exhaled a sigh of relief. Tomato and Hotsy were in a marksman competition, firing at cans and bottles.

"It's just Tomato and Hotsy messing around," Johnny said.

Paris relaxed her death grip on the bed sheets.

Then Tomato screamed at Hotsy for firing while he was stacking new cans and bottles. Johnny knew he had slept in later than usual, but the fact that Hotsy was up before him made him worry that he had slept the whole morning away. But he was relieved when he checked his watch. It was only eight thirty-two.

From the window, Paris watched Tomato and Hotsy's competition with great intrigue. She and Johnny joined them outside, and Johnny taught her to shoot. Hotsy offered to retrieve the Thompson submachine gun, but all three acknowledged that was a bad idea. They were deep in the woods, and even if a gunshot was heard, it could be passed off as hunting. But unloading a Tommy gun would bring questions, cops, and trouble. But even that fact changed on a dime. One moment, the gunshots echoed like sounds in a cave, and the next, they didn't even make it through the trees.

Paris missed her first seven shots, but each one was closer to the target than the last. It was obvious that she had grown up spending her time outdoors. She had no problem getting dirty. With each shot fired, she grew more comfortable having a killing instrument in her hands. She was competitive, not with Johnny, Hotsy or Tomato, but with herself. She wouldn't quit until she hit the can consistently, proving to herself that it hadn't been a fluke. Once she was satisfied, they went for a walk (Tomato adamantly insisted they drive, but once again, lost three votes to one) to a restaurant called Burger Barn. The owner of the place was a proud second cousin of Charlie Nagreen, a name that meant nothing to any of them. But before they could ask, the owner told them his cousin, Charlie of Seymour of Wisconsin, was the father of the hamburger, having sold them at the County Fair. If that was true, Johnny would shake his hand and buy him a drink. The damn meat patty was sensational. All three men wanted to order French fries, but Paris strongly encouraged (forced) them to order deep fried cheese curds. What marvelous, delicious things those were. The breading was crunchy and greasy, and the inside was a melted, stringy blob of cheddar cheese. Wisconsinites truly had figured out the secret to life.

Once again, they ate too much and gut rot took hold. The afternoon was filled with cribbage and walks, and in the early evening, Tomato and Hotsy went into town to get some soda pop, and to call Tomato's family.

When the two returned to the cabin, Tomato's mood had changed. Surely, he had gotten yelled at by Lorraine, but he had also spoken with his girls. The homesickness took over like one of his Old Testament hangovers. He sat on the couch, alternating between the drink in his left hand and the cigarette in his right, until Hotsy told everyone to get ready.

"Ready for what?" Johnny asked.

"Party in a barn," Hotsy said.

Johnny looked to Paris for explanation. "Is this a Wisconsin thing too?"

Paris only smiled on her way to the bathroom to ensure her makeup and hair were worthy of a public appearance. Then she went into the bedroom and changed into the dress she had worn to the movie palace.

No explanations were forthcoming on the vague phrase "party in a barn" on the car ride to wherever it was they were going, and it irritated Johnny more than the heat.

"Anyone care to explain?" he asked.

"We're going to a barn for a party," Hotsy said.

Johnny knew not to take it as a sarcastic comment. Hotsy genuinely believed he had provided clarity.

Tomato arched his head back toward Johnny. "Sam has a huge barn where he throws parties. Middle of nowhere."

"Who's Sam?" Paris asked.

"Our seller in the area," Tomato answered.

Johnny spent the remainder of the car ride envisioning what he was in store for—a barn filled with hay, cows, pigs, goats, and thirty different types of shit. In this heat, the manure must truly smell rancid. No need to worry about those attacks and not being able to breathe. The manure would see to that.

Minutes later, Tomato parked on a grass lot next to fifty other cars. It was nothing but country around—gravel roads, farm houses, and fields stretching to what seemed like the horizon. The barn's paint had faded so severely it was impossible to tell what color it had once been. Its doors were shut, something Johnny thought was meant to contain the smell of shit inside. They should have

235

left them open to air out the stench. But the whole area reeked of manure from the miles and miles of shit-covered fields.

Of all the times to not be able to breathe, now was the most ideal.

Tomato pulled open the thick, pine door. Johnny braced himself for the thick, stagnant manure-tainted air to violate his lungs. But he had never been more wrong about a place in his life. The barn only smelt of booze and cigarettes. There was not a straw of hay nor any farm animals to be seen. Golden lights were strung between the first and second levels. The mugginess had been mitigated by two large industrial fans. A rag-tag group of musicians—men and women ranging from seventeen to sixty—played music at the far end. Bottles of beer bathed in ice. Whiskey, rum, gin, and vodka bottles lined the long tables. An empty sixteen-ounce mason jar next to them was stuffed with dollars and change. The barn was self-serve. In Chicago, it would have never worked. People wouldn't have chipped in, and people would have stolen. But in a small Wisconsin town, the people were good and honest.

"Party in a barn…I'll be damned," Johnny said to himself, shaking his head.

Tomato removed a wad of cash and tried to stuff it inside the full jar. A woman, on the fresh side of thirty, smiled at him.

"Looks full," she said.

She grabbed a bottle of rum, an eighth-full, and brought it to her lips. She downed half of what remained and then pressed the bottle to Tomato's lips. When he finished, she slid his money inside the empty bottle, starting the next money jar. She left Tomato with a smile that told him it'd be in his interest to find her later.

Hotsy grabbed a bottle of whiskey and four coffee cups and handed them out to Tomato, Paris, and Johnny. He poured into the men's cups and stopped at Paris'.

"I forgot, you don't drink," Hotsy said.

Paris thought for a bit, then raised her glass. "What the hell."

"You don't have to," Johnny said.

"I know I don't. But when in Rome…" Paris said.

236

Hotsy cracked a wide smile. "Do as the Romans do, Paris!"

It took all of two songs to empty the bottle.

"Care to dance?" Hotsy asked Paris.

She took his offered hand. "Sure."

The music kicked in, and those brave enough (drunk enough) danced the Charleston. Hotsy was phenomenal, and each step and kick was a seed planted in the minds of every woman watching, one that would bear pure lust and longing, and take mere minutes to blossom. Dancing with Paris, an undisputedly beautiful woman, only helped Hotsy's case.

Sam, a man nearing six foot six and over two hundred fifty pounds, with forearms the size of most men's legs, plodded his way toward Johnny and Tomato, brushing off gratitude and praise from partiers. If he had been operating in Chicago, no one would have dared to be late with a payment. He had met Al Capone once, during one of Capone's Wisconsin retreats. Capone had asked him to move to the Windy City but had accepted Sam's wishes to stay in his hometown.

He exchanged pleasantries with Tomato and Johnny. Both offered Sam money to help with the liquor, but he shook his massive hand in refusal. Tomato insisted that the next time Sam made his way to Chicago, they'd give him the night of his life. Sam chuckled and nodded and then returned to making his rounds.

The barn was packed on both the ground level and the second level. In Chicago, bumping into someone would lead to a snarky comment or, at the very least, a sinister glare. But here, people only laughed and apologized profusely. Johnny witnessed an "argument" where each man blamed themselves for the blunder. Four rounds of apologies later, the two men toasted each other and went on their way.

When the song ended, Paris returned to Johnny and Tomato, a smile on her lips and sweat on her forehead.

"No courage to dance?" Paris teased them.

"I'm drinking it," Tomato said, raising his cup to toast her.

Paris shook her head in disbelief. "You two stormed out of a trench, but you're afraid to dance?"

"The Germans weren't laughing at us," Johnny said.

"No, they were only shooting at you," Paris said.

"Exactly," Tomato said.

But the sultry woman who had flirted with Tomato earlier was on the dance floor. Tomato would have to swim out into those shark-infested waters. After sipping two more glasses of whiskey and downing a third, he took a deep breath.

"Here we go," he said before bravely charging in.

Paris took Johnny's hand and dragged him ahead. Johnny finished his whiskey and set his cup on a wooden table they passed by.

Liquid courage better travel fast.

Hotsy thrust his hands up in celebration when he saw Tomato and Johnny. He was damp with sweat, sleeves rolled past his elbows, hair flopping about. The impromptu band discussed amongst each other, trying to get in sync and in the same key. Drums, guitars, saxophones, and trumpets filled the crowded barn with fast-paced music.

The golden blonde Tomato had met earlier cast bedroom eyes his way and took his hand. With Paris' encouragement, Johnny's confidence in his dancing improved until Hotsy flipped his dance partner in the air. It was part of the Lindy Hop, and many men had over-estimated their dancing prowess and had given their dates black eyes and bloody noses in their attempts. But Hotsy executed it flawlessly, drawing gasps and applause.

"I'm going to take a seat," Johnny said, equally dejected and embarrassed.

"Oh come on baby," Paris said.

Johnny rolled his eyes.

"No one's looking at you. They're all looking at Hotsy," she assured him.

"Great, that makes me feel loads better," Johnny said.

"Spin me," Paris instructed.

Under her benevolent guidance, Johnny continued dancing, but did little to distinguish himself from the crowd, which was exactly his goal. When the song ended, thunderous applause and whistling broke out for the band. Those who wore hats tipped them to show their appreciation.

Realizing their dancers needed a few minutes to catch their breath, the band's next song was slow. Hotsy had to make his choice of which woman he would dance (sleep) with and selected a woman with cat-like blue eyes, her ash brown hair styled in cootie garage braids. She was nearing forty and at the pinnacle of her beauty. She wore no ring, though that was hardly proof of her relationship status. Wedding rings, like all rings, could be nothing more than a fashion accessory.

Tomato made his move on the woman who had enchanted him upon entering. He pulled her close, discretely moving his wedding band to the other finger. Johnny pretended to not see it.

"Are you going to ask me to dance, half-breed?" Paris asked.

They were the only two so close to the band but not dancing.

Johnny pulled her close. "Dance with me."

"Are you asking or commanding?"

But they were already dancing, her hands draped across his shoulders, his hands wrapped around her waist.

"I'm pleading."

"You're sexy when you beg."

"Hang on now, I said *plead* not beg."

"Oh? A big difference, is there?"

"Titanic."

"You do realize you're using a ship that sunk to say that your statement holds water."

"I would say that a sunken ship holds a lot of water, wouldn't you?"

Paris arched her head back, laughing. "You're a strange man, Giovanni De Luca."

As they danced, everyone and everything around them faded away—the other dancers, the band, the people drinking, laughing, and chatting. It was just the two of them. His mind usually processed thousands of thoughts every minute, but now it had been wiped clean. The empty, calm mind he had longed for was his for those few minutes that the band serenaded them. It was only Paris on his mind. One singular thought. He'd never been held the way he was being held while they danced. He tried his best to reciprocate the warmth of that embrace. She hadn't been scared at what he had told her. She would listen to everything he said, if he but had the courage to tell her. He pulled her closer, her chest against his, his hips against hers. Their noses brushed against one another. It took nearly a minute for them to realize the song was over, and applause was breaking out.

Their gaze stayed uninterrupted until Hotsy dragged them, Tomato, and the woman he had been dancing with to the table for more booze. It was safe to say that after their second shot of gin, sobriety had left the barn. The sparkle in Paris' eyes told Johnny the alcohol was surging through her body.

"We'll see you later," Hotsy said, his eyes casting an invisible line at the woman he had danced with earlier.

When she caught his eye, he flipped his hair out of his face and strutted out of the barn. The brunette with cootie garage braids whispered to her friends, and to the dismay of envious admirers, followed Hotsy.

Tomato was dragged off by his dancing partner, and Johnny lost him in the crowd. The industrial fans had done an admirable job trying to cool the barn, but it was too jam-packed now, and grew muggier each second.

"You want to get some air?" Johnny asked.

He was drunk to the point where the barn was at a steep angle, spinning one way, and then another. He leaned on the table beside him for support, a wave of drunkenness leaving him off balance.

"Sure," Paris said, leaning into him in a way that told Johnny the barn was spinning for her too.

He kept his hand on her waist, escorting her through the droves of people and through the barn doors.

The fresh air outside was a godsend, and Johnny gulped it in. The music inside the barn was faint, surrendering to the sounds of nature. They left it behind, strolling alongside the corn fields stretching for miles. The tension between the two had only been postponed. She ran her fingernails across his chest, leaving behind goosebumps that not even the muggy, stifling heat could kill.

She balled the front of his shirt. "Are you going to ask to kiss me?"

"Kiss me," Johnny said.

"Are you asking or commanding?"

They drew closer, a whisper away.

"I'm pleading," he said, softly enough that it tickled her ear.

They pulled together, kissing under a canvas of stars. Paris entwined her hand with his, and they strolled back toward the barn. Halfway there, a man emerged from the corn field, tucking in his shirt.

"Hotsy?" Paris called.

Hotsy looked up, startled. "I was about to look for you two. Where's Tomato?"

Before Johnny or Paris could reply, a second figure emerged from the darkness, this time coming down the long driveway by the road. It was Tomato.

"Where were you?" Johnny asked.

"Clearing my head," Tomato replied.

Johnny glanced the way Tomato had come for the woman he'd danced with, but no other figures emerged from the darkness. He glanced at Tomato. His wedding ring was back on the correct finger.

"Where's your dance partner?" Paris asked.

"Turns out she's handcuffed," Tomato mumbled. "She broke down before we... and said her husband works on a train, gone for months. She gets lonely sometimes."

Tomato should have been relieved. He hated himself for cheating on Lorraine. But no relief came because it hadn't been he who had stopped it. The guilt was there, even if the act hadn't been committed.

"Wait..." Johnny said, turning to Hotsy, "where's your date?"

"Getting dressed," Hotsy answered.

"You left her in the corn field?" Paris asked, doing her best not to yell.

"Christ, kid," Tomato said.

"What? I found my way out!" Hotsy yelled out as Johnny ventured into the field and through its six-foot high stalks.

Tomato's fear of the dark wouldn't allow him to venture into that terrifying labyrinth. But Paris shook her head and hurried after Johnny, calling for him to wait.

They were hardly the first people to look for someone in a corn field, but they were among the first to feel its sobering effects. Corn fields evoked an innate fear in everyone. It didn't matter if you've never seen one before or lived right next to one. Wandering through a maze you couldn't see through or over is terrifying. That this labyrinthine passage was a physical manifestation of the maze in which Johnny kept memories, questions and answers, and truths hidden didn't help either. At any moment those memories, questions and answers and truths, wearing the faces of the men he'd killed and failed, would attack him. By the time they found the woman, Johnny was only slightly buzzed. The woman had her head between her knees, and she was sobbing.

And then it happened.

Johnny's chest heaved, the final breathes of air surging through his nostrils and mouth.

"Are you okay?" Paris asked.

"Yeah… Just get her out," Johnny said.

He had wanted to sound confident. Instead it seemed as though they were the first English words he had ever spoken. Paris reluctantly nodded and escorted the woman out of the corn field.

Johnny kept his gaze at the sky, holding onto a corn stalk. The memories, questions and answers, and truths rose from both shallow and deep graves and broke free from fragile and strong cages. Rotting corpses limped toward him. Distant screams and pleas wafted through the stalks.

"It's suffering."

Suddenly, a hand grabbed his shoulder. He reeled back. It was Paris. She held his hands, silently standing by him. Her strength and support warded off the haunting corpses, making them limp back into the cover of the corn stalks. Air flooded into his lungs.

And the attack passed.

They reached the barn just in time to see Hotsy's date give him a ringing slap on her way back inside. Knowing she would tell her friends and those friends would tell their male friends, brothers, fathers, boyfriends, and husbands—they decided it was best they leave immediately.

No one wanted to laugh about what Hotsy had done on the car ride back to the cabin. They wanted him to know that it had been in poor taste. But there was nothing funnier than something that shouldn't be funny. It was like being in church. When Tomato and Paris kept silent, it was Johnny who started laughing. When he was stoic, either Tomato or Paris broke out in laughter. On it went until all three couldn't contain their laughter and burst out into nearly mad guffaws.

"Paris, Johnny ever tell you about our getaway from the cops last winter?" Hotsy asked, shifting sideways to look at them in the backseat.

Paris laughed. "What do you think?"

"True," Hotsy said.

It was common knowledge Johnny wasn't a story teller.

"It was a week or two before Christmas," Hotsy continued. "We were delivering a case of premium whiskey from Canada. We had just gone by that prison near Prospect Heights, and this bright light turns on behind us. We're literally outside our drop. Tomato was driving, I was in the passenger seat, and Johnny was following behind us in his own car. Tomato pulled over, sweating bullets—"

"The hell I was!" Tomato yelled.

"He's praying the rosemary," Hotsy said.

"First off, it's the rosary. Second off, you're so full of—"

"Tomato, please. I'm the narrator here. I'm using the tools of the storyteller. I'm building tension."

"It's a good story. You don't need to flat out lie."

Hotsy dramatically put up his hand to silence Tomato.

"Like I was saying, Tomato's sweating bullets, praying the rosemary, rosary… whatever. Johnny pulls over about a block behind us. The copper gets out of his car, his flashlight lighting us up like we're on Broadway. It's obvious he knows what we're carrying. He aims the flashlight at both of us, trying to find which of us is more of a threat. He keeps his flashlight on me—the alpha. I'm thinking we're going to have to deck the halls with this guy's guts, but Johnny creeps forward, fires two shots into the air, and this cop, I swear makes a mess in his pants. He falls to the ground, going into the fetal position. We ditch the car and dive into Johnny's. We speed off, the cop gives chase. We're speeding through this city, ice-covered roads, thick snowfall the size of cotton balls. More police pursue us, I'm telling you it's like the United States Army on our ass like we were the Kaiser, Paris. There's police in front and behind. Johnny hits the brakes. We're surrounded. I'm loading my shotgun, Tomato, he's praying—"

"You lying sack of—" Tomato cursed.

"Tomato please. Fear causes people to remember things differently."

Paris failed at suppressing her laughter, but knowing she didn't buy Hotsy's embellishments kept Tomato quiet.

"Johnny floors it, going off road! We're bouncing up and down…" Hotsy mimicked jumping up and down in his seat. "The cops giving chase slam on their brakes. Now we're all confused, you know? You followed us this long and you just stop? That's worrisome, you know? Then I realize—"

"You realized!" Tomato yelled.

"I *had* realized before, but Tomato is the one who said it first, you know him, he always has to be heard," Hotsy said.

"Of course," Paris said, playing along.

"Tomato's flushed from color, now white as the snow on the ground. He looks up in horror and goes, 'We're on a frozen lake,' all solemn like."

Paris gasped, her eyes widened in actual fear.

"Johnny's speeding down this frozen lake, and the car starts to sink, we can feel the ice breaking. He floors it, hoping we can make it to shore before we go down. But the front end drops down, we all dive out and watch as Johnny's car sinks to the bottom. We're horrified you know—I mean we'd have been dead in a few seconds—and then, we just start laughing like three jackals."

"More like three jackasses," Tomato said.

"So you walked back into town?" Paris asked.

"Froze our asses off on that walk," Hotsy said. "We're laughing, walking like ducks, trying to make sure the ice didn't break. We had about two hundred yards to shore, and none of us could shut up. We feel the ice crack and tweak, and somehow, we're still laughing. We kept thinking about the cops slamming on their brakes! And how we all didn't know why!" Hotsy couldn't even finish before his stomach cramped from laughter. And to Paris, it was clear that life around these three would never be boring.

I Love You, Kid

The next day would be their last full day and night at the cabin. It was mostly cloudy, always threatening to rain at any moment, but it never did. All four agreed to abstain from any alcohol that day, Paris reminding them that she was no longer "in Rome." They spent most of the day playing cribbage and Sheepshead and eating every remaining snack they had bought during the week. When the sun fell, the gray blanket of clouds dispersed, giving way to a clear, cloudless sky. Tomato and Hotsy drove into town to fill up on gasoline and re-stock on snacks for the ride home the next morning.

"Come with me," Johnny said, holding out his hand to Paris.

She took it, following him outside. It was the coolest it had been since their arrival. A ladder, stretching from grass to roof, rested against the cabin. Johnny held it in place and nodded for Paris to climb. When she was on the roof, Johnny clambered up.

The green plaid blanket from the back of the couch was sprawled open on the roof. They crouched toward it. Years of uncontrolled growth had allowed the branches to hang and fall onto the roof. Johnny and Paris lay on the blanket and gazed up at the truly astonishing view. Every crater of the waxing crescent moon was visible in a clarity that, Paris—who had bounced around from one big city to another—had never seen. The Wisconsin summer sky glittered with every star the universe had to offer, a number that would take days to count.

"This is incredible," Paris said.

"It's like being back in that field in France… minus the bullets and explosions," Johnny said.

"Yes, I have to say, I'm better company than someone trying to kill you," Paris agreed.

"Well that depends on how many questions you're asking."

Paris hit his arm. "Watch it, half breed."

They gazed at the majestic black canvas stretched atop them.

"When you look at that, everything seems less important… you know what I mean?" Johnny asked.

"I do," Paris said.

At that height, with no other homes around, they could see all the way to the lake and to the road stretching to the cabin right until where the trees swallowed it up. Shooting stars blazed across the black sky, demanding their attention before the largest stars twinkled to regain their dominance.

A car sped down the long driveway, going too fast for any responsible driver—meaning it had to be Hotsy behind the wheel. Johnny could practically hear Tomato yelling at him to slow down. The car disappeared beneath the drooping willows and came to a stop in front of the cabin. The engine went dead, and two car doors slammed shut, one after the other.

"What if a deer would of jumped out?" Tomato yelled.

Johnny and Paris shared a laugh.

"What do you think brakes and headlights are for?" Hotsy countered.

Their bickering continued into the cabin where it soon became distorted and muffled. The glowing headlights had distracted Johnny and Paris from the sky, but the vividness of the oil black sky and the burning blue and blinding white stars could not be ignored for long. Yet, moments later, a second light claimed their attention—this time not emerging through the tree-covered road, but from the main street at least half a mile away.

Johnny and Paris sat up to look. Four cars turned from the street onto the long road. There was only the cabin on the road, and it was basically a driveway. During their week there, no car had ever mistakenly driven down it. The only way to go was forward, all the way to the cabin, or turn around. The section of the driveway engulfed by the drooping willow would have made someone turn around. The fact the cars continued forward was odd. But when the headlights shut off before the cars vanished into the dense tree cover, it changed from unusual to ominous.

"That's strange," Paris said.

They waited for the cars to emerge, but they didn't. Nor had they turned around and driven back onto the main road. A small, faint clunk echoed—the closing of car doors. The Wisconsin outdoors had its own acoustics, and a car door slamming should have echoed. The fact it didn't, meant whoever had exited the car wanted their arrival to be a surprise. The sliver of optimism in Johnny hoped Hotsy had struck gold in the form of promiscuous women. But the realist in Johnny told him whoever approached the cabin did so with malicious intent. Was it the police who had been directed by a tip from the men Johnny had beaten? Or had Mickey Diamond somehow found them?

"We have to get back inside. Now," Johnny said.

There was no time to downplay the situation. It would only cost time, and Paris wouldn't fall for any false sense of security anyway. She steadied herself and climbed down. Johnny held his composure, keeping his eyes locked at where he had last seen the four cars. It was impossible to guess how many people were inside them.

After Paris was safely on the ground, Johnny rushed down the ladder, jumping the last three steps. He kicked the ladder over and then grabbed Paris' hand and barged inside the cabin.

"There's somebody here," he said.

248

Hotsy and Tomato jumped up from their cribbage game. Tomato ran to the window beside the front door and peeked through the drawn curtains.

"What do you mean?" he asked.

"Four cars turned onto the driveway and shut their headlights off. Parked halfway down the road," Johnny said.

"They were sure to be quiet about shutting their doors too," Paris added.

"You're not expecting anyone are you?" Johnny asked Hotsy.

Hotsy shook his head.

"What did you tell that waitress or the dame you met at the barn?" Tomato asked.

"Huh? I didn't say nothing. She just wanted to know if I'd keep in touch, and if she could visit me in Chicago. She couldn't be the nark… we're two hundred miles from Chicago," Hotsy said.

But Mickey Diamond could have sent men, men who happened to have eaten at the same restaurant and had the same waitress who was "just being friendly," as Paris had put it.

"The guys we met on the way home from the movie house," Johnny said.

It was far more likely the self-appointed mayor and his cabinet had called for reinforcements.

"I doubt they're out of the hospital yet. Even if they were, they can't be that stupid," Tomato said.

"Someone at the party last night? Sam?" Paris asked.

"Nah, Sam's not a rat. Plus, he doesn't know where we're staying," Tomato said.

"Did I do something wrong, Tomato?" Hotsy asked.

"No, you didn't do anything, kid," Tomato assured him.

"Who else knew we were coming here?" Johnny asked.

"I don't know. I don't know who The Cardinal told," Tomato said.

"The Cardinal didn't know what city," Johnny reminded him.

Both Tomato and Hotsy stared at Paris. Though Paris was offended, Johnny knew the rationale behind their stare. She was the unknown variable. All three men trusted each other with their life. Period. Paris was the question mark.

"She didn't have time to tell anyone," Johnny said.

Strength filled Paris' eyes, but there was worry in them too. She was surrounded by violent men. Earlier, she had said a person's eyes reveal their true emotion, no matter what the mouth said. Tomato and Hotsy read her eyes and accepted the truth they conveyed.

"Let me answer the door. They're expecting three men, not a woman. Let me see if I can talk them into going away," Paris said.

It was a brave gesture all three men admired.

"Too risky. If it was the waitress or someone at the barn, they'll know you're with us," Tomato said.

"And if it's the guys from the movie house, they'll know too," Johnny added.

"If he's stupid enough to come, let him. I want to know if we should expect fists or bullets," Tomato said.

"I'll go outside, make myself known. We don't know it was them," Paris said.

"I'm not taking that chance. They see movement, they may shoot and verify later," Johnny said.

When Al Capone ordered a hit, his men scouted and ensured their target could be identified, and no innocent bystanders would be harmed. But Kowalski's royal screw up on the hit on Johnny proved Mickey Diamond didn't believe in gentlemen warfare.

Hotsy locked the front door. Tomato closed the windows. Johnny dashed into Tomato's bedroom and lifted the mattress and flipped it onto the floor. Three Thompson submachine guns, four pistols, and a shotgun were laid out on the bed frame.

Tomato and Hotsy ran in and chose their instruments of death—Tomato a Colt Police Positive Revolver and Tommy gun, Hotsy a shotgun and Tommy gun. In addition to his reliable M1911, Johnny also wielded a Thompson. The formidable weapon could fire fifteen hundred rounds per minute from its hundred-round drum magazine. It could light up a dark night like the Fourth of July and held the unofficial moniker of "Chicago Typewriter"—it was how business was settled.

Johnny hurried to Paris and gave her the very gun she had shot bottles and cans with. She took it, but not with the confidence with which she had held it earlier. Taking a gun to shoot a bottle was entirely different than taking a gun to potentially end a human life.

"Hide here," Johnny instructed her, pointing to the kitchen island.

The Wisconsin ground was covered in broken twigs—a valuable ally. They creaked and cracked, warning them that someone was approaching. Whispers came next. Johnny peeked through a crack in the curtain. The man outside wore a fedora and was far older than the self-appointed mayor or his cabinet members. And it was obvious he wasn't looking for a fist fight, but for a gunfight.

Johnny pointed to the door, signaling someone was outside it. Hotsy nodded, securing his grip on his shotgun. Johnny put his hand on the doorknob and, slowly and quietly, turned the lock. He nodded to Hotsy. He nodded back, then raised the shotgun. Johnny whipped the door open. The man outside, carrying a shotgun harmlessly by his side, looked up in shock, his eyes bulging, clearly not expecting to be greeted with a shotgun. A deafening blast echoed. The shell exploded through his chest, sending him flying backward. The birds in the trees fluttered away. Johnny slammed the door, and the three dove to the ground as the cabin was riddled with lead.

Since the War had ended eight years earlier, there had been many sights, sounds, and smells that brought Johnny back to France. But nothing brought him back to that trench quicker, more realistically than being shot at. But unlike with other smells, sounds, and sights that debilitated him, inflicting him with a temporary paralysis, gunfire brought out the solider, the survivor in him. It was the only time the world made sense. The only time he knew his purpose. The only time the questions, answers, and truths tormenting him left him alone.

"All these bullet holes will help that breeze get in, Johnny!" Hotsy yelled.

Tomato smashed the window above his head with his Thompson and fired.

Rat-a-tat-tat Rat-a-tat-tat Rat-a-tat-tat.

Gunfire erupted from the other side of the cabin. Johnny crawled to Paris. She was crouching with her hands covering her ears, and her head buried between her knees.

"Are you alright?" he asked.

She nodded. Her hands trembled—it was how every soldier reacted to their baptism by fire.

"Listen to me, Paris. I'm going to get you out. Trust me," Johnny said.

He squeezed her hand and wouldn't release it until she nodded to show that she truly accepted his words as a solemn vow.

Hotsy fired from the other side of the cabin, yelling and whelping like an Indian ready to scalp. The bedroom windows were smashed. Gun barrels protruded through. Johnny sprinted into his room and dove onto the floor, bullets ripping past where he had just stood. When the firing from outside paused, Johnny sent a flurry of rounds in retaliation, the end of the Thompson lighting up in a chain of flashes. A muffled scream rang out, barely audible over the deafening Chicago Typewriter. A smoke bomb rolled into the kitchen, hissing like a viper and releasing a cloud of smoke.

"Get upstairs!" Tomato yelled through a coughing bout.

Johnny called for Paris. The smoke was thick, granting him zero visibility. The gunfire was relentless. It was impossible to hear anything else, and he knew he had to physically find her. His hand grabbed hers through the haze.

"Stay low," he shouted, but with the deafening blasts, it was nothing more than a soft whisper.

The stairs led to an open space that would have made for a nice second level with bedrooms and a bathroom. But the work had never been completed. They half-crawled up the steps, coughing and hacking. Once free of the suffocating smoke, their lungs filled with air.

"We're surrounded..." Hotsy said. The usual thrill in his tone was gone. It was nothing but grave.

The windows were covered with years of grime and dirt. Tomato smashed the window closest to him and peeked outside. The gunfire had stopped, its sound replaced by chirping crickets and hooting owls.

"Is it police?" Hotsy asked.

"I don't know," Tomato replied.

"They would have given us a chance to surrender," Johnny said.

"Maybe they're crooked," Hotsy reasoned.

"Then they would have given us the chance and shot us as we walked out," Tomato said.

Paris looked into Johnny's eyes, seeking assurance initially, but ultimately the truth. He could only give her the latter and hope she knew how sorry he was for how it would end. He prayed that the men outside would honor the code of stand up men and spare her.

"They'll wait us out," Hotsy said.

"Somebody had to have heard those shots," Paris said.

"No one came before," Tomato reminded.

"But that wasn't like this. This is a goddamn warzone," Hotsy said.

Wisconsin had its advantages over Chicago. But had they been in Chicago, the shooters would have had to flee. Hundreds of people would have heard the shots and dozens of policemen would have been mere blocks away. But here, the cabin was the only sign of man's existence for close to two miles. The town most likely had a chief and a deputy. The two wouldn't be able to do anything even if they had heard the shots. During their stay, the surrounding woods had either amplified every noise, sending echoes through the trees, or it had completely swallowed sound, so not even a whisper made it out. What would the fickle forest do now? Would it swallow or sing? Their salvation or damnation was in the hands of nature. Would it extend a helping hand or clench its fist?

"If the buttons did hear, we need to be gone before they show up," Hotsy said.

Tomato fired out of the open window toward the ground at an approaching shooter. Shots were returned, ripping into the wall and through the window. The front door was riddled with holes and kicked open. Men dashed inside, firing up the steps as they took cover. Johnny and Hotsy returned fire.

Tomato was silent and still as a statue, contemplating something profound. He nodded, coming to some conclusion. His nod grew in confidence until he was adamant in his yet-to-be-revealed decision.

"I'll hold them off."

Johnny and Hotsy looked at one another, their hearts plummeting from a high mountain peak.

"Get onto the roof and try to make your way onto the trees. You find a car and get out of here," Tomato ordered.

He fired down the steps to keep whoever lurked outside the door outside.

"I'm not leaving you," Johnny said.

"Look at me. There's no other way. We don't have time to argue," Tomato said.

Hotsy, for the first time since Johnny had known him, was in shock. The color was gone from his face, and his charismatic smirk was now a grim straight line.

"I won't leave you," Johnny declared.

He'd left men behind too many times.

"There's no time."

Johnny shook his head. "I'm not leaving."

"Johnny, this is war. This here, it's a trench. You have to keep going. You have to. A man goes down, you push forward, you haul ass to that next trench. You keep Hotsy and Paris alive. You do that for me, Johnny."

"Tomato?" Hotsy said, hoping the cruel joke would end. He had never looked more like a boy.

Tomato guided Hotsy to the wall and out of harm's way. Johnny provided cover but soon ran dry on his Thompson and switched to his spare pistol.

"Listen to me... hey... look at me," Tomato said.

Hotsy forced himself to look up, tears swelling and falling from his eyes.

"My favorite thing about you, kid, is you. I love it all. You drive me nuts…
God, do you drive me nuts, but you're the son I never had," Tomato said.

Hotsy sobbed into Tomato's chest. Tomato lifted Hotsy's head and wiped
his tears.

"You tell my family I love them. Swear to me," Tomato said.

"I can't let you do this," Hotsy said.

"God damn it! If you ever listen to me, let it be now! You have to go. Swear
to me. You tell my family I love them, you tell my girls that their father is proud
of them, so damn proud of them, and that I love them with every fiber of my
being."

"I swear it… I swear it, Tomato," Hotsy sobbed out.

Somehow Tomato smiled. "Drive fast."

"What if a deer jumps out?"

"That's what brakes and headlights are for."

Hotsy handed over his Tommy gun, his tears so thick he could barely see.
Johnny was frozen. Tomato was a brother, not only in arms, but in life. To leave
him went against everything he tried to stand for. Had Paris not been there,
Johnny's feet would have grown roots in that cabin and not even a tornado
would have uprooted him. But Paris was there because he had asked her to
come. If he stayed, her death would be on his hands. She was innocent in all of
this. She didn't burn the distillery down or kill Kowalski. She had saved Johnny's
life, and he wouldn't let it cost her hers. But his choice would haunt him for the
rest of his days.

The smells, sights, and sounds of gunfire had brought France to him. But
faced with leaving Tomato behind, Johnny was truly back in that trench. There
was no mud, trench ladders or trench whistles. But that upstairs cabin was as
much a trench as the real thing. Once again, Johnny would have to leave a friend
behind. He stared at Tomato—a friend, a brother, a flawed man, just like him.
He was a human being full of imperfections. Leaving him behind would kill a
significant portion of what was left of Johnny's soul. But unlike in the trenches,
Johnny now had the chance to say goodbye. But he had no idea how to. What

do you say? What can you say? Twenty minutes ago, he had been stargazing, contemplating the wonder of the universe. Now, his heart pounded and his brain sent only two commands—fight or flight. Putting words together to articulate what Tomato meant to him was an impossible task.

Too often, there isn't the chance to say goodbye. Only reflection in hindsight provides the clarity of how to say goodbye. But in the actual moment, the shock is too severe. The animalistic impulses survival unleashed allowed Johnny to do nothing but stare.

But there was a peace in Tomato's dark eyes. His time in the trench was coming to an end. Time stopped while Johnny stood there, memories of Tomato and their time together cruelly replaying before his eyes like a film.

Let an attack come now. Remove the burden of choice.

He had fractured his soul in France, and now, he must fracture it even further.

"Giovanni," Paris called.

Johnny turned and found her eyes. She needed him, Hotsy even more. It was their dependence that snapped him into action.

He dashed to the opposite side of the room and smashed the window with his pistol. He shoved his head through, checking if there were men below— there wasn't a soul on that side of the cabin. How long that would be the case was a terrifying unknown. Johnny pulled himself through the broken window and onto the roof. He offered his hand to Paris.

Tomato fired down the steps, keeping the shooters rooted behind their hiding places. Johnny pulled Paris through the window. The over-grown trees had created a living bridge from roof to tree. Hand in hand, they tiptoed toward it.

"I'll be right back," Johnny whispered.

Paris nodded, and Johnny returned to the open window. Hotsy wiped his eyes so he could see Tomato clearly one last time.

"I love you, kid," Tomato said.

"I'm sorry, for everything," Hotsy said.

Tomato fired down the steps, then stormed to Hotsy. A man who normally had no patience now had all the time in the world while bullets zipped past.

"Don't be sorry for anything," Tomato said, "I have to do this. For Paris, for Johnny, for you... for me."

He nodded encouragingly at Hotsy. Both caught Johnny in their peripheral and turned to him. He wouldn't say anything, not daring to alert the intruders. He checked the ground behind and below him to ensure there was still no one there. Johnny and Tomato locked eyes, speaking through them.

Hotsy wanted to say more, but Tomato was back at the top of the steps firing down. Hotsy wiped his nose and pulled himself out of the window. Johnny forced him to climb into the tree first. He glanced one final time at the window, the gunfire light flashing through it like a strobe light. Then, hating every fiber of his being for leaving, he climbed onto the tree.

They scaled the tree carefully, testing each branch before stepping. Each snapping twig threatened to give away their position, but what the tree surrendered in sound, it made up for by completely absorbing all light. From the ground, the men could see nothing but black. Like circus performers on a high wire, Paris, Hotsy, and Johnny crept from tree to tree.

Johnny climbed down first, removing his trusty M1911 and scanning the surroundings before motioning to Paris. He helped her down without issue, but the branch Hotsy had been clinging to snapped, and he fell ten feet to the hard, unforgiving ground, twisting his ankle. He spit out a curse word, and another one after he tried to take a step.

"Leave me! I'll go back to Tomato!" Hotsy shouted too loudly.

Johnny and Paris looked toward the cabin, worried he had been heard.

The gunfire from the cabin continued, but the flashes of light were concealed by the forest. Johnny stood there, frozen. Every cell of his body demanded he go back, every thought commanded he return. All but one—a small, faint voice clinging to the belief that somewhere out there was a life for him. A place where he belonged. A place where he found purpose and meaning. A place that proved that the questions, answers, and truths in the maze weren't absolute. That they could be altered, that the path of his life could change.

While Johnny hoped to find that place, Tomato had found his. It should have been Johnny inside that cabin, not Tomato. But if he left now to return to the cabin, Hotsy would never make it. He wouldn't be able to walk ten feet unassisted. Paris may be able to support him, but it would be cumbersome and slow. She was a survivor; if he could get her to a car, she'd be fine. Leaving Hotsy in the middle of the woods would only nullify Tomato's sacrifice. Johnny would not let it go in vain.

He bent down and lifted Hotsy to his feet. With Paris' help, they draped Hotsy's arms over their shoulders and half-carried him.

The gunfire was sporadic and loud. Johnny forced himself to look only ahead. The longer the gunfire lasted, the more hope he had. Had Tomato managed to fight them off? But, seconds later, the gunfire stopped, giving way to an instant, eerie, heart-wrenching silence. Then two final gunshots rang out, the forest cruelly echoing them. The hope vanished like smoke. Johnny knew that the two shots were to confirm that a dead man stayed dead—one shot in the heart, one in the head.

Inside that cabin that had been built a hundred years ago lay a man who had lived to be only thirty-nine. Twenty minutes ago, Tomasso Capuano had been alive, yelling at Hotsy for driving too fast, filled with shame and guilt from his numerous affairs, and thinking ceaselessly of his wife and children. It would have been all too easy to give in to emotion. It was only human. But the War had destroyed that. It had given Johnny a coldness through attrition, pain, and devastation. The overwhelming emotions would come after the battle, during sleepless nights and absent-minded day dreams.

But Hotsy hadn't fought in the War, hadn't been cursed with such inhumane coldness, and he sobbed uncontrollably.

Tomato was dead.

The shooters were now well-aware that Hotsy and Johnny had escaped. If these gangsters or crooked cops knew what they were doing, they'd have left a man or two at the road entrance to cover any chance of an escape and to warn them if anyone was coming.

The trees through which they stumbled grew thicker and wider, signaling they were approaching the section of the road engulfed by the drooping willow leaves. The four cars were parked single-file, engines running. Johnny had his gun ready to fire. Two men stood there, smoking and holding their Tommy Guns uselessly by their sides. Johnny crept behind them, raised his gun, and fired two shots. Both fell face-forward onto the gravel road. He rushed back to Paris and Hotsy.

"Let's go," he said.

He and Paris helped Hotsy into the back seat of the last car. Johnny opened the door for Paris, and after she was inside, he picked up one of the Tommy Guns and laid waste to the other three cars. The power of the gun caused his arms to rise as bits of tire and metal flew into the air, leaving the cars smoking and hissing.

It would be days before they were drivable, and Johnny, Paris, and Hotsy would be back in Chicago by then.

But not Tomato.

Again, Johnny froze, this time in front of their escape car. He turned to look down the road toward the cabin. The trees blocked his view. But he didn't need to see to know that Tomato was inside that cabin, growing colder with each passing second. The shooters would be on their way to give chase in their cars. He could light up the road in machine gun fire and exact revenge. How many men would that be? He would have the element of surprise, and he could take out most of them before he was gunned down.

A fair trade.

He squeezed the handle of the Tommy gun, ensuring he had a firm grip, but a soft hand touched his shoulder. He turned. Paris looked into his eyes.

"Giovanni."

Somehow, she managed to put so many emotions into that word. There was pleading in there for him to hurry. There was understanding and compassion.

There was a reminder of what life could offer outside the world he knew. And there was a pledge that she would stand by his side to face the blizzard of bullets, should he choose it.

He turned once more, the inner conflict eating at him, consuming him. His grip softened, and the gun fell limply to his side and then onto the gravel road. He followed Paris to the car and took the driver's seat.

Tomato's seat.

He sped in reverse to the start of the road, then spun the wheel and raced off, his foot pressing the pedal to the floor, speeding them back to the Windy City.

Leaving the Trench

The headlights illuminated only a fraction of the outside world, the flashes of gunfire miles away and minutes ago.

The seconds before a trench whistle blew morphed time into a paradoxical entity. The *tick* of a pocket watch verified one second had passed. But it was also an hour. A surprising amount of thinking could be done in that second-long hour and hour-long second. Profound thinking. Thinking about family, regrets, reminiscing about great memories, and dwelling on dreams for a future you may never have the chance to live. But once you climbed out of that trench, your mind shut off, and once you made it safely through the devil's playground, it all washed over you—the carnage, the bodies, the near misses. And at last, you were left with the survivor's question—why me?

The cabin was an hour's drive north, Chicago a good five hours south. The drive, a once trusted friend, tormented Johnny now. Tomato filled Johnny's mind—his voice, laughter, mannerisms, and the conflicted emotions that clouded his face when he thought of his shortcomings. Now, he was just another specter to wander the haunted maze.

Johnny was so deep in his thoughts that if a deer had darted out from the roadside thicket, he wouldn't have noticed. Had he even stopped at stop signs? Only the sobbing from the backseat broke his trance. Hotsy would fall silent for a bit, a blank stare on his face, then continue sobbing for a few minutes.

Paris was silent, knowing the wound was too fresh to speak about. But she had a tremendous instinct for knowing when Johnny's thoughts descended to their darkest depths. And, when they did, she squeezed his hand.

Coffins and caskets had filled his mind since they had been to Al's, weeks ago. Now, one of his best friends would be put to rest inside one. And that's if the men who killed him didn't bury his body in a corn field or toss it in the lake. Tomato had survived miraculous odds in a war that had taken the lives of millions of men, only to be killed in a cabin over a dispute about booze.

"Did I do this? Was it the waitress, Johnny? The dame from the cornfield? Mad that I left her? Did I kill Tomato?" Hotsy asked.

Hotsy's limited life experience had always made him appear twenty years younger than Tomato. But seeing him cry like a child looking for answers made the age gap feel even more extreme.

"You didn't do this," Johnny said, trying to keep calm.

He was not in the mood to take care of a child. Everyone handled grief differently, and even if there was no right or wrong way, some ways were more annoying than others.

"Then who did?" Hotsy asked, desperate for an answer.

"I don't know!" Johnny shot back sharply, his patience gone.

"He's just scared, Giovanni," Paris whispered.

"I don't have answers, okay?" Johnny said.

The rest of the ride through Wisconsin and into Chicago was filled with silence. When he drove into the city, The Moonlight was deemed the safest place for Hotsy. Johnny pulled up front, and he assured Hotsy he would see him the next day. Paris walked Hotsy to the front door. She wiped his tears, hugged him, and then returned to the car.

The car pulled onto the barren streets. The city was an hour or two away from factory workers flocking to buses and trains to get to work.

Paris looked over several times to see if Johnny would speak, but his lips were tight. Even when he pulled alongside her apartment building, his lips didn't part.

"I'm sorry about what happened," Paris said.

"What happened… you mean Tomato being gunned down? Is that what you're talking about?" Johnny asked.

"You know, you can be a prick to me, but Hotsy lost someone he considered a father. You can at least show him a little sympathy."

"It was a mistake bringing you, Paris."

"I see…" Her tone suggested she had expected his comment.

"You stay with me, and you're going to get killed."

"You're hurting. I get that."

"Hurting? If I hadn't brought you, Paris, I'd be dead. There is no way I would of left Tomato. I would of stayed there and fought until I was out of bullets and blood. But because I asked you to come, Tomato died."

"You should thank God you did bring me. Most people don't regret not dying in a blaze of bullets."

"It's just borrowed time."

"*Borrowed time*? That's all any of us have. No one lives forever, Giovanni. We all go the way—"

"Of the dodo bird. Yeah, I get it."

"Do you know why you're a dodo bird? For one, you're stupid. And secondly, it's said that the dodo bird had no natural predators on the island they lived. Over time, they lost their ability to fly, to fight… everything. When the Dutch inhabited the island, the dodos lined up, too foolish to know they were marching to their death. The Dutch slaughtered them one by one until there was none left."

Johnny shifted in his seat, sighing annoyingly. "Do you have a point?"

"My point is death will find you, Giovanni. Don't line up for it like a dodo bird. Quit waiting to die and go live. You may find there is something out there to enjoy."

Johnny finally turned to face her. "Are you finished?"

"I guess I am." She opened the door and stepped out. "I am sorry about Tomato. Give my best to his family. Take care of yourself."

Johnny was beyond exhausted. He wanted to do nothing but sleep the next few days away. But his mind was far too busy replaying memories—the great, the awful, and everything in between—for him to even think about sleep. He drove aimlessly around Chicago until the gas ran low. When it did, he parked alongside the shoreline and sat on a bench overlooking the lake, listening to the waves crash onto the shore, their song a depressing lament. How cruelly different from the sounds of the beach he and Paris had frolicked on mere days ago. The melody of the waves coaxed Johnny to sleep but only for an hour. The period spent in the deep abyss of sleep, devoid of dreams, was the only time the pain and hurt were stifled. But upon waking, the cruel reality of his loss crashed over him like the morning tide.

Change of Ownership

Paris only managed to get five hours of sleep before she returned to The Moonlight. There had been opportunity for more, but a wandering mind did not tire. With so many thoughts crowding her mind, she had hoped it would be overloaded and temporarily shut down to let her sleep. Adding to the tumultuous memories of the cabin and the turmoil of her own inner maze was the unbearable heat, and the sun so bright it looked as though it was descending toward Earth like a crashing meteor.

Even though she had arrived at The Moonlight earlier than usual, she was well-versed in the hotel's long-tenured customers. The same city judges, police officers, congressmen, and senators returned nearly every weekend. The women of The Moonlight knew which of them were the most generous. But, in addition to the staples were new guests who had been referred by a friend or acquaintance. Then there were customers from the surrounding suburbs, or those in town from Milwaukee, St. Louis, or New York on business or adolescent boys looking to lose their virginity. But most often, apart from the high-prestige customers, the men who caught some breakfast before venturing off on their bootlegging businesses were Italian born. But that morning, there were fewer Italians in the hotel since Paris had started working there. The flux of new customers was so great that The Moonlight could have been more aptly called the "Midwest Ellis Island."

But men were men, all victim to the same weaknesses. The women of The Moonlight had two approaches for garnering men's attention. One was to dress to impress with an equally charming smile. Initiate conversation and flirtatious caresses or fondle the man's thigh, shoulder or hand. It was a slower and riskier process. One could flirt for an hour or even two, only to have the man leave. But the greater the risk, the greater the reward. Men liked to think their good looks and old-fashioned charm had enticed the woman. Feeling like masters of the universe, they tipped more generously.

The second approach was quicker and more straight forward. A woman sat silently at the bar, wearing a minimal amount of clothing to draw attention to her curves. Married men had to coax and almost bribe their wives for attention. The last thing some of them wanted was to spend hours competing for attention and having to pay for it. To some men, it was as simple as window shopping: Order a drink, scan the herd, and make your choice.

"Saundra," Paris called.

Saundra, who had been leaning against the bar and puffing on a cigarette, turned. She adjusted her dress, deceitfully doubling her cup size.

"What's going on?" Paris asked.

"Change of ownership," Saundra said.

"Valcoro sold?"

"Apparently. Don't worry, we've been assured our routine customers will still be routine." She rubbed out her cigarette on the ash tray.

"Who did Valcoro sell to?"

"I don't know. Some Polack."

Paris only knew Valcoro by reputation and from what she overheard at the bar. But even near-strangers knew The Moonlight was the love of his life. It was a lover offering great pleasure. It was a child—something he had created and watched grow with great pride. It was a loyal dog, never disappointing him, never judging him, always granting him security and protection. To Valcoro, selling The Moonlight wasn't selling a building—it was selling flesh.

It was easy to see Saundra didn't care, and Paris couldn't blame her. A week ago, she wouldn't have cared either. But she couldn't help but think the change in ownership was somehow connected with what had happened in Wisconsin.

The lobby and hotel had the same bustle as it had under Valcoro. No one had noticed or cared about the change in ownership. Drinks were served, the band played, and people danced, laughed, and ventured upstairs for an even better time. It was business as usual.

Paris scanned the dance floor and lobby for Hotsy and asked her friends if they had seen him. They each said no but told Paris to send him their way, for he was a good tipper and a great lover.

The sun set, and in the cover of darkness, the shy, bashful men could more fully shed their inhibitions. Her colleagues disappeared into the elevator, and were replaced at the bar by the next batch. Paris stayed there, nervously sipping her lemon-lime soda.

"Excuse me, can I squeeze in?" a deep, hoarse voice said.

Had she discovered a third method of attracting men?

Paris turned to face the man and slid over. "Of course."

The man was by no means attractive. Even his mother couldn't lie about that. He was overweight, a day or two behind with his shave, and his fat cheeks were covered with acne scars. A good smile could go a long way, but his didn't move an inch. Part of his lips curled up and the other curled down, forming a smile that was awkward and completely disingenuous. His teeth were crooked and stained yellow from years of dental neglect, coffee, and cigarettes, only adding to the smile's downright repulsiveness.

"How you doing tonight?" the man asked.

267

"I'm doing fine, and how are you?" Paris asked.

"Doing okay. Thank you for asking."

"Can I get you something to drink?"

"Sure, that'd be nice." He flashed another grotesque smile.

"What's your poison?"

"Whiskey as long as it's North Side. Not that rat piss from the South Side."

"First time at The Moonlight?"

"It is." He wore a guilty, embarrassed look.

"Well, you'll see that the moonlight shines on everybody here."

He had an energy about him. Though it resembled nervousness the most, his oddity was something intriguingly different.

"Any place we can go where the moonlight don't shine?"

Paris wanted nothing more than to stay perfectly visible in the spotlight. This had something to do with the fact the man was unattractive in every way. Even his conversation seemed fake and insincere. And his confident line had come out of nowhere. But more so, even though Johnny had said things were over, those words had come from a terrible grief. But she was in no financial predicament to refuse money. It was also the man's first time here, and he didn't look like he charmed women to bed. He had to pay for his pleasure, and pay well. Perhaps, he was a virgin, though that was doubtful given his age. Paris usually had a sense for the celibate. Men carried themselves different. Virgins and men cheating on their wives for the first time often talked for an hour before anything happened in bed. Something the hotel girls called a "therapist fee." These men were also fooled into believing an inflated tip was standard.

"Plenty of those places, but it could be a while before you get a drink," Paris said.

The man raised his hand and the bartender ignored ten others to serve him.

"The good whiskey on the rocks. And for the lady?" the man asked.

"Old Fashioned. Sweet, but make it a virgin," Paris said.

"Right away, sir," the bartender said.

Having the bartender ignore everyone else in line to serve you a drink was a power few had, something that only added to the mystery clinging to him like cigarette smoke.

"*Sir?* So what are you, a prohibition agent or police captain or something?" Paris asked.

The man's scoff neither confirmed nor denied her question. He didn't give off the vibe of someone who upheld the law. His knuckles were in the very early stages of healing, like Johnny's knuckles had been after fighting those men in Wisconsin. And judging by the crookedness of the bridge of his nose, it had been broken at least once.

The bartender served them their drinks and assured him the round was on the house before the man had even reached for his wallet.

"Now about that place where the moonlight don't shine," the man said, holding out his hand to gesture to Paris to leave the bar.

The man put his hand on her waist and escorted her to the elevator. The position of his hand was too low to be a gentlemanly gesture, but too high to be sexual. His touch was equally dichotomous. Not a soft guide, not rough, but it steered her where he wanted her to go.

"After you," the man said when the elevator doors *pinged* and opened.

Paris stepped inside first, the man followed, hitting the button for the seventh floor. Everyone who was remotely acquainted with The Moonlight knew Valcoro lived on the seventh floor. Had he moved out? The ride up the seven floors was slow and uncomfortable. The man's hot breath was foul and only enhanced the oven-like temperatures. The elevator *pinged* and opened once more.

"You must know someone in some really high places to get this suite," Paris said.

She had never been in it before. Valcoro didn't care for her race, and she didn't care that he didn't either. Valcoro was not as good a lover as he boasted to be and was stringent with his tipping. But most of the girls had been inside the suite and had described it vividly and often enough that nothing inside the room came as a surprise. But like with anything, seeing something in actuality led to a whole new perspective. The view of the Chicago skyline visible through the tall glass panels was simply breathtaking.

"A jungle out there," the man said.

The words broke her gaze.

"Should we be expecting Mr. Valcoro?" Paris asked.

She had a strong guess what his answer would be, but she was trying to piece together the facts herself.

"No, we have the run of the place. Just don't go breaking anything," the man said, casting another stomach-churning smile.

"Trying to impress me?"

"Is it working?"

"Maybe." She flashed a phony smile of her own.

"Good. You were recommended by Mr. Valcoro himself."

Paris continued her fake smile in response to his lie.

"Usually, people who want me have particular tastes."

The man shrugged. "I have those tastes."

He took a sip of his drink, watching Paris do the same with hers.

"I never got a name," Paris said.

"Do you always get a name?" the man asked, leaning against the kitchen island.

Up here, his nervousness (the only word that seemed to fit his demeanor at the bar) was gone. Paris had been right in judging its genuineness.

"Not always. And when we do, some are fake," Paris said.

The man chuckled. "I imagine. Can you tell when you get a fake one?"

"I like to think so."

"Okay. Let's make a game of it. I say a name, you tell me if I'm lying."

"Stakes?"

"A gambler? Looks like I'm not the only one a victim to their vice." He raised his drink with an approving nod.

She returned his toast. "Makes things more interesting."

"It most certainly does. How do you prove I am who I say I am?"

"I guess I'll have to take your honest word."

"You have my word that I will be honest if you guess correctly."

The man held out his hand to shake on it. Paris shook it. His grip was powerful, almost savagely so, and his hands were dry and callused.

"Shall we begin?" he asked.

"When you're ready, darling."

The man finished his whiskey, shook his glass to get to all the liquid trapped under the ice cubes and sipped what was left.

"Doug Jones," he said.

"Liar," Paris said.

The man smiled. "Very good... let's see... Bobby Thomas."

Paris studied his face. It was impossible to read. His beady, gray eyes revealed nothing, and his face was too fat to show any nuanced expression.

"And where is Bobby Thomas from?" Paris asked.

"St. Louis. In town for a work conference."

"What do you do?"

"Financial consultant."

"Is Bobby Thomas married?"

"He prefers not to say."

Paris studied him for a moment.

"Convincing, but the name is a lie."

"What gave it away?"

"If you were in town for a work conference, your company wouldn't set you up at The Moonlight. It's too scandalous. You'd be at some hotel on the Magnificent Mile."

The man smiled again. Paris finished her virgin Old Fashioned. The last sip was the best part, containing all of the orange and cherry juices. The man grabbed her glass and filled it a second time.

"My name is Edward Saunders from Milwaukee. My friends call me Ed, my wife calls me Eddie. I am a zoning commissioner in town to talk my friend here into taking a bribe to ignore that these buildings are outdated, in violation of code and in need of repair."

He handed Paris her refill. It tasted entirely of whiskey. Had he forgotten she had ordered a virgin? Or did he not care?

"Convincing back story, but no."

"And what gave it away this time?"

"You spoke before about South Side whiskey being rat piss. You seem to have a strong dislike of the South Side. I highly doubt you'd risk your job for a building making money for the Capone Gang."

The man smirked between sips of his whiskey. "You are like one of those women in the court with a type writer."

"A stenographer."

"That's it!" he said, snapping his fingers. "… hmm, let's see…" He paused to take a drink. "My name is Doyle McNaulty. I was eight when my parents brought us here. I am a reporter for the LA Times and writing an article about corruption. I have developed a reputation for exposing the truth, something that causes even gangsters to fear me."

Again, his face betrayed no lies. But his hands and mouth had.

"A fallacy," Paris said.

"Why do you say that?" he asked.

"A journalist would know the word *stenographer*. And your hands… you don't get those calluses from a pencil. Nor those swollen knuckles."

The man stared at her with an uncomfortable severity. But he cracked a smile, cast an approving nod, and finished his refill of whiskey.

"Let's get serious, shall we?" he said, before setting his empty whiskey glass on the counter behind him.

"Please do," Paris said.

"I am a bootlegger from Chicago. I deliver booze to those who need it. I am also the muscle who gets the local businesses and shops in line when they are considering not supporting the cause. I do what they say when they say it.

Doesn't matter what it is. These hands," he said, holding them up, "lay down the law of booze. I am married with two little girls."

"Hmm… your best one yet. And the names of your daughters?" Paris asked.

"Mary Louise and Gretchen Marie."

The names were oddly familiar. She searched her memories, but it was as if the names had been spoken by an unknown voice in an unknown setting.

"And your name?" Paris asked.

"Tomasso Capuano."

Her stomach plummeted. The glass nearly fell from her hand. The shock of what he had said paralyzed her. She did her best to hide her emotions, but she knew she had failed.

"Am I lying?" he asked.

"Yes…" Paris answered.

He had been difficult to read before, but it was obvious it had all been a game for his amusement.

"How do you know that?"

"Because he is dead…"

The man smiled genuinely for the first time. "Busted. Let me try again. My birth name is Quintu Di Salvo, but most people call me Hotsy Totsy on the account of my boyish good looks. I have slept with almost every woman in this place. Do you believe that?"

Paris shook her head, her eyes bulging. Her hand shook so much that the ice in her glass threatened to rattle and pop out like jumping beans.

"It's the good looks part, right?" the man asked.

She wanted to look to the elevator, and in her head, she played out how much time she would have before he caught her. Could she make it in time? Would the doors shut before the man stuck his callused hand through?

"My name is Giovanni De Luca. But I am called Johnny. My mother was a *boche,* and my father a *wop.* I'm a hired gun who kills because I'm told to. A man who murdered a faithful husband and father with two young girls of his own. After killing this devoted family man, I scurried off like a rat to a cabin in

273

Wisconsin with two of my friends and a nigger hooker I met at The Moonlight Hotel. Do you believe that?"

Paris couldn't even shake her head, let alone speak—the fear surging through her veins was too great.

"You are a tough one... alright... My name is Michael Dimonkowski, but people know me as Mickey Diamond. I owned the distillery Valcoro had Capuano, Di Salvo, and De Luca burn down. My brother-in-law, Earl Kowalski, was murdered by those three. I had to explain to my sobbing, heartbroken sister why her husband was dead. Why her children's father was gunned down. Capuano is dead, but Di Salvo and De Luca are still roaming around Chicago. Do you believe that?"

"Yes," Paris said, finally summoning the courage to speak.

"I gave you my word that I would tell you the truth if you guessed correctly. I am Mickey Diamond. Now it is your turn to tell me your name."

"Paris."

"I am glad you told me the truth. I do not like being lied to. Now, my sister identified your boyfriend and his friends to the police. That was a mistake, because a man nicknamed The Cardinal told your boy toy and his deviant dogs the buttons were looking for them. And the four of you fled to Wisconsin. I told my sister to tell the police she was mistaken, that those weren't the men who took Earl. Do you know why?"

"So you can find them yourself..."

"That's right. I don't want the police to arrest them. I decide their fate."

"What do you want?" she asked, steadying her shaking voice.

"I want to know where Di Salvo and De Luca are."

"I don't know. I haven't seen them since we got back."

Mickey Diamond stared at her and then smiled. "Now it's my turn to judge if you are lying. A bit more nerve-racking from that spot, is it not?"

"I'm not lying," Paris said with a sure voice.

She had spent years of her life in fear of dominating men, and she wouldn't fall back into that pit again.

"I think you are being honest with me. I will be asking this question again and again. I will know when you are lying. And if you do, I'll string you up a tree and hang you like was done with your nigger ancestors."

He dug his finger into her glass, pulling out one of her maraschino cherries. "Thanks for the company."

He tossed two quarters into her glass. They sunk like two torpedoed ships. And with that, Mickey Diamond left.

Saying Goodbye

S aying goodbye is never easy. Johnny had gone to dozens of funerals for his grandmother's friends. In such gatherings, he had always heard a certain quote: "It was their time." Johnny never believed that. He was selfish with those he loved. He wanted them here. But even if he accepted that rationale for the gravely sick and old, it did not apply to the hundreds of young men he had personally seen die. Anyone who said "It was God's will" to him would have had their face introduced to his fist. Those men had been too young to die in France, and Tomato had been too young to die in Wisconsin.

It would only take a blank stare from Johnny for Tomato to know what nightmare visions were playing out behind those blue eyes. Most would think Johnny was daydreaming. But Tomato knew the truth. He knew it wasn't a daydream filled with a beach, a hot sun, a cold drink, and a beautiful woman. It was a nightmare. A nightmare of mud and grime, of bullets and barrages, of screams and whistles, of standing at a ladder in a trench, waiting for a whistle to signal devils and demons it was time to feast on flesh. A site of Armageddon.

The Bible had quotes for every event, and growing up attending church two to three times a week, Johnny had many memorized. But there were so many that he couldn't appreciate as a child. For instance, Isaiah chapter 13, verse 9: *"Behold the day of the Lord cometh, cruel both with wrath and fierce anger, to lay the land desolate: and he shall destroy the sinners thereof out of it."*

That day had come, and not just once, but every day from July 28 1914 to November 11 1918. 1,567 days of carnage. 1,567 days of genocide. 1,567 days the devil roamed free.

Tomato had recognized the demons living behind Johnny's eyes because they had lived behind his too. He didn't need to ask, "Something wrong?" or "Why are you so down?" An encouraging nod from Tomato was a hand that yanked Johnny out of the trench. It was the ship ride home. It was the comfort in knowing that whatever Hell he had faced, Tomato had too. And now, that comfort was gone.

Grief and guilt were two snarling beasts locked in battle in Johnny's stomach. They were two titans, but far from the only emotions fighting for supremacy. Overshadowed by the behemoths were dread and worry—two small, but venomous snakes. He had to tell Lorraine about Tomato. That toxic thought slowly destroyed all others.

Over there, there had been plenty of jobs no soldier wanted to do. Digging trenches at the risk of enemy fire was a suicide mission, but he'd rather dig a hundred trenches than have to deliver the news that a mother's son or a wife's husband had been killed. An astounding total of 116,516 American mothers and wives had had to be told their beloved son or husband had been killed. Notification officers had only to drive up the street to deliver the next heartbreaking news. News delivered in seconds that would have a lifetime's impact. Johnny didn't have the courage to do it even once.

For over an hour, he sat in the car in front of Tomato's apartment building. The heat inside was hell fire, but to Johnny, it was penance for his sins.

Hotsy sat in silence, his arm hanging out of the open passenger window, a blank expression on his face. Three stories up, Lorraine Capuano and her two girls were oblivious to the fact that the man they loved was dead.

"You okay?" Hotsy asked.

"An ocean away from okay," Johnny answered.

The subtext to Hotsy's question was, "Are we going to do this?" But if Hotsy was waiting for Johnny's courage to show, he would die of heat stroke. And yet, they had promised they would be the ones to break the news to Lorraine. A simple creed came to his mind: *Death before Dishonor.*

They had vowed they would tell Lorraine, and Johnny's honor meant more to him than his cowardice.

"You need to keep yourself together when we get up there," Johnny said.

Hotsy nodded, trying to show he would. But everything about Hotsy said otherwise. His eyes were puffy and bloodshot with bags under them from hours of missed sleep. He was gaunt and pale with disheveled hair.

"What are you going to say?" he asked.

Johnny shook his head. "I don't know."

He had never given a speech in public. Never said anything in private that would qualify as a speech either. He'd rather jump in front of a train. But if he had to, he would rehearse until every line was memorized. But saying out loud that Tomato was dead even once would destroy him. He couldn't repeat it.

Johnny opened the car door, and he and Hotsy lumbered inside. Only a couple of weeks earlier, Johnny had been bleeding out, pulling himself up a different set of steps. So much had changed since then. Changes that should have been spread out over years, not days. That crawl up Paris' steps was painless compared to this. With each step, his mind wandered, bringing him back to all the times he and Hotsy had come over for dinner. Times when they had hopped up the steps, two at a time, in order to enjoy Lorraine's meals. But now, he only took one slow step at a time.

Johnny had hoped words would come to mind eventually. But when he stood in front of apartment number 313, his mind remained blank. It was as if his heart, knowing what pain was in store for it, had taken control of his arm and was not allowing it to knock on the door.

But Tomato had been brave. He had stayed behind to face a blizzard of bullets, and if he had the courage to do that, Johnny could knock on a goddamn chunk of wood. He took a deep breath and rapped on the door. Nervousness hit him in the chest like a baseball bat. Emotion curdled in his throat.

"Just a minute," Lorraine called from inside.

Hearing her voice made his heart leap into the pit of his stomach. Hotsy's stare bore into him, but Johnny didn't dare acknowledge it.

The door opened. Lorraine was a tough woman with natural good looks, but she had stopped trying to impress Tomato with lipstick and eyeliner years ago. He wanted her "dolled" up, but a nude face was a small way to get back at him for all of his offenses.

"Good morning, it's about time you came back," she said, pushing the door open further. "Come on in."

Johnny and Hotsy stepped inside and removed their fedoras.

"Did he send you two to report on what mood I'm in? It's early, the sun's out, and I'm feeling great, but there's always time for him to ruin that," Lorraine said, half-joking.

Johnny and Hotsy gave no reaction, and her welcoming smile vanished.

"Where's Tomasso?" she asked.

Mary and Gretchen were reading in the living room, but once they saw Johnny and Hotsy, they sprinted into the kitchen.

"Welcome back Uncle Johnny and Uncle Hotsy. I read two chapters this morning," Gretchen boasted.

"Two? That's not that good. Keep trying," Hotsy said.

It was a performance worthy of accolades and awards.

"Jerk. I bet you haven't read more than a headline in a week," she countered.

"Are you stopping for supper tonight? You cheated in our last competition of who could blow bigger milk bubbles," Mary asked.

"Competition? I thought it was a friendly sparring contest," Hotsy said.

"Is father at work already?" Gretchen asked.

"I miss him," Mary said.

"Girls, can you go to the store and get a gallon of milk and some cheese. I'll need it if you want macaroni for lunch," Lorraine said.

"Can't Hotsy and Johnny take us?" Mary asked.

"No, your legs aren't broken," Lorraine said.

"Here," Johnny said, holding out a few dollars.

"I have money," Lorraine said.

"It's nothing," Johnny assured.

Please take the money. Let me do one good thing today.

Mary Louise grabbed her younger sister's hand and the cash from Johnny's hand, thanking him.

"If you see my daddy, can you tell him to please come home? We miss him awfully much," Gretchen said.

She and her sister skipped out of the apartment. Lorraine brushed her chestnut brown hair away from her eyes. The bun she had tied it up in had come loose during a morning of cleaning. Johnny and Hotsy sat at the kitchen table. He wouldn't even gesture for Lorraine to sit. She didn't take orders, not even suggestions. On her own accord, she sat. The moment had come for Johnny to speak, but the words and the strength needed to utter them continued to evade him. Images of Tomato filled his mind, tightening his chest like it had been put in a vice.

Lorraine's face was grave, tears pooling in her eyes. But she refused to let them fall. She knew where the conversation was headed.

"Lorraine…" Johnny started, but the words curdled in his throat.

"I got to tell her, Johnny. I made a promise," Hotsy said.

His eyes looked strangely broken. He turned to her, looking like a boy in grief. "He's gone, Lorraine…"

"How'd it happen?" she asked, her lip quivering, her stoicism breaking.

"At the cabin in Wisconsin. They came for us, I don't know who. We were cornered. Tomato… he… stayed behind so we could escape. I promised him

I'd tell you how much he loved you and the girls. It's my fault," Hotsy said, now through anguished, unfettered sobs.

"It isn't your fault, Hotsy," Johnny said.

"His body... is it still in Wisconsin?" she asked.

Johnny nodded, brimming with shame. He was the reason everything had happened and why he was at Tomato's table, telling his wife that he was dead. Everything could have been avoided had he just accepted dying on that sidewalk, staring at a sewer grate. But no, he had to see Paris, see something of beauty before he faded into history.

Hotsy bawled into his cupped hands.

"It should have been me, Lorraine. I'll never be able to change that," Johnny said.

"No. He chose his fate. He loved you Johnny. And you, Hotsy... God he loved you both. And he loved the life... more than he ever loved me," Lorraine said.

"That's not true, Lorraine," Johnny said.

Lorraine shook her head at his comment, the truth she knew threatening to overwhelm her. She took a deep breath choking at the devastating task that lay ahead of her. "I... I have to... tell our girls. It's best if you're not here when they return."

Hotsy sobbed uncontrollably. Lorraine reached over and pulled him close, pressing his head against her shoulder.

"You save those tears. You hear me?" she said.

"Yes mam," he said.

He wanted nothing more than to do right by her. But his tears fell like rain.

"We're going to find who did this, Lorraine. I'm going to make this right," Johnny vowed.

"And what are you going to do, Johnny? Make someone else tell a wife that she just became a widow? Force another mother to tell her children that their father is dead? Murdered over a few crates of booze? I guess us mothers can only hope we can tell our children that it was the good stuff. Aged and properly barreled."

She rose from the table.

"Can I have one more word?" Johnny asked.

She glanced to the front door, silently counting the seconds to when her girls would return.

"Can you give us a second, Hotsy?" Johnny asked.

Hotsy nodded, but before leaving, he hugged Lorraine a final time, whispering an apology and pleading for forgiveness. He stumbled to the door and stepped outside. Lorraine stared at Johnny, impatiently waiting for him to speak.

"Tomato wanted you to know that he was sorry… for everything. The booze, the crime… the women. He loved you, Lorraine. The other women… they didn't mean anything to him. In that cabin, he told us you were the thing that kept him on orbit, and without you, he would of spiraled through space out of control. Lost and alone. You were his gravity."

A lone tear trickled down Lorraine Capuano's cheek. Over the course of her life, she had cried rivers for Tomasso Capuano, but there was too much pain now, and she was too proud a person to shed more than a single tear.

"I'm happy he had you. You two had a bond he and I could never have. The War ate at him. He never said a word about it. As far as he was concerned, the years 1917 and 1918 never existed. But he found comfort in being around another soldier. He was always better when he was with you and Hotsy," Lorraine said.

Johnny's stoicism was a submarine. An unfathomable forced pressed against him. If he allowed one crack, one tear, it would be the end of him. But sadness was overpowered by a feeling of self-loathing. He was ashamed, sickened of who he was.

"If you need anything, I mean anything…" Johnny said.

"I know. You were his brother, and Hotsy the son I never gave him. Tomasso had his shortcomings, but he made sure we'd be taken care of," Lorraine said.

Johnny rose from the table, glancing about the place. It would be less of a home now for the Capuanos… and for him.

"You take care of yourself," she said.

Lorraine sat on the couch, waiting for her girls to return, searching for the words to tell Mary and Gretchen they would never see their father again. Lorraine had told him to leave before they got back, and Johnny didn't have the courage, the strength or the heart to hear her tell them their father was dead. Their crying would destroy him. He knew it would.

Johnny slouched to the door, his head hung low. Outside, Hotsy was seated at the top of the stairwell, his head buried between his knees. Johnny put his hand on his shoulder. Hotsy looked up and wiped his tears.

And without warning it came.

He squeezed the railing, stopping himself from tumbling down the steps. He had to get out of the building, away from Tomato's home. He wasn't mad the attack had come. He deserved it. It was a comfort, even if he couldn't breathe. It meant he had some humanity left in him. He was assailed with clairvoyant hallucinations of Lorraine telling Mary and Gretchen about Tomato's death, torturous views of them sobbing.

Let that final breath leave my lungs. End this hell.

When the sunlight massaged his face, the hallucinations vanished, and air returned to his lungs.

And the attack passed.

They drove to The Diner hoping to catch The Immortal at lunch. Neither were in the mood to eat and only ordered Colas to avoid being accused of loitering. It was well past The Immortal's normal lunchtime, but Johnny needed him to be there, and if fate ever needed to be amenable, it was now. He was in desperate need of guidance. Hotsy had looked to Tomato for it, and now, that burden had been passed to Johnny, who had no words of comfort to give. The Immortal had thirty-some years on Johnny, but in those thirty-some years were two lifetimes worth of experience.

But the Immortal was a man of routine, and his normal booth was occupied by a group of geriatric women talking over a bland breakfast of oatmeal and black coffee.

Johnny and Hotsy stayed for a second cola, and having gone twenty hours without food, human grief was temporarily usurped by animalistic hunger. They ordered a slice of meatloaf with mashed potatoes—Hotsy taking it with gravy and Johnny with butter. Needing to eat was only natural, but it always disgusted Johnny that a person could eat after suffering such a loss. It sickened him that while he ate meatloaf, Mary and Gretchen were sobbing in great agony. And it sickened him that after men had stormed out of a trench, and a majority had been killed and/or maimed, the survivors would eat.

After the hunger had been dealt with, the same emptiness descended and settled heavily at the bottom of his stomach alongside the subpar meatloaf. When they were back in the car and had driven every block of the Chicago shoreline, Johnny only knew of one place to go, a place where he, Hotsy, and Tomato went for business and pleasure—The Moonlight. The sun dropped low into the horizon, its white center surrounded by a starburst of blinding orange painted on the cerulean lake.

The exterior of the hotel was lined with smokers, people who had consumed too much and had to vomit along the walls, and those who needed a breath of fresh air. Both sides of the streets had zero open spots to park, forcing Johnny to park further away than normal. They usually had a space saved, but it wasn't uncommon for some politician, policeman, or prohee to take it. He and Hotsy sought the solace of a torch on their walk to the hotel three blocks away. Johnny's only plan for the evening was to consume enough alcohol and reefer to forget who he was and what he was.

Normally, Hotsy would gallop like an excited horse to the hotel. But now, he trudged forward with pained struggle. There had always been excitement, even jubilation, hanging in the air around the hotel. But now there was only dread. Johnny prepared himself for another gut punch at the memories that would come when he stepped into the hotel, but before he could cross the street to the hotel, someone grabbed him. Johnny clenched his fist, ready to deck someone, but when he turned, it was Paris.

"Turn around and follow me. Both of you," she ordered in a grave tone.

Johnny wasn't arrogant enough or dumb enough to think that this had anything to do with her feelings for him. Paris had more dignity than that.

"What's going on?" Hotsy asked.

"Wait until we're in the car. Move quickly," she said.

She pulled Johnny's arm, forcing him into a sprint.

Instinctively, Johnny looked behind them to see if someone was tailing them. Another instinct forced him to sprint past the driver's seat. It was Tomato who always drove. Realizing his mistake, Johnny hurried back around the hood of the car and into the driver's seat. Hotsy was in the back seat, while Paris waited impatiently in the passenger seat.

"Where am I going?" Johnny asked when they hit the first stoplight.

"Just drive," Paris ordered.

"Talk to us, Paris!" Hotsy pleaded.

"The hotel has been sold," Paris said.

Johnny's eyes darted to Paris. "Sold? To who?"

"Capone take it back over?" Hotsy asked.

It was the only thing that would make sense.

"Mickey Diamond owns the hotel now," Paris said.

Johnny's head revolved like an owl to see Hotsy's expression. His dumbfounded look belonged in a cartoon.

"Is Valcoro dead?" Johnny asked.

"I don't know…" Paris said.

"Paris, if Valcoro is alive and sold The Moonlight to Mickey Diamond…" Johnny said.

Hotsy looked from Johnny to Paris, still not connecting the dots.

"That means that Valcoro could have told him where we were in Wisconsin," Paris said.

"What are you saying? That Vencini betrayed us? Why would he do that?" Hotsy asked.

"He hates me, Hotsy. Ratting me out would be easy for him," Johnny said.

"We've been nothing but loyal. We don't take more than our cut! I sat in the jailhouse for three weeks! I could of ratted for a deal!" Hotsy said.

"Diamond offered him his life for the hotel and our location," Johnny said.

"I need to hear it from him, Johnny. If he got Tomato killed, I'll end him," Hotsy said.

Johnny had always had the most reason to dislike Valcoro. Tomato had been wise enough to not trust him. Of the three, Hotsy had the most respect for Valcoro, since he had everything Hotsy hoped to have in thirty years—the power, the wealth, the women. He was also naïve enough to think Valcoro cared about him. The fact Hotsy had vowed to kill Valcoro if he had any hand in Tomato's death spoke volumes of the love he had for Tomato.

"The police won't be looking for you anymore. Diamond had his sister tell the police she was mistaken. He wants to be the one who finds you," Paris said.

But Mickey Diamond would still have the resources of the police at his disposal. They would still hunt for them, only now they wouldn't bother bringing handcuffs.

Johnny ran through the events of the last week—he and Paris on the cabin roof their final night, the barn party, the game of Spin the Bottle beside the fire, the beach where they had made love, fighting the self-appointed mayor and his cabinet, the movie house, the fish boil, cribbage, arriving at the cabin, the gas station in Milwaukee, and...

"Paris, we stayed at the Nettesheims' cabin," Johnny said.

The color faded from his face. His dread was mirrored by the worry in her eyes. Johnny's foot turned into a cinder block, smashing the gas pedal to the floor.

"Cilly ratted us out?" Hotsy asked.

"No, I don't think that's the case," Paris clarified.

Johnny was too nervous to answer. His right arm was draped over the wheel, the fingernail of his left thumb sandwiched between his teeth.

"If she didn't rat us out, then what are you… oh…" Hotsy said.

The dots finally connected.

Revelations

Johnny sped out of the city, and soon the Chicago skyline was a blur in the rearview mirror. As they pulled up to the Nettesheims' apartment building, Johnny's worry morphed into anger. He was out of the car before it had even stopped rocking. He dashed across the street, Hotsy and Paris right behind him. Johnny leapt up the steps and whipped open the front door. He pounded his knuckles on the Nettesheims' wooden door hard enough to leave a dent. It was late, and he hoped that no one answering and no light pouring through the crack in the door could be attributed to them sleeping and not the morbid alternative. His mind filled with how they could have been killed—Clarence shot dead in his favorite chair, Cilly fearlessly defending her family before being shot down. And poor little Wally, the man of the house, defending his fallen parents.

But the deadbolt lock lifted, and the door was pulled open.

Wally was half-way through a yawn, his eyes nearly glued shut. "Johnny!" he exclaimed.

"Wally." Johnny exhaled. "It's great to see you."

It took less than five seconds for Cilly to be beside her son. No mother would be okay with their child answering the door this late at night.

"Everything alright?" she asked.

She was well-accustomed to late visits from Johnny, but being snapped out of sleep was always alarming.

"Can we talk?" Johnny asked.

Cilly knew this was his way of saying that it wasn't a conversation Wally should hear.

"Time to go back to bed, Wally," she said.

"Mom!" Wally said, putting up a fuss.

"Wally, you will be one crabby monster in the morning if you don't go to bed now," Cilly said.

"I'll stop by later… and by later I mean the afternoon," Johnny said, making sure Cilly knew not to expect a knock at two thirty in the morning.

"Fine…" Wally said.

Johnny looked at Paris and Hotsy and breathed a sigh of relief. After Wally had sulked down the hallway, Cilly nodded for them to sit.

"I know you're standing there listening! In your room, now!" Cilly shouted.

Wally groaned from the hallway before his bedroom door closed.

"I know you're still out here!" Cilly called out.

The bedroom door opened once more and then shut. A mixture of maternal intuition and experience gave Cilly the confidence that Wally had indeed gone into his bedroom.

Cilly crossed her arms, a sudden chill sweeping over her. "What's wrong?"

"Cilly, did anyone come here asking about us? After we left for Wisconsin?" Johnny asked.

"Someone did stop here."

Paris and Hotsy shifted further onto the edge of the couch, rigid as wood.

"When?" Johnny asked.

Cilly shrugged. "I'm not sure. A few days after you left."

"Do you know who it was?" Hotsy asked.

289

"He said he was your boss and wanted to make sure you were safe," Cilly said, her eyes darting to all three of them, trying to gauge what was going on.

"Did he threaten you?" Johnny asked.

Cilly shook her head, her eyes swelling with fear now that she knew she had been in a situation that could have been harmful for her, but more importantly, for her husband and son.

"No… I told him where you were because I've heard you mention his name before. Vincent… no… Vencini, that's it."

Johnny ignored Hotsy's volatile scowl.

"Do you still have Clarence's service pistol?" Johnny asked.

"Somewhere, yes…" Cilly said, her eyes the size of silver dollars.

"Just a precaution, Cilly," Paris said.

She slowly nodded, only half-believing.

"Can you get it?" Johnny asked.

Cilly wanted to ask more questions but was too unnerved to form words. Instead, she hurried down the hallway as asked. She came back moments later, the gun dangling from her hand as if it were a poisonous snake.

"Can I take a look?" Johnny asked.

She was more than willing to hand it over. It was a standard issue M1911, holding seven rounds, and the same model Johnny carried. But to Cilly, it was the weapon Clarence had carried when the shellshock had taken him. To her, it was a black magic relic containing part of his soul.

"Hotsy, can you make sure this is in working order?" Johnny asked.

Hotsy took the gun like a seasoned snake wrangler, sat at the kitchen table and started dissembling the weapon.

"How's Wally doing?" Johnny asked.

It was a sincere question but also one that he hoped would stop her wandering mind.

"He's good…" Cilly answered, but her eyes were on Hotsy cleaning the weapon.

Even if it weren't for the fact that Johnny had just asked her to prepare to defend herself with a pistol, her answer was far from genuine. But it was hardly a matter for small talk and deserved its proper moment to be discussed in earnest.

Hotsy cocked the pistol. "It's ready."

"You know how to use it?" Johnny asked Cilly.

Cilly nodded. "My father and I used to hunt… years ago."

"If someone does stop by looking for us, you tell them the truth, okay? Don't lie for me. You need something, you let me know. Anything," Johnny said.

Cilly nodded, not because she was okay with the situation but because it was a nervous habit.

"Nothing is going to happen," Johnny assured her.

Cilly nodded again, more certain this time. Not because of Johnny's words, but because she wouldn't allow anything to happen to Clarence or Wally.

The ride back to Chicago was a silent one. A million thoughts spiraled through Johnny's head, and surely the same could be said of Hotsy and Paris.

"Go to my place. It will be best if you two stay off the grid," Paris said.

Johnny wished there was an alternative. He had already involved her enough. But there was none. He wanted somewhere Hotsy could be safe, and Paris would win any rational argument about there being an alternative.

Johnny's blood had stained the carpeted stairs of Paris' apartment building. Walking up the steps, it was impossible not to imagine how much better off everyone would have been had Johnny never made it up those stairs. His death in place of Tomato's was more than a fair trade, and the Capuano household, no matter what Lorraine said, would take the trade without hesitation.

And, yet again, Paris knew exactly what was going through his mind and cast him an uncomfortably strong gaze. When they reached her floor, Paris opened her door, gestured at Hotsy and Johnny to step inside, and told them to make themselves at home.

Hotsy went to the window sill and lit a cigarette to stifle his emotions. Taking a puff of her Lucky Strike, Paris studied Johnny who was standing half-way between the kitchen and the door. Johnny dug his hand into his pocket for his own torch. The action lessened her worry that he would leave, and she went down the hallway to her bedroom.

Free from her watchful eye, Johnny dashed out of the room, descending the steps three at a time. Where he was going… what he was going to do, he would do alone. There was only one way his night could end. Only one way he would allow it to end. He would barge into The Moonlight and pierce Vencini Valcoro and Mickey Diamond with lead. His life would end too. But that was alright. It was a price he was willing to pay to ensure the safety of Paris, Hotsy, and the Nettesheims. Tomato had been loyal to Valcoro, had worked for him for years. What Valcoro had done, even if he had not meant for Tomato to be killed, deserved to be repaid with justice. The justice of Valcoro encased in his own pine box.

Johnny pushed open the glass entrance door and hurried to his Chevy. He brought the engine to life, the car sounding like an annoyed lion woken from its nap. He put it in drive, but before he could speed away, the passenger door opened, and Paris climbed in. Johnny turned to look at her, waiting for a speech, but she remained silent.

"What are you doing?" he asked, squeezing the wheel in irritation.

"What am I doing? I'm stopping *you* from doing something stupid," she replied.

"You have to get out of the car, Paris."

"You first."

"I'm just going for a drive."

"Good. I could use a drive."

"Paris, just go."

"I know where you're going."

"Yeah?"

"Yes."

"And where's that?"

"To The Moonlight, so you can go out in a blaze of glory trying to kill Vencini or Mickey Diamond or maybe both."

"Tomato's death doesn't go unavenged."

"That's not what I'm asking."

"What are you asking? That I just sit here and let the people around me be at risk? No, I'm not okay with that… You need to get out of the car."

"I won't do that."

She was annoyingly calm and non-confrontational, patiently staring ahead. Johnny bit his lip.

"Get out of the car," Johnny ordered again.

Paris repositioned herself on the seat. "Drive."

"What? Just get out of the car and go back inside."

"Drive."

Johnny hesitated. Knowing the sun would rise before she would leave the car, Johnny had no choice but to go back inside or drive. He couldn't stand being cooped up in apartment like a bird in a dangling cage, so he turned the car onto the street.

"And where am I driving to?"

"Drive to the lakefront."

Paris had all the power. She knew Johnny wouldn't put her in harm's way. But that didn't mean he had to like the situation he was in, and he stayed silent on the drive to the lakeshore.

Johnny parked in a vacant lot overlooking the now black-marble façade that was Lake Michigan. Paris was silent, allowing the waves to fill the car with their methodical, almost hypnotic, music. Why they were there, he hadn't a clue. Was it to remind him of their night in Wisconsin? Was it to take him to the coldest spot in Chicago and get him away from the unrelenting heat? Or was it merely to keep him away from The Moonlight?

Paris broke her long silence. "You asked me about my step-father…"

Johnny turned to face her, neither upset nor annoyed. She had always been quick to change the subject whenever her past was mentioned. Whatever had happened was something that had affected her profoundly and still affected her.

"What I'm about to tell you I've only told my mother," Paris said.

The significance of that statement was not lost on him. The fact that she was going to reveal something deep in the inner-level of her own maze that she had revealed only to her mother meant she trusted him with her words, with her memory.

She looked into Johnny's cobalt blue eyes. For the first time since he had known her, her eyes, which had always been a fortress, had lowered their drawbridge, raised their gates, and what had once been utterly impenetrable, was now completely vulnerable.

"When I was thirteen, my mother, my step-father, and step-siblings went swimming in the lake. A beach like this one. It's funny how nothing has changed, you know? It's twenty years later but looking at the water, it seems like it was minutes ago. Anyway... I... I had to use the bathroom. I was the only one. My step-sister, Credence, was the type who had to go every twenty minutes, and I would have to take her, but when I had to go she didn't, and I would have to go alone. But my step-father offered to walk with me. The beach had one of those poorly kept, seldom cleaned restrooms, you know? He came in with me. I thought it was odd. I was thirteen, not three. He stood outside the stall, and when I came out, he asked if I was clean. He insisted on helping me wash. He said that the beach had a strict hygiene policy..."

She paused, granting herself a small reprieve.

"He put his hand down my bathing suit and forced two fingers inside me. He broke my hymen. I bled, I was in pain... scared... shocked. So many emotions fought for control over how I responded that I just stood there. After he removed his fingers, he splashed water on me to clean me. Then he told me it was okay to be embarrassed, and that he wouldn't tell anyone that I had gotten my period. He made me think that I had done something wrong, and that he was being this great man and father figure by not telling anyone," Paris said.

294

He had never been more drawn to Paris than he was at that moment. Not because of her heartbreaking experience but because of the strength in her voice. There was a time when speaking those words out loud would have caused her voice to crack and tears to swell in her eyes. A time when the mere sight of a beach would have devastated her. A time when memories haunted her and drained her happiness from her like a black hole. But Paris had picked herself up over and over again. Paris had found her way out of her trench, and now, it could do her no further harm.

"What did your mother do when you told her?"

"Nothing. I think she believed me, but she had lost one husband, and Josh, my step-father, had a good job. You have to understand that being a single mother is already difficult. It's nearly impossible when you're colored."

His eyes were locked onto her. He wouldn't let anything he did make her think he didn't want to hear what she was telling him. He would do nothing to break her trust.

"I didn't understand that at first," Paris said. "I don't think I really understood until quite recently. Maybe I'm just understanding now. The worst thing is... I thought I was in the wrong for so long. I thought I was disgusting. And then, when I realized I had done nothing wrong, I hated myself for allowing it to happen. I was furious I let him force his fingers inside me. I hated my mother, I obviously hated him, I hated his children, I hated men his age... I hated the world for what it had done to me. And from that self-loathing, that terrible dark place my mind had wandered to came a promise, a pledge, a vow. I would not let that moment define me. Wouldn't let it make me live half a life, be afraid, be hateful. He took so much from me, I wouldn't let him take more."

"Is that why you can do what you do?"

"Any man that touches me, it's because I allow it. The thing that had kept me in that dark place... I use it for my gain. I am choosing what happens in my life."

"What are you trying to tell me?"

His eyes remained fixed on hers. Paris grabbed his hands.

295

"I wanted revenge, Giovanni. I thought of killing him. If I did, I'd be in prison right now. My life would have been over. He stole something from me. Something I'll never get back. My childhood… my innocence. He changed who I was. I'm a different person because of what he did. The little girl I was… she died in that bathroom. But I let his actions of two minutes take years of my life. I wouldn't give him the whole thing. And I won't let you give yours."

"Vencini ratted us out because of my heritage."

"Would you quit that? Vencini's actions are his and his alone. Most people learn that the sun doesn't revolve around them, but I guess you missed that."

That last jab caused a slight smile.

Paris had said she wanted to help people cope with things they had experienced. And now, he knew why. Paris had done it alone and knew how difficult that was.

"I don't want you to work at The Moonlight anymore," Johnny said.

"Why? I thought we were finished?" Paris asked.

"Because you have my heart, and I want yours. But you have to promise me, Paris, even if it's a false promise, that you won't get hurt because of me."

Paris gently cupped his face with both of her hands. "Would you ever hurt me?"

"I'd tear my own heart out first."

"Then everything else is out of your control."

Even in the darkness, Johnny could see her eyes. How one person could exude so much strength he didn't know. She had made it out of her trench with no one to help her. No one to confide in who had shared the same fate. No family. No friends. Without question, Paris Dawson was the strongest person he had ever met.

"Should we head back?" she asked.

"Nah, the sun will rise soon."

Losing

To counter the questions Hotsy would most likely ask, Paris and Johnny returned with maraschino cherries and oranges to sell the lie that they had gone to the store.

While Hotsy and Johnny were caged inside her apartment the next day, Paris insisted on returning to The Moonlight to gain information. Johnny was adamantly against the idea, but Hotsy was eager to know what was going on. Not that it mattered what the vote was. Paris could have been out-voted a thousand-to-one, and it would have made no difference. She had her mind made up, and no one was going to change it. It irritated Johnny, but he admired her stubbornness all the same. But if she was allowed to leave, Johnny was more than willing to leave the apartment and try to catch The Immortal at the diner, banking on the hope that his daily dinner time hadn't changed, and Johnny's relationship with him was unknown to outside parties.

Being cooped up was just a small fraction of the reason Johnny wanted to see him. In a few days, The Immortal would leave Chicago, and Johnny was willing to risk his life to say goodbye. No one had given Johnny better advice during his time in Chicago than The Immortal. The Cardinal had given great counsel, but it had all been on behalf of Valcoro. Hotsy would have gone to him. Johnny liked to think The Cardinal didn't know about Valcoro's betrayal, and if he had known, he would have advised against it. Not because he was a pacifist by nature, but because Johnny, Tomato, and Hotsy were members of a brotherhood. Brothers who held their silence when words could have incriminated, declined bribes when money or power was offered, and who had shot and been shot at for defending Valcoro.

Upon entering the diner, Johnny and Hotsy scanned the room not only for The Immortal but also for men who looked suspicious. Johnny didn't know any of the usual suspects of the diner by name but had seen them enough to know they were there for a meal and not a hit. A sense of comfort swept over him when his eyes fell upon The Immortal at his habitual booth. It wasn't right that soon he would never sit there again.

Johnny and Hotsy slid into the seat in front of him. His plate was empty apart from his used napkin, which was neatly folded beside it. And while most people made a newspaper look like it was a thrashing lake trout, he had it folded so neatly that only the article he wanted was visible.

"I heard a lot of rumors. I'm happy to see not all of them were true," The Immortal said.

"But some were," Johnny said.

"Some were," The Immortal agreed, knowing what it meant.

The waitress returned to clear his plate and silverware and asked how everything was. The Immortal assured her everything had been fantastic.

"I'm sorry about Tomato. He was an honorable man," The Immortal said after she had left.

It didn't seem like there would ever be a time when it was easy to talk about what had happened. People would say it had only been days. But the War had been eight years ago, and that wasn't any easier to talk about now than it had been on the ship ride home.

"It was Vencini who ratted us out," Hotsy said.

"Ratted you out?" The Immortal asked.

"He gave our location to Mickey Diamond," Johnny said.

For the first time since Johnny had known him, The Immortal looked confused.

"Mickey Diamond killed Two Shits. Vencini would never make peace with him. This whole thing escalated because he couldn't understand that death is part of the business. Everything was personal," The Immortal said.

"We have it on good authority that Vencini was asking around where we were," Hotsy said.

The Immortal took a sip of his coffee. How anyone could want to drink something hot in this godforsaken heat was beyond Johnny's understanding.

"Vencini or a man *claiming* to be Vencini?" The Immortal asked.

Johnny and Hotsy looked at each other, both feeling shocked and stupid. Why hadn't they asked Cilly what the man looked like?

"Listen, I have had my differences with Valcoro. He never liked me because of my heritage, but the man wasn't a traitor. He loved Two Shits like you loved Tomato. You wouldn't make peace with Mickey Diamond if he had a gun to your head, offered you a million dollars and the chance to sleep with Gloria Swanson," The Immortal said.

"What are you saying?" Hotsy asked.

"Has anyone heard from Valcoro?" The Immortal asked.

"He sold The Moonlight," Johnny answered.

The Immortal had brought his cup to his lips but paused after hearing that. "Sold The Moonlight? That place is his home. To say that is suspicious is putting it lightly. None of this seems right."

Johnny nodded.

"Just be careful. Keep your head on a swivel," The Immortal said.

"Can you give us a moment?" Johnny asked Hotsy.

Hotsy nodded and stood. "We'll see you later, Jack," he said before heading for the exit.

"When do you leave?" Johnny asked.

"Tomorrow after breakfast," The Immortal replied.

Johnny was silent, deep in thought.

"Say what's on your mind, kid," The Immortal said.

"Can you do me a favor?" Johnny asked.

Johnny preferred visiting the Nettesheims without Hotsy and Tomato. Alone, he could trick himself into thinking he lived a normal life. But The Moonlight wasn't safe, and asking Hotsy to go back and sit in Paris' apartment was like putting a dog in a kennel on a bright, sunny day.

When they arrived, the neighborhood baseball game was already under way. Written in chalk on the sidewalk was a column tallying the innings, runs, hits, and errors. Currently the "A" team was up 4–3 in the fourth inning. Johnny stopped his Chevy well short of the Nettesheims' apartment building. Wally was out in center field, slapping his hand into his glove, attempting to fight off boredom. The street was narrow, and since the left and right field was responsible for stopping the ball from hitting any windows, the taller kids were forced to play those positions.

The freckled, red-headed batter hit a weak grounder to third and was thrown out, ending the inning. Wally jogged over, wearing his newsboy cap on his head and a proud smile on his face.

"Stay out of center field today, will you?" he said.

"You got it," Johnny said.

"How you doing, kid?" Hotsy asked.

"Not bad. We're in a tight one. I'm scheduled to bat fourth this inning, so if someone can get on, you can see me hit," Wally said in a "if you're interested" sort of way.

"Wouldn't miss it," Johnny said.

Johnny and Hotsy sat on the stoop. With the sun blocked, they removed their fedoras and hung them on their knees.

The first two batters did not give the pitcher much of a fight unless you counted him having to dodge and duck when the batter inadvertently let go of the bat.

"Should have parked further away," Hotsy teased.

The third batter managed to rip one past the short stop and advanced to the chalk-drawn first base. Wally held up his hand for a pause, and, holding the bat like it was William Wallace's greatsword, dashed over to Johnny.

"How's this?" he asked, taking his stance.

"Tuck in your left elbow a bit more. Make sure you move your hips into your swing," Johnny said.

Wally nodded and retook the batter's box.

"If this pitcher strikes him out, I'll steal his chewing gum," Hotsy said.

The first pitch sped past. Wally hacked at it, slicing nothing but air. The second one faired marginally better. Johnny wanted to see Wally send one to Northbrook, not only for Wally's sake—striking out was embarrassing even if it was part of the game—but also for the poor pitcher and his gum.

The third pitch came. Wally swung, grunting from the torque. The bat connected with the ball. It whistled through the air, soaring over the pitcher's head...past second base... toward the outfield. Wally's eyes lit up like two stars as he watched the ball soar like a comet through space. But the comet crashed toward earth and fell into the center fielder's glove. Wally dropped the bat in frustration and threw his cap against the pavement.

"I suck! I can't do anything," he said.

Johnny stood from the stoop and went to Wally.

"Hey..." he said in a soothing voice.

"I can't do it, Johnny. It's so hard to learn how to hit listening to a radio. I need to see it," Wally said.

"That was a great hit, Wally."

"Were you even watching, Johnny? I flew out!"

"You swung at the wind on that first pitch, almost got the second. But you were in an O-two count. The fact that you even connected on the third pitch is impressive. You get a bit more patient, get the pitcher behind in the count, you get an even better ball to hit."

Wally reluctantly nodded.

"You can't always be at your best—" Johnny said.

"But you can always give your best," Wally said.

"Now, go back out there, and let it go."

Wally nodded and jogged out to center field.

Johnny returned to the stoop. Cilly was there, an appreciative smile etched on a melancholic face.

"Can I speak with you?" she asked Johnny.

Johnny nodded. Hotsy rose from the stoop without being asked and strutted down the sidewalk toward right field.

Cilly and Johnny sat on the stoop. She was silent for a while, staring across the street. But like Johnny, it wasn't the street or the baseball game she was looking at. There were a hundred thoughts bouncing back and forth in her head.

"I'm sorry about last night, I didn't mean to involve you," Johnny said.

"You didn't add any more worry than I already have," she said.

But those were not the words she had come outside to deliver. He could only wait patiently until she spoke what was truly on her mind.

"I'm losing him…" Cilly said.

"Who? Clarence?" Johnny asked.

She shook her head. "No… I'm afraid I lost him years ago."

It was the first time he had ever heard her show any signs of abandoning hope. Had it been a recent conclusion? Or something she had realized a year back? Or had it been a truth she had accepted the moment she had first hugged Clarence when he had returned home from war? The moment her eyes had met his blank, almost lifeless ones? Maybe that truth was what Cilly had buried in the center of her own maze. Like Johnny, she had ignored, denied, and refused it for as long as she could.

"You can't think that, Cilly," Johnny said, almost begging her.

Cilly turned to look at him, looking as if she hadn't been holding in tears for minutes but, years. Because she had been.

"Your strength gives him strength. You hold onto hope. You haven't lost him. He's in there," Johnny said.

"I wish you could have known him before, Johnny. He could command a room with his silent, mysterious demeanor. And what a dancer he was. There wasn't a night we didn't dance. I'd be doing the dishes, and the record player would start playing. I'd turn around, and he'd be standing there, offering his hand... and his smile..."

It was a bittersweet recollection that brought joy and heartbreak. Johnny could only look on with sorrow. The past and future had always been tormenting and terrifying to him. They attacked him from behind, from the front, from every conceivable angle, and he was powerless against their onslaught. His past had hardly been exemplary. It represented missed opportunities, regrets, mistakes, and great, profound memories. Memories that had shaped the man he'd become—the good and the bad. Memories of things that could never be again. Of people who had passed away. But so much of his past he longed to forget.

To some, the future was an exciting slate of infinite possibilities, a promise of better things to come. But to Johnny, it was only a reminder of his shortcomings, of all he had failed to do, of the fact that nothing had changed. The thoughts he had hoped would leave his head hadn't and wouldn't. If it wasn't the past that afflicted him, it was the future, and vice versa. Their attacks were relentless and as a result, Johnny was never able to live in the here and now. Paris had spoken about how life was like a car ride, and her description couldn't have been more accurate. She understood what harm the past could do more than anyone else, except for maybe Cilly. She was haunted the very same way, and it had created an unbreakable bond between Cilly and him.

"I'm losing Wally," Cilly delivered in a truly heartbreaking, matter-of-fact way. "He doesn't understand why his father isn't normal. And soon that will turn into contempt, even hatred. What happened the other day...Art E Lee... it broke my heart. He can't think back to how Clarence was, like I can. He can't draw on those memories to get him through. He never knew the man his father was," Cilly said.

Memories are treacherous things. They have the power to cause pain or relief. Bring joy or sorrow. Comfort or torment. Cilly had thousands, maybe millions of memories of Clarence Nettesheim. They powered her through the tough days, and God knows there were many. They comforted her when she cried herself to sleep. They allowed her to dream of a day when Clarence would once again be the man who had enchanted her and made her fall madly in love. It was a hopefulness and respite her son was not afforded. He had no great memories to dwell on. His memories tormented him, embarrassed him, and brought him to tears. Memories of having to throw his baseball against the brick wall rather than playing catch with his father, of having to learn how to swing a bat by listening to the radio, of shivering in bed because there was no one to get the heater working in winter. Cilly was a phenomenal mother. All children deserve such a mother. Her sole purpose was Wally. Everything she did was an attempt to better his life. When everyone in Wally's class had gotten yoyos, Cilly had scraped every cent she had to buy him one, so he wouldn't feel left out. When food was short, it was Cilly who went without. But raising him while taking care of Clarence had taken a toll. She looked ten years older than she was. She spent her days exhausted but was offered no relief with sleep. There were too many things to worry about for her to have that comfort. Stress had eroded her joyous smile, wrinkling her face. The wedding photo hanging on the wall behind Clarence's chair was of two people who no longer existed.

"You're not losing him, Cilly. He just doesn't understand right now. He will," Johnny said.

Cilly looked to him, wanting to say something but deciding against it.

"What is it?" Johnny asked her gently.

"Would you talk to him? Not today, but soon?" she asked.

There was fear and worry in her eyes. Johnny had never seen that level of desperation in her. Not even when she had been starving and facing eviction.

Money was a necessary evil for Cilly. Money was the end goal of so many people, but once someone you love is taken from you, money becomes nothing more than paper. Cilly only wanted her son to be happy. It was a motive Johnny never questioned, and for that, he trusted the Nettesheims on a level he did few others.

"I will. I promise."

Paris Blitzed

The Moonlight was packed in the middle of the afternoon, not surprising considering it was a Saturday. It had gotten busier quicker than normal, and bands that normally played for only hotel staff and a few "lifers" of the hotel now played to a packed house, going from opening act to headliner.

Paris stood by the bar, sipping from her glass of lemon-lime soda. The high sun poured through the window across the room, warming her skin in a relaxing sunbath. But the sunlight vanished. She turned to see what had caused this sudden disappearance. A gigantic man blocked every bit of light the sun could provide. He ordered a pint of beer, his voice a mile deep. The pint looked like a shot glass in his hands. Paris couldn't help but stare. He was a man who could have been employed to wrestle a bear.

"You work here?" the man asked in a thick Irish accent.

It was no surprise her staring had not gone unnoticed.

"I do," Paris answered.

"What's your name?" he asked.

"Paris," she replied.

"Sean O'Malley," he said, extending his gigantic hand. His forearm was as thick as a python after it had fed.

Paris shook his hand.

"You work for Mickey?" she asked.

O'Malley nodded in the middle of his gulp of beer. One gulp equated to half the pint. Was there enough beer in Chicago to get the man drunk?

"How much did he need to fork out to buy this place from Vencini?" she asked.

"Let's say he got a bloody good deal on it," O'Malley said with a grin.

Even though he was a foot taller than Diamond and had every right to be more intimidating, his grin was more genuine and humane.

Paris tried to hide her worry with a smile of her own. "He let Mickey keep everything in his room too. Must have been a persuasive conversation."

"Aye, best negotiator in the city."

A posse entered the hotel through the revolving door. Somewhere in the middle, wearing a white fedora with a red trim and a King of Diamonds playing card pinned to it and a fat cigar tucked in the corner of his mouth was Mickey Diamond.

Paris had been told Diamond usually didn't arrive at the hotel until well after seven, and she consulted the clock behind the bar to see if Diamond was early or if she had lost track of time. It was only twenty after five. She had intended to get as much information as she could and be gone before Diamond arrived. That plan had failed. She wore a svelte black dress, colorless in comparison to the reds, greens, blues, silvers, and golds of her counterparts. But she was the only black person in the room, making her, in an ironic switch, the only person in color in a black and white lobby. She had hopes O'Malley would continue blocking her from view, leaving her free from the sun's glow and hidden in the darkness of space. But the man set his empty pint down and was at Diamond's side in four strides. The sunlight which had been a safe blanket, a welcomed friend, now betrayed her, and was nothing more than a spotlight.

"Ms. Dawson," Diamond called out.

Paris summoned her nerve, turned and forced a smile on her face. "Mr. Diamond."

"Sean, will you see to it that Miss Dawson is treated well in my room. I will be up there shortly," Diamond said.

O'Malley was surprised to find that the woman he had been chatting with was of some importance to his boss. But his hand, which had given her a shockingly soft handshake, now grabbed her shoulder like the jaws of an alligator and forced her toward the elevator bank. When they were inside, his broad shoulders nearly stretched end to end. He leaned back, bending his legs to avoid bumping his head on the ceiling.

"What does he want?" Paris asked.

O'Malley ignored her comment. However irrational it was, she half-expected some unfathomable monster to be waiting for her when the doors opened. But the elevator opened to an empty suite.

Hygiene did not appear to be a priority for Mickey Diamond, so she had expected the room to be filthier than it had ever been under Valcoro. But, to her shock, the suite was probably the cleanest room in the hotel. It smelt of a mixture of cigar smoke, citrus, and lavender.

O'Malley stood in front of the entrance, blocking her escape, but he allowed her to walk about the room. Paris considered the idea of retrieving a knife from the knife block on the kitchen counter, but O'Malley pulled a pistol and held it by his side. She would be shot dead before she even got within stabbing distance. Even if he didn't have the gun, killing him would require a miracle. She couldn't reach his neck or even his heart. It would take multiple stabs to kill him, but only one strong punch from him to knock her out of the fight.

She was trapped inside. She waited and waited by the kitchen island, the nerves in her stomach like bees fleeing their hive. It was after six when the elevator finally *pinged*. The doors opened, and unlike before, the monster she had expected was real this time. The mobster stepped out and entered the suite.

"Sean, would you see to it that Mr. Valcoro joins us?" Diamond asked.

"You got it, boss," O'Malley said.

He disappeared into the elevator. O'Malley assuredly wasn't the tallest man in the world. Somewhere in the uncharted areas of the world were men tall as trees, but here in Chicago, no one compared to him in size. The fact he worked for Diamond and not the other way around was unnerving.

"What do you want to talk about?" Paris asked.

Her voice was steady. It came as second nature. If a woman of The Moonlight couldn't hide her true feelings, men would limp out of the hotel, dejected and embarrassed, and never return.

"Oh, I think you know. I have to say, I am disappointed you did not take my threat seriously. Very disappointed," Diamond said, removing his fedora and setting it on the kitchen island.

The chicken pox and acne scars on his face were more pronounced without his drooping fedora covering half of his forehead.

"I haven't seen them," Paris said.

Diamond revealed his yellowing, rotting teeth with a disgusting smile. He stayed silent. How long the silence lasted was hard to say. Realistically, no more than a minute, but to Paris, it was a decade. She hoped anything would break it. And something did—the elevator. It *pinged* and opened a third time. A long white sheet-covered cart was pushed into the room. Food service wasn't an uncommon thing, but the hotel had dozens and dozens of waiters and waitresses to do that. The fact that O'Malley was pushing it told Paris it wasn't fresh lobster and biscuits under the white cloth. Once the cart was inside the room, O'Malley yanked off the white covering, revealing a pine box.

"Come here," Diamond ordered Paris.

She had little choice, but she'd rather walk on her own than be dragged. With each step, the lightheadedness setting in worsened.

"Put your ear to it," he ordered.

She refused, shaking her head and stepping back. He grabbed her by the back of the head and pushed her face against the casket.

"Do you hear it?" he asked.

Paris heard nothing but her own heartbeat thumping inside her throat. But then there was a faint *knock*. Whatever or whoever was inside was pounding on the lid. Paris screamed, her stomach leaping into her throat. But her shock morphed into fear, worry, and—though she would have been ashamed to admit it—intrigue. She wanted to know, needed to know who was inside.

"Open it," Diamond ordered O'Malley.

O'Malley obliged, grabbing a crowbar from under the cart and prying it open. After it was loose, O'Malley lifted the cover off. A fetid smell flooded out like a poisonous gas. Rising out of the coffin like a reanimated zombie was Vencini Valcoro.

"Tough night of sleep?" Diamond asked.

Valcoro gasped for air. Though he coughed violently and thrashed about, he looked as though he had already died days ago.

"Hotel occupancy has been a hundred percent since Mr. Diamond took ownership, so Valcoro's been staying in the coffin for the last few days. Don't worry, we check on him every hour or so to make sure he's still breathing," O'Malley said.

The stench radiating from Valcoro was putrid. He had a mess of his own making in the casket, and the smell of stale urine and ripe feces attacked her senses. It was enough to make her gag.

After the shock of the smell settled, she was able to fix her eyes on Valcoro. His face was swollen and bruised, masked in shades of blue and purple, his lips were cracked, and his left eye, swollen shut. When he gasped for the ever-evasive breath, she could count at least two missing teeth.

"Let me tell you something about my sister," Diamond said, "She is a strong woman. I see that sort of strength in you. Maybe we have nigger blood somewhere back in the family. Who knows... Now, I never particularly liked Earl. You know, as a protective brother, I don't know if I would have liked anyone being with my sister. He was weak, soft hands, virgin face. But he allowed Ellie to be strong and run the house. I could respect that. He was always asking about working for me, but Ellie wouldn't have it. He was not meant for this life.

He was not made of stone or steel like most of us. He was made of butter. But they was tight on money, and he did not want handouts. I respected that most of all. He wanted to do right by me. And he was a good father, a damn good one. When your boyfriend and his pals burned down my distillery, I was rightfully upset. It was no secret I wanted them dead. Earl asked me, just short of begged me, to let him deliver the retaliation. Bless his heart for asking, but I honored the wishes of my sister. But Earl took matters into his own hands. Do you know what your boyfriend and his friends did to him?"

Paris stayed silent, her gaze locked onto his maniacal gray eyes.

"They broke his cheek and jaw… he was missing teeth. If I had to guess based on my experiences, they used a blunt object—a bat, a crow bar, tire iron, golf club, something like that. Then they shot him in the chest a handful of times. I could not get down to the morgue before my sister did. She was sobbing on his cold, lifeless chest when I got there. She had called me after the police… right after your boyfriend and his friends took him… called me up sobbing, barely speaking English, reverting back to the old language. I promised her I would find the men who took him, and I would put them in the ground. Now I have fulfilled thirty-three percent of that promise. I am here for the other sixty-seven."

Paris remained quiet, but only a person who was dead inside couldn't be moved imagining Earl Kowalski's widow weeping over his lifeless body. Women could be equally malicious as men, but Kowalski's children, like all children, were pure and innocent. What a terrible thing it was for a young child to have to mourn over a parent's lifeless body.

"You stay the hell away from my men!" Valcoro growled.

He had finally found his breath. He grabbed the edge of the coffin with both hands, steadying himself.

Diamond smiled, admiring the resolve of the old dog. "Even De Luca? I hear you don't like mutts, Vencini?"

"He may be a *boche*, but at least he ain't a Polack like you," Valcoro said.

Diamond grinned again, his breath as foul as the casket.

311

"You don't have none too many loyal men left. I do not see anyone storming the castle to save you. That four hundred pound sack of shit you had on that stool? Worms will feast on him for thousands of years, and your little Cardinal? He'll never fly again neither," Diamond said.

Valcoro spat in Diamond's face. Diamond simply wiped it away with his dirty hand with as much indifference as if lake mist had kissed his face.

"You are making me feel bad for framing you, Valcoro. You sold me this place. It was you who ratted out their location in Wisconsin. We paid De Luca's pets a visit. The retard, his dried up old lady, and the young twat in Cicero. Told them that I was Vencini and that I wanted to make sure my men were safe," Diamond said.

"You kill me, you Polish prick. There's enough cops who come here and a big enough price on your head that they'll arrest you and take the promotion that comes with it," Valcoro said.

"Kill you? As in murder? Oh, no, no, no… You died in a tragic accident. Grieving over the death of your pal Two Shits and the guilt of betraying your own men. You drank a bottle of Panther Piss and rode the air down."

Valcoro started to speak but a long hose was shoved deep into his mouth causing him to gag. O'Malley held it in place while Diamond poured a bottle of whiskey into a funnel connected to the hose. Whiskey may have been the desired liquid inside that bottle, but it was mostly industrial alcohol and paint thinner. O'Malley's hand kept Valcoro's head from moving, and with the other, held the hose in place and plugged Valcoro's nose. Valcoro had no choice but to drink. After the whole bottle had been poured, O'Malley ripped out the hose. Valcoro leaned over the edge of the coffin and vomited a blend of bile and whiskey. It splattered onto the floor, narrowly missing Paris.

"I didn't get this batch quite right, did I? Paint thinner was not diluted enough, was it?" Diamond taunted.

He dug his fingers into Valcoro's mouth, grabbing the back of his bottom teeth, and dragged him out of the coffin and onto his feet.

As soon as Valcoro was able to stand on his own, O'Malley drove his stone-like fist across Valcoro's face, sending him and three of his teeth back to the ground, the former landing like a rock, the latter scattering like pebbles.

"Let's turn the clocks back to yesterday, Ms. Dawson," Diamond said. "You spent most of your shift outside, pacing about nervously, smoking four of your Lucky Strikes. Giovanni De Luca and Quintu Di Salvo were seen walking toward the hotel as expected. You went out to meet them. Some went as far as to say you *ran* out to meet them."

Paris' lips formed a guilty curve. Clearly, she had been watched. Diamond knew the truth. She wouldn't even attempt a lie. She would not cater to his demand of falling victim to fear.

"I told you I wanted them. And I told you there would be consequences for lying," Diamond said.

He wound his hand back and slapped her—a noise that went echoing across the suite. It was hardly the first time she had been slapped, but he had a raw, primitive strength in him, and the pain exploded throughout her face. Then he sent a backhand across her face, knocking her to her knees. He dragged her by her hair to the glass table and pinned her against it with his left forearm. With his right hand, he tore her dress and underwear. Clumsily, he unclasped his belt with his free hand and wrapped it around Paris' throat and tightened it. He violently forced himself inside her. She repeatedly tried pushing him off and resisting, but each time she did, he rammed her face against the glass table and yanked the belt tighter. She gasped for breath, her face turning blue.

"Look at that, you turn any more blue, you won't be a nigger no more," Diamond taunted.

Valcoro stumbled forward, striving to help, but O'Malley grabbed him by the neck of his shirt and swung him over the kitchen island. Valcoro collided with the wooden cupboards. The glasses and dishware inside fell to the floor and broke into a dozen pieces.

Diamond's breath was thick and vile. He knew how repulsive he was, but it was the power that got him off. He wouldn't pay for sex. He didn't like consent.

He wanted to feel the fear of the woman he was forcing himself into. He grunted out exhausted breaths, bits of spit hitting her face. Finally, he climaxed with a grotesque grunt. Then he smashed Paris' face through the glass table. She flipped over, landing on her back. Shards punctured and sliced her skin. But there was no respite yet. He drove his boots into her stomach with vicious kicks. Summoning the fight of a wounded animal, Paris grabbed a jagged piece of glass and sliced his leg.

He cursed and kicked her face, putting her in a temporary stupor. He spit on her, then lifted one of the nearby chairs above his head, and drove it down across Paris' back, snapping the chair in the process.

"Where are they? Huh? Where are they hiding?" he yelled, continuing to beat her with his fists and feet.

The blinding sunlight pouring in through the tall, wide glass windows turned to blackness, abandoning Paris. Diamond wound up for another kick but stopped. Paris was unable to even defend herself anymore, and once that happened, it was no longer fun for him.

"Bring Valcoro here," Diamond ordered.

O'Malley grabbed Valcoro by his leg and dragged him to Diamond. Valcoro had been stuffed inside a coffin for days with little water and no food. He had no strength to fight, and even if he had, his prime fighting days were twenty years behind him. But even in his peak physical state, he would have been no match for the Irish giant.

"You could have just sat here in your castle and kept your head to the ground. But no. You wanted my piece of the kingdom. You should not have crossed me," Diamond said.

Valcoro summoned his last bit of strength to raise his head and with a mouthful of spit and blood yelled, "Go to hell!"

"I had hoped that you would realize the depth of your mistakes. But you know, sometimes we don't do that until we have reached bottom. My bottom was having to let my grieving sister punch me in the chest until she couldn't punch no more. And when she couldn't, she cried until she couldn't cry no more. That was my rock bottom. Now it is your turn find yours."

He grabbed Valcoro by both the neck of his shirt and belt and forced him toward the window and shoved him through it. The glass shattered into a thousand pieces with a deafening crescendo. Vencini Valcoro seemed to plummet forever toward the hot, hard concrete.

Escape

How long she lay face down on the carpet Paris didn't know. Its bristles were soft and smelt of citrus, coaxing her into a false sense of comfort. Had it all been a vivid dream? A palpable nightmare? Something or someone lifted her, the movement causing the glass shards to dig deeper into her flesh. Her body had been in a comatose state, mercifully granting her respite from the torturing pain. But now it shot through her body with an uncontrollable tenacity. Her bruised, swollen and cut face ached and throbbed from the kicks, punches, and cuts it had received.

The wind whistled in through the open window and with it came a wave of clarity. No one had lifted her. She had done it herself. The room was empty, but Diamond and O'Malley would return. And they would use her as bait. She would not allow that. She crawled to the kitchen island, grimacing and grunting from the pain. Once there, she pulled herself to her feet. Her head throbbed, the room spun, her legs were weak, threatening to collapse. She was Atlas with the world's weight pressing down on her. Each step was like trudging through knee-high snow.

Even if Diamond and O'Malley took their time in returning, she was not willing to hope time was on her side. Sometimes, the difference between being a victim and a victor was acknowledging you were on your own. Time, faith, grace and luck could never be counted on.

An unknown timer ticked down. Did she have an hour? Minutes? Seconds before someone came up to investigate? Even pushing the elevator button caused pain. When the doors opened, she stepped in and hit the button for the basement. She prayed that the elevator didn't stop at any floor, least of all the lobby. But she clenched her fist, ready to defend herself if the doors opened.

Victim or victor.

She made it to the basement level without the elevator stopping. The hotel basement was dark. Washing machines and dryers lined the back wall. Bins were filled with dirty sheets, towels, blankets, and wash cloths. Shelves were stacked with clean and freshly folded linens. Voices carried from different sections of the basement. Paris crouched behind the hanging sheets and bins of dirty towels on her way to the exit, using the latter as a walker to help her in her weakened state. Opening the door required every ounce of strength she had, and even on a windless day, it seemed as if a massive gust off the lake had tried slamming the door shut on her. Her right arm hung uselessly by her side, and the twelve steps up to street level stretched endlessly before her. She used her left arm to pull herself up, the steps themselves feeling slick as ice.

Her whole body pulsated from the pain. She knew she had minutes before she passed out again. Once she was set on crossing the street, there would be no stopping for oncoming traffic. Once she set her body in motion, it could not stop or there she would stay. Annoyed drivers blared their horns, but their annoyance changed to shock when they saw the condition she was in. She stumbled forward, her left arm outstretched, grasping at air. Two men approached her, their faces indistinguishable. Then her remaining strength drained away in a flash, and Paris fell face-forward on the unforgiving asphalt.

A Solemn Vow

For the second time that day, Johnny found himself at The Diner. It had been Hotsy's decision to meet there at eight forty-five. That was too damn late for supper for Johnny. But Hotsy would be up until four in the morning. Though Johnny didn't plan on staying up until then, he most likely would be. But it wouldn't be on purpose. His mind hadn't shut off at all over the last few days.

Johnny was on time, being punctual by nature. But it was not uncommon for Hotsy to run ten to fifteen minutes late. But he was going on twenty minutes, and with each passing minute, Johnny's annoyance changed. During the zero-to-five-minutes range, all was forgiven. Six to ten minutes late was annoying. Eleven to twenty minutes was irritating. Twenty-one to thirty minutes was infuriating. Anything longer was only worrying. But given all that had happened the last few days, the worrying started in that first window. Somewhere between twenty-five and twenty-six minutes, Hotsy came up to the glass windows with a frantic look on his face. Johnny had seen him right away, but Hotsy saw only his reflection cast back at him. Johnny knocked on the window to get his attention. Hotsy turned and gestured at him to come outside. Johnny rose from his booth and crossed the distance of the diner in ten strides and stepped outside.

"What's wrong?" Johnny asked.

"Vencini's dead," Hotsy said.

A coldness filled Johnny's chest.

"Was it you?" Johnny asked.

Hotsy shook his head. "No."

"Who then?"

"I don't know."

He was nervous, even scared. Hotsy should have looked relieved for what he had said, but his demeanor told Johnny he hadn't said what he had really come to say.

"What is it? What's wrong?" Johnny asked.

Hotsy turned to face him, struggling to find the words to speak. "It's Paris…"

The words drove a knife into Johnny's back, through his heart, and out his chest.

"Diamond got to her… she's alive," Hotsy added, trying to lessen the devastating blow he had delivered.

"Where is she?" Johnny asked.

"She's in rough shape—"

"Where is she?"

"Provident Hospital."

Johnny was in his Chevy before Hotsy had finished speaking. Provident Hospital wasn't the closest hospital to The Moonlight. Not even in the top five. But it was the only one close that treated Negros. In the War, the wounded were treated. It was as simple as that. It didn't matter what God that person prayed to or what the color of their skin was. Doctors took an oath to treat and help those who needed it. But outside war, that Hippocratic oath was loaded with hypocrisy and asterisks.

Provident Hospital was the first American hospital owned and operated by African Americans. Bless the men and women who worked there or only God knew how far Paris would have needed to go for help.

Johnny drove south, laboring to keep the contents of the maze hidden, caged, and buried.

Please don't let Paris be added to the center of it.

"Rough shape" left so much open to interpretation. Yet, his mind filled in the blank spaces with vivid detail and left no room for hope. Paris was in a hospital because of their relationship. He knew the danger he was putting her in, but his greed had overcome his better instincts. Like with all addictions, it was only a matter of time before the desire became a need, and all sense of reason was abandoned. Paris was his vice, his addiction, his sin.

Johnny pulled alongside the entrance of the hospital, leaving his car parked in front of it. What security did with it he didn't care. He stormed to the front desk.

"Can I help you?" the heavyset Negro woman behind the desk asked.

"I'm looking for someone. Paris Dawson," Johnny said, speaking so fast he couldn't blame her if she missed the name.

"Relation to her?" she asked.

The woman studied Johnny. He had only one possible answer, but he had delayed too long for it to be believed.

"I'm sorry, only spouse or immediate family," the woman said.

"Please… I have to know if she's okay," Johnny said.

"Sir, I'm sorry, I can't," the woman said softly.

Johnny did his best to stay calm, the thoughts in his head growing darker, more depressing, and more desolate.

"Listen to me, I need to know," he pleaded.

"Norma, I'll speak with him," a man said.

Both Johnny and the receptionist turned to see a man in his sixties. His once raven black hair and beard were now salted white. Johnny hurried to him. He crossed his arms and nervously stroked his chin with his left hand.

"I'm Dr. Bukater," the man introduced himself.

"Johnny... Can you tell me something, anything, please?"

The doctor stood there, silently debating his course of action. Would he uphold the policies of the hospital or uphold compassion? If hospitals could refuse service to Negros, and in essence, fail to uphold the Hippocratic oath, then a doctor should be able to help someone who clearly cared about the patient in question without facing repercussions.

"Follow me," the doctor said.

Perhaps he had gone through the same thought process as Johnny and had come to the same conclusion. Johnny followed him through a set of doors, up the stairs to the third floor and into the hallway of patient rooms.

"She has severe bruising on her face and torso," the doctor said. "Her right arm is broken... there's more, but it's not my place to tell. We've given her something for the pain, and she's resting now. I can ask her if she'd like to see you, if you'd like?"

Johnny nodded, the doctor's words temporarily eliminating his ability to speak.

The doctor turned toward the closed door. Behind it, bloodied and beaten, was Paris.

"Hey, Doc," Johnny called.

The doctor turned back to face him, his hand resting on the door knob.

"Thank you," Johnny said.

The doctor inclined his head ever so slightly. The blinds were drawn shut, and the doctor slipped through a crack in the door, offering Johnny no view inside the room. The coward in him was thankful for that.

Everyone dislikes hospitals. But they affected Johnny more than the average person. They turned his thoughts toward death and kept them there for weeks. The smells, the polished floors, the bright lights, the white uniforms, he hated all of it. In every room, someone was having the worst time of their life. Standing in that hallway induced a claustrophobic feeling that demanded he race toward the exit.

Nurses moved with a frenetic pace no one moved in when all was well. They dashed in and out of rooms, grabbing clipboards, administering medicine, and answering calls.

And then it came again.

The lights blinded him, reflecting off the polished floors, nearly burning his eyes. He tried to inhale, but all he could take in was the strong smell of industrial cleaning products. He closed his eyes, shielding them from the overpowering lights. But all he saw behind closed eyes were the faces of dead men lined in No Man's Land, his parents' graves, Tomato in that cabin, and now, Paris in that hospital bed.

Breathe in. Breathe out. Breathe in. Breathe out.

The door opened once more, and the doctor ducked out.

And then it passed.

"I'm sorry, but Ms. Dawson doesn't want to see you right now. She's tired," the doctor said.

Johnny glanced at the door, foolishly expecting to be able to see through it and gauge why Paris would say that.

"She calls me Giovanni, can you tell her that?" Johnny asked.

"You're welcome to wait in our waiting room, but I'll have to escort you there," the doctor said, gesturing toward the doors they had come through.

The doctor had shown Johnny remarkable courtesy in revealing Paris' condition, and Johnny wouldn't make him regret that kindness. He followed the invisible line the doctor's hand cast outside where the doctor put a soothing hand on Johnny's shoulder. "She'll come around, son."

Johnny nodded. His mind was on the maze and would divert no cognitive function for speech. He sat on the bench along the wall, staring blankly into the distance the very same way Clarence did.

Did Paris blame him? Did she feel betrayed? Was he now held in the same breath as her stepfather? A million and one questions ran through his mind like the running bulls in Pamplona, each more destructive than the last. He hated every minute of sitting on that bench. But he stayed, hoping a nurse or doctor would emerge from behind those doors and tell him Paris would see him. But even that wasn't good enough. *Would* meant little more than she was willing to tolerate it. What he wanted to hear was that she *needed* to see him, that something deep inside her required him to be in that room. Just like Johnny had needed to make it up those stairs to her apartment. But each time the doors opened, it was only a cruel tease. At midnight, after he had gotten nervous glances from every member of the staff, Johnny rose from the bench and left the hospital. He stormed down the walkway, the horrible feeling of having betrayed Paris' trust turning to hatred for the entire world, but mostly hatred for himself. His Chevy was in the lot. Some Good Samaritan from the hospital had parked it. Stopping halfway between the hospital and the parking lot, he lit a torch and took a long, smooth drag.

He had meant what he had said about Paris ending up hurt if she stayed with him. And here they were. Paris was better off without him. But she had been betrayed and abandoned her whole life. He wouldn't be the next to do it. If she didn't want to see him, he would face that. But it would be her choice. He wouldn't let her think he had left so easily.

He flicked his cigarette to the ground, squashed it under his foot, and with long strides, headed back to the hospital. But not its entrance. Paris was up on the third floor, and he would get to her if he had to climb the building. And climb he did. His side pulled, but he didn't care. He was prepared to have it ripped open, prepared to plummet to the ground.

The third floor window was ajar. Paris was behind the billowing white curtain. He pushed open the window further and pulled himself inside.

"Who's there?" Paris cried out.

Johnny stood tall, a silhouette illuminated by the first quarter moon's light, she a shadow of black and gray. The covers were up to her neck, her fingers squeezing them for an illusion of safety.

As Johnny stood there, their eyes met in the darkness. She knew it was him. He took off his fedora and squeezed its brim. From the distance, none of Paris' wounds were visible.

He had never expected to feel the level of fear he had experienced in that trench again. It didn't seem possible. From trench to trench was over four hundred yards, a distance covered in mines, barbed wire, hedgehogs, and a torrential onslaught of machine gun fire. The distance to Paris was less than ten feet. No machine gun fire, no mines, no barbed wire or hedgehogs stood between him and her. But there was something more powerful, more destructive, and more valuable at stake. It was love—no matter how trite and foolish that sounded. Johnny couldn't pretend to call it anything else. He had spent his life believing his own lies. But he wouldn't be able to believe that one. From the distance, his emotions were safe. One step forward, and the security darkness provided would end. With each step, he would be forced to face regret, pain, failure, and ineptitude. But also with each step, he would shed the cowardice clinging to him like a life-sucking parasite. He would be consumed with an unquenchable thirst for revenge, but more than that, he couldn't pretend what he felt for Paris was anything else. He would stand in front of her, all his flaws and weaknesses fully on display. Maybe that was the scariest thing of all.

Unlike the trench, there would be no whistle springing him into action. But something did. The strength, the confidence normally radiating from Paris' eyes was gone. Replaced by uncertainty and utter vulnerability. Wounds visible to the eye would heal. But Johnny knew what damage unseen wounds could inflict. What thoughts ran through her head? One sentence sprung him forward like he was back in that trench, whistle shrieking.

Does he not love me now?

She had once told him that she had a constant feeling of not being wanted or good enough, and at this moment, broken and beaten as she was, she must have felt that more than ever. Her confidence, her self-respect, her self-worth and her emotional well-being meant more to him than his own cowardice. She meant more.

He stepped forward, the moon's light casting him in a gray hue. His legs were weak. With each step forward, the details of her face took shape. She turned away from him, hiding her mangled face. But Johnny just stood there, a stone gargoyle.

"What are you doing?" she asked.

"I'm not going anywhere," Johnny said.

"I'm fine."

"I know you are."

A temporary silence fell.

"I don't want you to see me. Please leave."

"Why?"

"Just go."

"Not without a reason."

"Because I don't want you to seek revenge... not for me."

Johnny reached for her hand. Only her finger tips were visible, the rest of her hand and arm already wrapped in a cast.

"Let me see you," Johnny said.

Paris slowly turned. Her once smooth, immaculate creamed coffee skin was now covered with crimson cuts and purple and blue bruises. But bruises and cuts couldn't lessen her beauty. Beauty isn't limited to the flesh. Beauty is not defined solely by appearance. It wasn't just her voluptuous form, her piercing eyes, her knee-weakening smile or smooth skin. It was so much more. It was how she treated others—people above her and below her, friends and strangers. It was her compassion, knowledge, strong moral compass, and her conviction. And it was her strength. Mickey Diamond's fists could never take all that from her. Time would never lessen the ineffable, immaculate, *immortal* beauty of Paris Dawson.

"Let it go, Giovanni. You need to leave Chicago. He won't stop until you are dead. You shouldn't be here. If he knows I'm at this hospital, he'll come knowing you'll be here," Paris said.

Johnny shrugged off her warning. "Don't worry about anything."

Paris sat up the best she could. "I don't want your death on my conscience."

"What did he do to you?"

But he knew. How, he couldn't say. But the moment the light had caught her face, he knew she had been raped. There was a fear, a pain permeating from the depths of her soul. Paris had made a living off of sex. When the world offered her nothing, when businesses wouldn't hire her because she was colored or female or both, she did what she had to do. God had blessed her with remarkable looks, and she had used it to her advantage. But each man she had slept with had been her choice. It should always be a choice. Never forced, never rushed, never pressured, never guilted into.

"What was done… was done to me, and I get to decide how to respond to this," Paris said.

"And respond with what?" Johnny asked. "Doing nothing? He did this for a reaction. If this doesn't get one, what's next? He goes after Cilly and Clarence? Wally? Comes back around and kills you? He killed Valcoro even after he ratted us out, you think he'll grant any of us mercy?"

"It wasn't Vencini."

Confusion contorted his face.

"Vencini didn't rat you out. Diamond framed him and then killed him. He died defending me. He died defending *you*."

Johnny had never had respect or admiration for Valcoro. Johnny was a flawed man, many of his flaws unforgiveable, but no one could blame him for this one. Valcoro had degraded him daily. But the fact Vencini Valcoro hadn't ratted him out, hadn't caused the death of Tomato, meant more to him than he had thought it could. Seemingly impossible though it was, guilt bubbled inside his gut. He had instantly accused Valcoro of being the rat. Yet, Valcoro had died defiantly in support of his men.

"Thank you for telling me that," Johnny said.

"He spoke of someone else too," Paris said.

"Who?"

"I don't know. He said something about a cardinal not flying anymore."

Johnny knew what it meant in an instant.

"What?" she asked.

"The Cardinal. He's the one who tipped us off and told us to leave town, and it cost him his life," he answered.

If not for him, Johnny would be wasting away in a jail cell or rotting in the ground.

"I'm sorry," Paris said.

Johnny nodded, not wanting to speak about it. The Cardinal's death needed to be processed later. It was easier that way. Johnny wanted to bury it in the center of that maze, if there was any free soil to bury him with.

"You promise me right now that you won't sneak off when I'm sleeping. You stay. All night," Paris said.

Johnny's eyes dropped to their entwined hands. "I promise."

Paris freed her hand and raised his chin. "Look me in the eyes."

Johnny obliged.

"You look me in the eyes and swear to me," Paris said.

"I promise."

"If you break this promise, you'll hurt me worse than he ever could. And you promised you'd never hurt me. You'd tear your own heart out first…"

If tearing his heart out could take back the pain she had endured, he'd tear it out with his bare hands.

Paris raised her eyes to him. "It's not just your heart you keep now…"

Johnny stayed with Paris all night, sitting in the chair and either staring out of the window or watching Paris sleep. But Johnny could have been laying on a cloud, and no sleep would have come to him. As usual, it was too damn stuffy, but Johnny had barely noticed the heat. He was awake, but his mind had transported him to a place where his senses were dulled. No longer was he aware of how numb his ass was from sitting in that rigid, unforgiving chair. He toiled over thoughts, over memories, over questions and answers and over truths he had tried to bury deep in the expanse of his mind. The contents of the maze ran unchecked, each thought freeing the next like the passing of a key from one shackled prisoner to the next. And once free, they could never be locked back up, never buried, never hidden again.

327

Paris woke every half-hour or so, calling his name or reaching for his hand to verify he was still there. When morning came, and after Paris had eaten her breakfast, Johnny squeezed her hand and rose from his chair.

"Where are you going?" Paris asked.

"I have to meet Jack. He's leaving Chicago today," Johnny said.

"You promise?"

He bent down and kissed her forehead. "I will be back in less than two hours. I swear it."

Offers & Propositions

B reakfast falls between the large window of four and ten. But The Diner had its own tier of timings. First Breakfast, for factory workers and early risers, fell between four and six thirty. From roughly six thirty to eight, the diner saw a significant lull before the Second Breakfast phase of eight to ten, for those on banker's hours and the late risers. It was during the tail end of the second breakfast that Jack would stop in for a final meal. A baker's dozen worth of people were inside, including the hostess, waitresses, and cooks. A simple glance at the few other customers sufficed as a scan for any potential threats.

"One final conversation over breakfast," The Immortal said when Johnny sat in front of him.

He looked Johnny over. Johnny didn't need a mirror to know he had bags under his eyes and crow's feet, and that his skin had that sickly grayish dullness to it from lack of sleep.

"You look like shit," The Immortal commented.

"They got to Paris," Johnny said.

The Immortal's joking mood shifted immediately.

"Who? Diamond?" he asked.

Johnny nodded.

"Is she okay?"

"Broken arm, cuts, bruises. There's more, but—"

"You don't have to say it."

He leaned back, shaking his head, his face showing he knew what those unspoken words were.

"Jesus Christ. Where is the honor? Johnny... I want to help you... but my time in Chicago is at an end."

"I know, but there is a way you can help." He slid a paper bag over, the top folded over to keep it shut.

"I take it you didn't pack me a lunch."

"There's cash inside. Can you do me a favor?"

"I'll do whatever you need me to."

"My time in Chicago is over too. I'm taking Paris, Hotsy, and the Nettesheims, if they're willing, to Los Angeles. There are good doctors there that could help Clarence. Can you get a place on the beach? Big tall windows. Enough space for all of us. Telegraph the address to me?"

"Beachside... that's a hot ticket with a bunch of numbers."

"Check the bag, let me know if I need more."

The Immortal ensured no waitresses were on their way to his booth. Then he unrolled the top of the bag and glanced inside. He lifted the stacks of bills. Decades of holding, delivering, and picking up cash had given him the ability to read amounts of money with his hands like it was braille.

"That's enough. I'll make some calls to my contacts there. I should have an answer tonight."

The Immortal set the bag down on the seat.

"Your time in Chicago is over?" The Immortal asked.

"Over."

"And Capone... he's aware?"

Johnny only shrugged.

The Immortal nodded, a grim look on his face. "I'll see this done."

"Good luck... and thank you... for everything."

"You take care of yourself."

He rose from his favorite booth one last time and tossed enough cash to cover his bill and leave a generous tip. He nodded toward the door. "Your guest has arrived."

Johnny's eyes followed The Immortal's nod. At the entrance, a man ran his hand through his slicked-back black hair, looking far too nervous to be worried about the quality of eggs and pancakes.

"Take care," Johnny said.

"And you," The Immortal replied.

Their hug was brief. It was uncommon anyway for two men to do such a thing. Johnny tried to convey his deep respect and admiration for him with a final, firm pat.

The Immortal grabbed the paper bag, sauntered to the door, said a quick word to the nervous man standing beside it, and left his favorite restaurant in Chicago for the last time.

The nervous-looking man watched The Immortal walk past the diner before approaching Johnny. He sat at the booth, keeping his hands on his lap, not wanting any of the filth to get on his bare skin.

"That's the man they call The Immortal, huh?" the man asked.

Johnny nodded.

"I hear you want to talk to me," the man said.

His dark brown eyes fixed themselves on Johnny's. If his skin wasn't so pale, he could have passed for Italian, but instead he looked more like a vampire.

"You're Arthur Nash," Johnny said.

"You're Giovanni 'Johnny' De Luca. Now that we have the introductions out of the way, why don't we get down as to why I'm here?" Nash said.

"You're a corrupt agent."

"You're a violent criminal."

"I never claimed to be a good man."

"Is that why you invited me here? So we can make claims and accusations over some eggs and bacon?"

"I know you gave that address to Mickey Diamond."

Nash leaned back dismissively. "What address?"

"You know which one."

"Tell it to Sweeney." Nash looked about the diner, annoyed.

"You gave the name and location of George Dillert to Mickey Diamond. You knew he'd kill him. And his mother... an innocent woman's death is on your hands."

"I was told she was out of town. I never would have given that address had I known she was at home."

Johnny didn't have to question his sincerity. The regret showed in his eyes. And regret was like weeds—it never really goes away.

"And Dillert? You may not have thrown the rope over his neck and strung him up or shot his mother's brains out, but you killed them," Johnny said.

"You pass judgement on me?" Nash said, leaning toward Johnny. "Are your hands clean? North Side. South Side. Irish. Italians. You're all the same. You own Chicago. What happens to us agents or police officers who are just trying to do our job? You gun us down. Do you think if I raid one of Capone's speakeasies or factories I'd walk away with my head? I do my job, I get killed. My family gets threatened. And I'm supposed to put my family through that? And for what? A twenty two-hundred dollar salary? I play by their rules, *your* rules, I get that amount in three months. More importantly, my family stays safe. I didn't hang Dillert. I didn't shoot his mother. Don't sit there and criticize me for playing the game you and your pals created."

"You take a vow to be above it all."

"You're speaking to me about vows? I hear the Italians are getting a little stricter in their recruiting. Soon there may not be room for a mutt in the ranks."

"You became an agent in 1920, right? How long were you honest?" Johnny asked.

Nash shook his head at Johnny's audacity. "You smug bastard. I didn't vote for Prohibition, but it was my job to uphold the law. Why don't you pick up a sign and protest instead of blaming me? We've got three hundred agents in Chicago and over ten thousand places selling and serving alcohol. We have enough agents to cover a few measly blocks of this city. You sit on that side of the table thinking because you grew up in the dirt, it's okay for your hands to be filthy. I saw what happened to those who tried to uphold the law, and I saw what happened to those who let it go. Those who tried are either on the wrong side of the dirt or piss poor, and those who didn't are living better than what that salary pays for."

He fell silent when the waitress stopped by to offer him coffee. He politely refused but asked for water. There was a moment's pause as she filled it. Nash thanked her and took a sip.

"Since you're so high up on giving me my life facts, allow me the same courtesy," Nash said. "I know you're a suspect in New York for the murder of a police officer. I'm not sure how that fits into your holier than thou view—"

"I killed him," Johnny said. "I'm not hiding behind my sins. I'm not pretending I'm a good man. I'm not."

It was clear by the look on Nash's face he had intended to level the playing field. Nash had done nothing but defend his actions. It startled him when Johnny didn't do the same. He took another sip, unsure of how to proceed. The power dynamic had shifted.

"So are you going to tell me why I'm here?" Nash asked.

Both the water and the moment's pause had assuaged his agitation.

"You're going to help me take down Mickey Diamond," Johnny said.

Nash laughed artificially. "You wasted my time for this?"

Johnny only stared at him, no remnants of any smile or smirk on his face. Nash met his gaze, waiting for "the catch." When none came, he leaned forward again, suddenly paranoid that they might be overheard.

"Okay, let's say Mickey Diamond doesn't shoot me the moment I pull out my cuffs, why would I risk death?" Nash asked.

"Because if you don't, evidence of your crime will make its way to 'Decent' Dever and Superintendent of Police Collins," Johnny said.

"What evidence?"

"The note you wrote Dillert's address on. It won't take much to compare the handwriting on that note to yours."

"Handwriting? You think that'll hold up in court?"

"Whether it holds up in court or not, I don't care. The papers will print it. The people will make up their own mind."

Nash cast him a dirty look and took another sip.

"I just came from a hospital because Mickey Diamond assaulted the woman I love," Johnny said. "She had no part in any of this. Say what you want about me, about the men I ride with. We never involve families. It is always business."

"Right… you're just some noble, gallant knight forced to kill in the name of honor and justice. You never involve families? For every man who is killed, there is a wife or mother who needs to be told. Children who drench their pillows with tears. Listen, I go to church on Sundays, so if I want a sermon or a confessional, I'll take it from Father Kuhr, because you or Capone or Jack McGurn aren't any better than Diamond. I was at the flower shop after O'Banion was killed. I had to hold back his wife, I had to wipe his blood off of her heels. I'm sorry about your girl. I am. That's truly awful. But don't sit there and act like you're any better than Diamond or the North Side."

Lorraine Capuano flashed in Johnny's mind.

"No one's innocent," Johnny conceded.

Nash nodded his appreciation of the truthful comment.

"There's a price and a cost," Nash stated.

"Fifteen hundred," Johnny said.

Nash leaned back and finished his water. Sweat dripped down his cleanly shaven face. It wasn't the heat from the kitchen or the sunshine pouring through the window, it was the thought of crossing Mickey Diamond that made him sweat.

"That's the price. And the cost?" Nash asked.

334

"I'll worry about the cost," Johnny said.

"Say I agree to this... I arrest him on some minor offense. He is out in six weeks, and we have matching bullets in our foreheads and the promise of worms feasting on our flesh until we're nothing but bones. And that is a best case scenario. Worst case scenario, that cave man O'Malley beats us to death with a mallet. Then he kills my dog, my family, and the woman you love."

"He won't get out."

But it was too confidently stated for Nash to simply accept.

"How do you know that? Mickey Diamond has quite the reach, and Hymie Weiss... you think Diamond is ruthless? If Weiss cares about Diamond at all, he'll kill us and everyone in this restaurant for not killing us first."

"Weiss won't get involved."

"Since our lives are on the line, you'll indulge my asking how you know that."

"Because Capone isn't seeking retaliation for Valcoro's death. Sometimes things are personal. Sometimes, it's the cost of doing business."

"Why? Why should I do this?"

"Tell your kids to do the right thing? This is the right thing. You get fifteen hundred dollars for doing the right thing."

"Because doing the right thing always benefits the person doing it, right?"

"George Dillert's mother. I believe you when you say she wasn't supposed to be there. But she was. I see the regret in you. I won't lie to you and tell you that Mickey Diamond going to jail erases that. Take it from someone who knows. But I can tell you it will keep that pain from growing."

Nash stared out the window, deep in thought. "What's your plan?"

Voluntary Discharge

The front desk worker at the hospital hadn't exactly cast Johnny a friendly smile when he had left earlier, and her lips didn't curve into one upon his return either. Johnny had every intention of walking by, but she cleared her throat loud enough that it was impossible to ignore. Johnny stopped, keeping his eyes on the door separating him from Paris.

"Is Giovanni De Luca a common name?" she asked.

"I don't know," Johnny said, unsure of how to answer. It wasn't like he had a phonebook handy.

"Listen, rules are put in place for the order and safety of everyone. Family or spouse. You've been granted permission to stay, but that name isn't a ticket that you can slide under the fence once you're inside."

More riddles. Johnny exhaled, growing more irritated every second. "What?"

"One of your friends stopped in to see Ms. Dawson earlier. His name was Giovanni De Luca too," the attendant said.

The annoyance was instantly replaced by worry. His stomach free-fell like an elevator cut from its connecting cables.

"What did he look like?" Johnny asked.

Now it was the nurse who was uneasy. Johnny was a poor actor and had buried his worry under a few shovels of loose dirt—most of it was still visible.

"Tall as a tree," the attendant said.

O'Malley fit that description. But he didn't bear fruit or colorful leaves. He bore nothing but malicious intent.

"Is he gone?" Johnny asked.

"I turned him away. Rules are rules. Why? Did he have something to do with what happened to her?"

"Doesn't sound like anyone I know," Johnny said.

He hoped his lie would be believed. But the attendant's cold gaze saw through it. If the police were called—even the ficklest of gamblers would bet the house the heavier-set attendant would call them—it would take only a flash of a badge for the hospital's rules to disappear. The police couldn't be trusted. A large number of them were on Hymie Weiss' payroll, and an unnerving portion of them had loyalties to Mickey Diamond. A loyalty not bought with money but fear—a loyalty more unwavering. Paris would be arrested and taken into their custody and hand-delivered to Diamond.

Johnny hurried through the doors and to Paris' room.

"You're back," Paris said, exhaling her relief.

"We have to go," Johnny said.

Her relief at his return was cruelly short-lived.

"Why? What's going on?"

"They were here. Can you move?"

Paris nodded. She pulled herself to a seated position and swung her legs to the floor, groaning as she did. Her body was so badly beaten that even a light breeze brought fresh pain.

"Grab my clothes from the closet," she said, her breath shortened.

337

Johnny flung the door shut and rushed to the closet to grab her clothes from the hangers. He balled them in his hand and tossed them onto the bed.

"Do you need help?" Johnny asked.

"Offering to help me put my clothes back on?" Paris asked with a grin.

Johnny returned it. "And, again, you thought I wasn't chivalrous."

Paris dressed as quickly as her condition allowed and attempted to walk to the door. Her legs were brittle as glass, each step threatening to shatter them. But she was too proud to ask for his help. He wouldn't make her, and instead, put a secure arm around her for support if she needed it. Johnny opened the door and peeked out to make sure Mickey Diamond and his giant ogre thug weren't storming down the hallway. When he had made sure that there were only doctors and nurses outside, they stepped out.

It was a testament to either how busy the overwhelmed nurses were or how incompetent they were that no one noticed Johnny and Paris slipping through the corridor to the stairwell. But Paris was no longer wearing her hospital gown which would have stood out like a flashlight in the dark. In her street clothes, she looked like a visitor.

The stairs were loud, sounds of their descent echoing up and down the flight like clapping hands. For Paris, the stairs were a sheer drop from a mountain side. She had been confined to a bed, so her legs were nearly useless. Johnny wrapped his arm around her waist and gently held her hand. They came to an exit at the back of the building. He guided Paris to a dumpster.

"I'll bring the car around… I'll be right back," Johnny said.

Paris nodded, catching her breath.

Johnny was gone all of six minutes before he pulled alongside the building. He sprinted out of the car and scooped Paris into his arms.

"Are you making sure I don't have to walk on this filth?" Paris asked.

"I told you. Chivalry," Johnny said.

He helped her inside the car. Paris closed the door before he had to. She despised her current state as a damsel in distress and would do everything she was able to—which was everything until proven otherwise.

The open road brought a moment's respite from the constant state of worry, even downright paranoia, they had been in since returning from Wisconsin.

"Where's Hotsy?" Paris asked.

Johnny turned to her and shook his head. It was a coward's play, but he didn't want to breathe any life into the ember of fear sparking in his stomach.

Paris met his gaze. "We have to find him before they do."

Midnight Motel

The whiskey numbed every muscle but the one he wanted it to. Hotsy prided himself on being able to perform his manly duties with his nighttime fling even after imbibing copious amounts of alcohol. But that night, he would test his limits. To his intoxicated gaze, the whole city of Chicago was a revolving merry-go-round, and Hotsy ping-ponged off the stone building and the woman beside him. He grabbed her arm for support. When he stared hard and forced himself to focus, her raven-black hair stayed firmly perched on her head instead of flying all around it. She wore a fair amount of make-up but pinpointing it as lipstick or thick eye liner was, at the moment, impossible. Though his eyesight failed him, his sense of smell had no problem picking up her intoxicating jasmine-citrus scent, and his lust demanded he sober up. But the sting of loss that had taken an unwelcome stay in his chest still throbbed painfully. He knew only one way to try to numb it, and he raised a bottle to his lips to do just that.

"You better be careful with that bottle. If a copper or prohee catch you with that..." the woman warned.

"Baby... don't you worry... nothing," Hotsy slurred.

"Oh, boy. Let's get you checked in, handsome," the woman said.

She helped Hotsy into the passenger seat of a Chrysler Model B-70 and then took the driver's seat. The wind rushed at Hotsy's face and into his lungs. Many would have their own words to describe the phenomenon of Hotsy going from a sip of booze away from blacking out to a gulp of water away from being only buzzed. Plainly stated, like a starfish that regrew a lost leg or a lizard that regrew its tail, Hotsy regenerated.

But that didn't mean his manners also regenerated. He waited in the car as Amelia or Shawna (he was fairly certain one of those names was correct, although if it turned out to be Lila, Rose or Lucy, he wouldn't be shocked either) checked into the familiar motel. He must have told her about the motel earlier that night. She stepped out and shook the key in her hand with an excited smile. Hotsy stumbled out of the car and followed her to room fourteen, gulping fresh air like a fish returning to water. The parking lot was bare, nothing that Hotsy found strange. It was a place people rented for an hour or two rather than the whole night. It was mostly used as an opium den and a quick bedroom.

Hotsy's list of women he had slept with was longer than a child's Christmas wish list. And with such a number, not all of the women were what he called "front door" material. Some needed to be snuck out the back. And there was no better place for that than the opium den moonlighting as a motel. Before working for Valcoro, Hotsy had frequented the motel, but it had been years since his last stay.

The motel gave off a musty smell, and luckily for Hotsy, he was too drunk to think of how disgusting the sheets were. The maids came less than the police. His sybarite senses were consumed by Amelia or Shawna's perfume and the way her cleavage revealed how desperate her breasts were to be free of her dress.

"Let's get you some water, handsome," Amelia or Shawna said, strutting to the bathroom.

"Water? I'm fine, baby," Hotsy said.

She returned seconds later with a glass filled riskily to the top. It was a confidence only waitresses had. She sat on the edge of the bed next to Hotsy.

"You're fine, huh? Hmm… how about we play a little game then?" she asked.

"I like games," Hotsy said.

He wrapped his arm around her shoulders like a python and leaned in for a kiss, but she dodged it.

"I will ask a question. If you get it wrong, you drink the water."

"And barring some miracle, what do I get when I answer correctly?"

"I remove a button."

To prove her commitment to the game, she undid the top one, freeing more of her cleavage. Hotsy had never been more of a supporter of emancipation. Lust was a counter-drug to alcohol, and he sobered up even further.

"What's my name?" she asked.

It was a dreaded question he knew was coming. He should have gone to the front desk with her, where there could have been a chance of getting her real name while booking the room. Hotsy had never been accused of having a great memory. While greater minds had a database filed by date, location, name, and event, Hotsy's mind was filled with tiny notes taped to every nook and cranny. Dates were on one note, names on another. It worked for him, but when he was drunk, it was like a tornado had gone through, leaving behind a debris field of scattered notes. Hotsy could do nothing but pluck one from it.

"Shawna?" he said with as much confidence as if he was guessing the translation of a foreign word.

"Is that a question or an answer?" she asked, sounding equally amused and offended.

But the fact she hadn't hurled the water in his face gave him confidence he had guessed right.

"Statement, baby," Hotsy said.

"You deserve half a button for your hesitation," she said.

But she unburdened another shackle all the same, and Hotsy had to refrain from smiling and grabbing a handful of her bust.

"You were talking to my friend at the bar too…"

Had he had a chance of leaving with both of them?

"…what was her name?"

If he hadn't remembered there was a second woman, he sure as Hell wouldn't remember her name.

"Hand over the water," Hotsy said.

Shawna smiled, enjoying watching him sip.

"That was a small button," he said in defense of the sip and not gulp. "And besides, who can remember anyone else with you looking like that?"

She smiled, loving his compliment.

"What drink did I order at the bar?" she asked.

"An alcoholic one," Hotsy said, then nodded to the two remaining buttons.

"Nice try, Hotsy Totsy."

"You were taking swigs of Panther Piss with me."

"Please, I have class you know."

The disgusting motel walls sneered at her comment, privy to all the secrets and diseases the room held.

"Let's give you a simple one. What's your name?" she asked.

Hotsy scoffed. "Now who's drunk? You just said it."

"Hotsy is a nickname, silly. You expect to charm me into this bed without me even knowing your real name?"

"Quintu."

"*Oooh*, I like that. Quintu what?" She tickled his chest with her long fingernails.

"Di Salvo." He ran his free hand across her smooth arm.

"Mr. Di Salvo."

She removed the penultimate button. Hotsy's eyes found her exposed cleavage, and like a shark that had found its prey, his eyes flashed black, pupils dilating.

"If I finish that glass of water, will you unburden that button desperately trying to free itself?"

She arched her eyebrows to stoke his lust. "Maybe."

Hotsy kept his piercing gaze on her, bringing the glass to his mouth. He finished it in one continuous gulp and then tossed the glass behind him.

"Now, as the descendant of a Union solider, and on behalf of all who died for freedom, I cannot sit back and allow you to enslave those any longer. President Lincoln wouldn't stand for it and neither will I."

She undid the button, deliberately slow. By now, Hotsy's lust could power a city. She rose, removing her black, buttoned Veronique dress with its golden swirls and spirals, and allowing it to slither off her body and coil to the floor. Hotsy's hands rose to her breasts, but she entwined her fingers with his to stop him.

"I have to get ready. Give me five minutes," she said, twirling his hands in hers.

He released her hands. "You have thirty seconds."

It wasn't an idle threat.

"Have a quick smoke, I'll be out before it's done."

With a seductive slither, she sashayed into the bathroom, making sure Hotsy had a good view of her profile. Hotsy kicked off his shoes and had his pants and shirt off in less than ten seconds. He grabbed his pack of cigarettes and lit one, annoyed at how long she was taking.

He lay on the bed, taking relaxing, sobering puffs from the cigarette, watching the smoke seductively dance to the ceiling.

"Your time is up!" Hotsy shouted.

In a flash, the door flew open, and two men, one giant and one stout, stepped in with Tommy guns raised. The cigarette dangling from Hotsy's mouth fell onto his chest, burning his flesh. But his body couldn't register the pain because it was too preoccupied with the pain that would overwhelm it in a fraction of a second. Hotsy made a motion to dive for his gun lying uselessly on the mocha carpet.

O'Malley and Diamond unloaded their guns. A rapid, deafening stream of *Rat-a-tat-tat-rat-a-tat-tat* filled the room. The pillows burst, sending feathers floating in the air, the white walls looked like Swiss cheese, the lamp and mirror exploded, sending shards of glass everywhere. But the room took nowhere near as much damage as Hotsy. From thigh to neck, he was struck with at least thirty bullets. His blood splattered onto the white walls and ceiling. His hand hung limply, inches from his gun. Blood dribbled off his fingertips, collecting into a pool on the carpet.

Smoke wafted off the barrels of the Thompsons. O'Malley stepped forward and prodded Hotsy's body, ensuring he was dead. Satisfied with the result, O'Malley spit on him. Diamond wiped the sweat from his forehead, handing over his Tommy gun to O'Malley.

Shawna stepped out of the bathroom, neither surprised nor shocked. She briefly examined her dress for blood before putting it back on. She paused to look at Hotsy.

"Such a shame," she said.

"I thought you were going to put on a show," O'Malley said.

"That wasn't covered in Mickey's fee," she said.

O'Malley smirked.

"The fee did include a ride back to my apartment though," Shawna said.

Diamond tossed a King of Diamonds playing card and a hand-written note onto the bed.

"We should go," O'Malley said.

Diamond admired his work a few minutes longer before nodding. The three of them left the motel, leaving behind Quintu Di Salvo's body hanging off the bed with smoke rising from his bullet holes and the remaining blood in his body dripping out onto the mocha carpet.

Wishing & Praying

No Chicago street was safe, but Johnny would search every block to find Hotsy. Paris shared the same passion, but her body was just too weak to carry out its pledge. Even if she insisted she was fine, she needed rest. There was only one place and one family with whom Johnny would entrust her.

No cars drove the streets of Cicero because they were all parked along the curb, bumper to bumper. The clubs, gambling halls, and brothels were filled, their music wafting out like the cries of ghosts. The streets were so filled with cars that even the front of the Nettesheims' apartment building had no open space, meaning the driver and passengers had a good half-mile hike to the center of vice. Each owner would only be able to leave if the first or last car in the row left. Johnny cursed when he saw that the closest spot was over a block away. He considered dropping off Paris, but he wouldn't let her out of his sight until she was safely inside.

After accepting he wouldn't find anything closer, he parked. Then he hurried to help her out of the car, but Paris' pride demanded she do it alone. Her self-reliance was both commendable and heartbreaking. Rides could make anyone stiff, but for Paris, every bump and stop had been another punch and kick. In the darkness, it looked as though the bruising on her face had faded. But when they stepped under the streetlight, the swollen blacks, blues and purples stood out like mountain ranges on a map.

Those three steps up the stoop might as well have been Mount Everest for Paris, but she gripped the railing and ascended on her own. Johnny opened the entrance door for her, assuring her he was only being a gentleman when he kept a supporting hand on her lower back. Paris leaned against the wall, while Johnny delivered a round of knocks on the Nettesheims' door. After a second round of knocks, the door opened, and the barrel of a pistol greeted him.

Johnny flung his hands up in surrender, and the pistol fell to Cilly's side. "Johnny," she said, exhaling in relief.

She set Clarence's pistol on the stand beside the door, and crossed her hands over her chest—fear had a way of causing people to shiver. But before relief could take over fully, she gasped at Paris' appearance.

She flipped the door open and then hurried to the couch to remove the decorative pillows so Paris was able to lie down.

"I'm sorry to barge in," Johnny said.

But Cilly ignored him. "Paris? Oh my God, are you okay?"

"Just sore," Paris said.

"Is it okay if she stays here?" Johnny asked Cilly.

"Where are you going?" Paris asked.

Cilly's eyes darted between Johnny and Paris, pleading, demanding to know what was going on.

"You're the only people I trust, Cilly. I have to find Hotsy before Mickey Diamond does. Please. I'll explain more later," Johnny said.

"Of course. Go," Cilly said, shooing him like a fly.

"I'll be back before sunrise," Johnny said.

He allowed Paris to gaze into his eyes, so she could gauge the truth in his words.

"You promise?" she asked.

"I promise."

Johnny gestured his appreciation to Cilly and then hurried out and down the steps. If he allowed Paris any time to think on it, she would join him, and he couldn't risk that. He jogged to his car and sped out of the city at a speed not suited for streets, but highways.

Hotsy had spent nights in every part of Chicago. He had stayed at The Moonlight most nights, but Johnny knew the cesspool Hotsy had frequented prior to that. It was only after Tomato and Johnny called the place "a box of syphilis" that Hotsy finally stopped going there.

Johnny kept the car window down, allowing the wind to drift across his face. There was something comforting about daylight. Everything was seen. Everything was known. Darkness only increased every worry, every paranoia. Johnny ensured his M1911 was ready for action. He parked a block away, killing the engine and shutting his door without a sound. He crept out of sight of the blinding neon sign spelling out "MOTEL" on nights that the "L" had lit up. Currently, it spelt "MOTE," but flickered between that and "MOT."

The place was a fossil. The parking lot was barren except for dandelions pushing their way through cracks in the pavement. The overhead light posts flickered like fire flies, but no light came from the dark front desk. It had been too long since his last visit for Johnny to know who owned the motel now. When he had first visited, the rooms had been packed. Was it common now for the motel to be a miniature ghost town? Had the police shut it down for selling opioids? Or had the city health department shielded it shut for a thousand years until it would be safe for human occupancy once again?

Johnny pushed open the glass door of the front office, gun held at the ready for anyone hiding. The parking lot lights cast enough glow to show the silver room keys hanging on the panel behind the desk. All of the hooks had accompanying keys except for one—room fourteen.

Johnny crept outside and dashed across the parking lot to room fourteen. The lights betrayed his location, but there was nothing but darkness surrounding the motel. An eerie silence filled the grounds. Even the bugs circling and buzzing around the parking lot lights stopped to watch him.

Not surprising, the room door was locked. The curtains concealed the window and everything inside. After ensuring he was still alone, he kicked the door open, splintering the frame. The door collided with the wall with a bang.

He hit the light switch, preparing himself to unload his clip in case he had walked into an ambush. But the lights revealed a horror that wounded him more than a thousand bullets ever could.

Hotsy was face-down on the bed, his limp arm reaching for his gun. Blood was everywhere, varying in color, scarlet for the blood still dripping from his body and sangria for blood dried on the walls, ceiling, blankets, lamp shade, and carpet.

The outstretched gun in Johnny's hand fell limply at his side. He stared, horrified, at his best friend's lifeless body. It was the perfect time for an ambush, but he didn't care.

He crouched down beside his fallen friend and stared into his blank eyes. Eyes that had glimmered with an insatiable love of life. Hotsy had enjoyed every second of a day. The annoyances that hindered Johnny rolled off Hotsy's shoulders. Tomato and Johnny were irascible, Hotsy carefree.

Johnny wanted to cry. He should have cried. Ten years ago, he would have. But it wasn't time that had numbed him but experience. He honestly couldn't even estimate how many young soldiers he had seen dead on a field, open eyes no longer seeing. Johnny had given in to cowardice before, and the coward in him demanded he look away now. But he forced himself to gaze at every bullet hole in Hotsy's once flawless form.

He couldn't take Hotsy with him, but he couldn't leave him hanging off the bed like that. Hotsy couldn't be at peace in such a position. Gently, Johnny lifted him back on to the bed and rested Hotsy's head on the pillow. He traced his fingers down Hotsy's eyes to close them. He stared at the man. A man with a usually devious smile now expressionless. A man who loved to laugh, but was now silent. A man who had loved to dance, but was now permanently still. A man who would have died for Johnny… and had. Hotsy had loved the life. Getting him to leave it behind would have forced him to turn from the only thing he ever knew. There was too much about it he loved, too much he was addicted to. Hotsy would have never left Chicago.

Johnny kissed Hotsy's forehead and folded one hand over the other. The room was stifling, even ten degrees hotter than the nighttime air outside. But Hotsy's hands were like buckets of ice. His body was already starting to turn. Hotsy would never allow himself to smell. He prided himself on his masculine scent—a musky, mint fragrance. But now his flesh was ripe with rancidity.

Too preoccupied with his friend, Johnny had noticed neither the white stationary note at the foot of the bed nor the King of Diamonds playing card. He took the note in his hands, knowing who it was from.

What a pretty boy laid to waste.
But he chose his friends in poor taste.
The Taker reached for his hand
A final song played by Heaven's Band.

There was more to the poem, but Johnny had no desire to read it. He had made a promise to return to Paris by sunrise and if he finished that poem, he would break that promise. And he wouldn't do that because he had been goaded into foolish action.

He removed his lighter and set the poem aflame, watching the fire destroy Mickey Diamond's painful jest.

A single memory was a rain drop. Reflecting on not only Hotsy, but Tomato too, those rain drops swelled into a tsunami crashing upon him.

When the waters receded, he snapped out of the painful paralyzed state he had been in. He wouldn't let Hotsy's body rot in that swamp of a room for God only knew how long. He staggered to the front desk. The memories attacked his motor function, twice he almost tripped. Inside the office, he dialed the police.

A million memories tormented him. Tomato and Hotsy had been his family in Chicago, and now, they were gone. Over the years, he had dreaded the spontaneous attacks. But since that shootout in Wisconsin, those attacks had been rare. It was because he was at war again. Those attacks would come on the ship ride home.

He drove away from the motel, the wailing sirens of the oncoming police breaking the muggy silence. Whenever the young die, shock is the hardest emotion to comprehend. Here one minute. Gone the next. Johnny was immune to shock. He'd been too close to death, knew all its tricks, to be shocked by it. Death is a poison. Sometimes slow moving, sometimes fast. A poison we are all born with. A poison that will take us all. The only question is when.

Though Johnny was immune to the shock, the pain in his chest was like a smashing anvil. The strings holding a heart in a place are strong and thick. But loss cuts and tears at them, and now, Johnny's were nothing but threads. There had been a time when Johnny would have hated something or someone rather than face the truth. He hated Woodrow Wilson for getting involved in a European affair. He hated the crooked cops for taking advantage of his parents. He hated Valcoro for the way he treated him, hated the rising sun and despised it when it left him. But Johnny could no longer hide the truth through anger. He had to accept truths and do away with the lies he'd been living for years.

The open parking spots in Cicero remained an endangered species. He was forced to park three blocks away but stayed seated inside his car, staring blankly out at the black expanse. Was this what each day was like for Clarence? Staring out of a window but not seeing? Only replaying the horrors he had witnessed? The loss, the carnage, the mayhem, the soul-destroying terrors of war? No matter where in Chicago, Cicero or Wisconsin they were, every night brought them back to France. There was never a true tomorrow.

As the clock turned, and night transformed into dawn, the cars lining the streets drove off, leaving Cicero like an evacuation had been ordered. The black sky was met by a blinding blend of yellow and orange. Johnny had promised he would be back before sunrise, so he pulled back onto the street and parked the car along the now deserted street directly in front of the Nettesheims'. He collected himself the best he could, but it was as futile as collecting water with a net.

Paris opened the Nettesheims' door on the first knock. It was clear she hadn't slept a wink. A wave of guilt swept over him for her having to rise from the couch to get the door.

"Did you find him?" she asked. She tried to look past Johnny, hoping to see Hotsy standing behind him.

Once again, Johnny's cobalt blue eyes revealed everything. There was no need for him to say anything, and for that, he was grateful. Her warm chocolate brown eyes filled with sorrow, mirroring the grief they saw in Johnny's.

"Oh, Giovanni…" she gasped. She pulled him into a hug, stroking his face. "I'm so sorry," she whispered.

It was a kind phrase, a nice gesture but nothing more. He'd heard it before at funerals, he'd said it to soldiers who had lost friends, but it provided little relief. But in most cases, it was all a person could offer. But the way Paris held him exceeded all expectations of comfort a person could bring. She made him stronger by allowing him to be weak. In her arms came a calming peace he had given up hope of ever finding.

"I'm going to be outside for a bit," Johnny said.

Paris nodded, squeezing his hand as he stepped outside.

The stoop seemed as good a spot as any to sit, and somehow, the hard stone was soothing. The street he gazed upon was much the same he had looked upon back in Brooklyn. So many memories on one block. Children spend so much of their lives gazing down the road at what's next, failing to realize some of the best moments of their life would be spent on the very block they were looking past. Johnny's parents and grandmother would always warn him to be careful. Careful of the traffic, of strangers, of other children. But the real dangers of life came after you left that familiar street behind.

His immersion in nostalgia only broke when the door opened, and Wally bounded down the steps. He sat next to Johnny with a cross between a groan and a sigh.

"Paris said you were out here," Wally said.

"Hey Wally," Johnny said, trying to look and sound normal.

He could count on one hand the number of hours he had slept in the last few days, but he was far from tired, at least in terms of sleep. But Johnny had been wearing a mask for years.

"How come you're sitting out here? Is it the goddamn heat?" Wally asked.

The last thing Johnny had expected to do was smile but, somehow, he did.

"Something like that," Johnny said.

"You seem sad."

"I am."

Children could be ruthless. They could find any insecurity, even the ones you weren't aware you had and destroy you with them. But they also had the ability to be incredibly kind. Wally was genuinely saddened by Johnny's depressed mood.

"I get sad too. You have the same warning signs as me. My mom calls me out on them all the time. It's annoying. I don't want her to know when I'm sad because then she gets sad too. She has enough to worry about and the fact that she gets sad makes me feel bad."

"What are my warning signs?"

"You're staring blankly. It's like your body is here, but your mind is someplace else. Is it in Schönfeld or Mirabella Imbaccari?"

"No, not there."

"Montfaucon-d'Argonne?"

"Sometimes… a lot of the time. Sometimes on a country road. Where do you go?"

"I guess nowhere… Sometimes I just think about if things were different."

"Me too, bud."

"Mom tells me to pray. I don't know if that's the same thing. I mean I wish for things, you know? That's what prayer is, right?"

"I think a wish is something you'd like. You know? A new glove, new bike. I think a prayer is something you desperately need. It's a plea to God."

Wally nodded, taking in the new information. "I like that."

He allowed a moment's pause.

"So what are you doing? Wishing or praying?" Wally asked.

"Accepting," Johnny said.

Wally nodded again, finding some truth in Johnny's words.

"Johnny, I've been doing a lot of thinking. About what's best not just for me, but for my mother too. You know I have to take care of her."

"You're a good son, Wally."

"You know, I thought I was wishing, but I think it's something I really need. So I guess I was praying. I want you to be my father. I know you're with Paris, but you could still marry my mom. You can just pass on the lovey dovey stuff, you know? We can't afford a child running around anyway."

"Wally, you have a father."

Wally turned to Johnny. "He doesn't do anything the other fathers do."

"Wally, you know your father loves—"

"Everyone says that! 'You know your father loves you.' How do I know that? He doesn't say it. He doesn't give me hugs or kisses. He doesn't help me with stupid arithmetic or spelling. He doesn't play games with me. He doesn't play catch in the summer or go sledding in the winter! It's... it's not fair!"

His anger morphed into sobs. Johnny put his arm around him. Wally buried his face into Johnny's chest, his tiny shoulders bobbing up and down with each sob. Sobs that weren't shallow, caused by falling down or being denied dessert or a new toy. These sobs originated in the pool of his soul, formed over a short lifetime. Tears of a caliber no child should ever have to shed.

"It isn't fair, Wally," Johnny said, gently raising Wally's face. "I can't argue against that. Life... sometimes it doesn't go our way. Most often it doesn't... it's cruel you had to find that out so young. The hurt you feel, that unrelenting pain... that should never happen to someone your age. It shouldn't happen to anyone. Life and death... they're not always different, you know? Death takes things right away. Life... it's a gradual loss. You're always saying goodbye to someone or something. You're too young to understand the sacrifice your dad made."

"I am the man of our house. I have to help with everything. I've sacrificed too."

"I know, Wally. You've had to grow up much quicker than a person your age has any right to. And you've done so much. But your dad wasn't always like this."

"I know. My mom says that all the time," Wally snapped back.

"It's true," Johnny said softly.

"How do you know? You didn't know him."

"No, I didn't. But I knew men like him. Wally, war is… it's awful… it… it breaks you."

War was inexplicable. Only someone who had experienced it could truly know its horrors and the compunction it brought afterword. Detailing its horrors to adults was nearly impossible. But how do you explain war to a child? How do you relay the horror of something without describing its graphic sights, its terrifying sounds, and its putrid smells?

"It didn't break you," Wally said.

"It did though, Wally," Johnny said. "The country asked me to fight so that people like you and your mom would be safe. There was a lot of fear about people in the States getting hurt from what was going on in Europe. A chance that you and your mom could be hurt. And you know what your father did, Wally? He signed up right away because he loves you. If there was any chance of you being hurt, he was going to fight to stop it. Without hesitation. I know you think those medals your dad got are just scrap… but one day, you'll hold those in your hand, and you'll be consumed with pride."

"I want him to be normal!" Wally bawled into his hands. "I don't wish it, Johnny. I pray for it. I desperately need it."

"I know. There is hope with the doctors. It takes time, Wally. But your dad understands what you say. He may not show it, but he knows. He knows when you tuck him in at night, when you refill his lemonade, when you read to him, when you help him in the bathroom. He knows all of it."

"Why can't he be like you? You're not like him."

"Your father is a better man than me, Wally. Much better. War destroys the good in people. Your father had so much goodness in him, that it took almost everything. Everything but the love he has for you and your mom. Me, I am not a good person, Wally. War took a lot from me, but it couldn't feed off of me the way it could your father."

Wally wiped his tears on his arm. "Do you really think he knows all the stuff I do for him?"

"I know he does. You keep being strong for him like he was for you. Strive to be who your father was and who he is. Can you do that?"

Wally nodded, sniffing.

"I knew you could." He rubbed Wally's head affectionately, leaving a patch of hair standing like an antenna.

Wally collected himself for a few moments until his breathing settled. "I'm sorry, Johnny. You came out here because you were sad, and I rambled on about my problems."

Pure and kind down to the last bone.

"It's better than having you drill me with a ball."

"You cost me a round bagger."

"Maybe if you got some height on the ball."

They rose to their feet, Johnny's shadow stretching across the road and Wally's barely leaving the sidewalk. When they stepped inside, Paris was on the couch, Clarence in his favorite chair, and Cilly at the sink washing and drying the breakfast dishes.

"Cilly, can I talk to you? In private?" Johnny asked.

She wiped her hands and looked at him for a moment before answering. She had worn that look too often recently, and Johnny's stomach pushed aside the grief, worry, and remorse it was filled with to make room for guilt.

"Follow me Paris, I'll show you the hallway," Wally said.

Paris smiled. "A hallway tour, how exciting."

Like an usher at a majestic theatre, Wally linked his arm with hers and regally escorted her out.

"Everything okay?" Cilly asked.

Based on the fact that she continued to wipe her hands with the towel long after they were dry, she was obviously nervous.

"Me and Paris have to leave Chicago. It's not safe," Johnny said.

"Okay…" Cilly said, unsure of how to respond.

"We're going to California. I want you, Wally, and Clarence to come with," Johnny said.

"California?"

"There are doctors out there who can help Clarence. A fresh start."

"Oh, Johnny, we don't have money for that."

"Don't worry about money. I have a place right on the beach. Enough room for all of us. Wally will have a blast. Clarence will have a great view looking out at that ocean sunrise, and you will leave the debt collectors here in Chicago."

Cilly looked around her apartment. She wore a look Johnny hadn't worn since he had come home from France. Cilly was home. Sure there were a thousand things that needed fixing, and appliances and furniture she didn't have or needed replaced, but it was home. And what an indescribable luxury that was. Fond memories dwelled in every room. But there was also pain lurking behind every corner.

Wally's room was home to tickling fits, his laughter fuel for her soul. But it was also a place where Wally cried himself to sleep, his sniffling audible through the thin walls.

Holiday dinners, tables bowing under the weight of turkey, potatoes, corn, and stuffing. Barren tables with only a few boiled potatoes. Dancing with Clarence in the living room while he sang. And now, Clarence imprisoned in a chair, eternally silent.

"Good doctors?" she asked, a subtle plea in her voice to be convinced.

"The best. They follow the method of a British doctor named Hurst. He's had great success in treating men like Clarence," Johnny said.

And it was true. Arthur Hurst's treatment had been transcendent, "curing" men in as little as one session.

Cilly nodded—indecisively at first, then with greater conviction. "When?"

"Today."

Her mouth dropped. She looked around, eyeing all that needed to be packed. "I have to talk with Wally."

But in reality, if she didn't agree to leave today, she most likely never would. The whole morning and afternoon flew by. Cilly, Wally, and Clarence sat at the kitchen table, Cilly detailing the proposed move. At first, Wally was against it. But realizing how much his mother needed a new start and the prospect of doctors helping his father, he warmed up to the idea and was soon overcome with excitement. He was sure to pack every last toy and stuffed animal he had and insisted those boxes be taped shut last. There were twenty-three boxes in all. By the time they were loaded into the moving van, the sun was on its last legs, hunched over the horizon.

"We won't all fit in the van, not five of us," Cilly said.

"It's just the four of you. I've got some things to finish up here," Johnny said.

Paris' gaze shot at him like a bullet. "What things?"

"Don't worry, I'll be there. I have to stop by Goma's. Things that need to be settled," Johnny said.

"Do you need me to stay?" Wally offered.

"No, I need you to make sure these two women don't get lost along the way," Johnny answered before Cilly had to.

"Best way to do that is to let me drive," Wally said.

"I tell you what, if it takes six years to get to California, you can park the van in the driveway when we get there," Cilly said.

Wally rolled his eyes. "Not funny, mom."

Clarence was in the passenger seat, mouth agape, staring out of the open side window. Johnny rested his hands on the door, staring into Clarence's raven black eyes.

"You're going to get out of that trench, Clarence."

Clarence had spent too long in his trench. His tour was over. Maybe it was the sunshine pouring into the van or maybe Johnny's eyes weren't working well from all the sleep deprivation, but for the first time, there was a glimmer in Clarence's eyes.

Johnny rounded the front of the van to Cilly, Wally, and Paris.

"Drive safe," Johnny told Cilly.

"See you soon," she said.

She hugged him. It was the first time she had. A "thank you" for all the envelopes of cash that kept the apartment heated during the brutally cold winters, kept food on the table, kept them in their beds, kept the swarming debt collectors at bay and covered the medical bills, and for everything he had done for Wally.

"See you soon," Johnny repeated.

"You leaving tomorrow morning or night?" Wally asked.

"I'm hoping morning," Johnny replied.

"You'll want to leave before the rush hour traffic. I hear that can be a real son of a bitch," Wally said.

"Wally! How many times do I have to tell you not to use words like that!" Cilly yelled.

"I'll be sure to leave before the traffic sets in," Johnny said with a grin.

"Do you think this dam… blasted heat will follow us the whole way?" Wally asked.

"You make sure your mother goes above the speed limit or it may," Johnny said.

Wally smiled and held out his hand for a gentleman's shake, but Johnny crouched beside him.

"You remember what I said?" Johnny whispered.

Wally nodded. "I'll strive to be the man you think I can be."

"You already are. Remember you can't always be at your best…"

"But you can give your best."

Wally wrapped his thin, gangly arms around him, squeezing him in a strong hug.

"They play baseball in California?" Wally asked.

359

"Thinking of hitting some balls into the ocean?" Johnny replied.

"I plan on sending a few to Hawaii."

"Hawaii? Why don't you start by clearing my head first?"

"Yeah… yeah. Round bagger, Johnny. A round bagger." He flicked his wrist dismissively at Johnny's jest before stepping into the van.

There was only one more goodbye—Paris. She had given Johnny his moment with the Nettesheims. Now, she would have hers. Johnny eliminated the distance between them, taking her hands in his.

"How are you feeling?" he asked.

"Don't worry about me. I'll find my way up," Paris said.

"I know."

He'd never been more certain about anything in his life.

Paris massaged his fingertips, squeezing them and taking in their heat. Her eyes locked onto his, warm brown against icy blue.

"What is it you have to do? What you *truly* have to do?"

"I have to make sure Mickey Diamond doesn't follow us."

Paris stared into Johnny's eyes. Impossibly, her eyes reflected both anger and sadness. How she could level him with a glance while fortifying him at the same time defied logic. It was spellbinding.

"Your piercing eyes are ripping into my flesh. Relax. I am working with a prohee," Johnny said.

"A prohibition agent? Why is he helping you?" she asked.

"I've got some info on him that could ruin his career. He gave the location of a witness to Diamond. Diamond killed that witness and his mother."

"And this agent, he's going to do what? Arrest Diamond?"

Johnny nodded.

"On what charge?"

"We're still planning that bit out."

"Seems like a lot of heat that agent is willing to put on himself. Diamond will get out and have a new target."

"Well, that will be his problem, won't it?"

Paris studied his eyes. Johnny locked in on hers.

"I'll go with you."

"Paris, you need to rest. Don't worry about all this. It's just paperwork."

"I don't want you to kill him... I know what he's done, what he's caused. But I know you, Giovanni. I know how much the killing has eaten at you. I don't think you can handle tearing your soul like that again."

Johnny only listened, tracing his fingertips across her palm.

She lifted his chin, their eyes mere inches apart. "Why do I feel like this is goodbye?"

He ran his fingers through hers, taking in her smooth skin. "Your hands are cold again."

"You don't have to do this alone. I am willing. I understand the risk."

Johnny stared, his mind tracing every line, every curve of her face until it had filled every crevice of his mind.

"I need you to promise me you'll get in that van, and you'll go to California. If you don't, you'll hurt me worse than he ever could," Johnny said.

"I'd rather tear my own heart out," she recited.

"Promise me, Paris."

"I promise."

He kissed her like he had on that beach in Wisconsin when it had only been the lake, the trees, and them. When they might have been the only two people in the world. Before everything had gone horribly wrong. When Johnny had still hadn't accepted certain truths, realized and disproved the lies, and answered the questions.

Neither wanted the kiss to end. Both were wordlessly communicating their love, their hope, and their pain through their kiss. Holding onto youth's naivety and ignoring the sobering realization brought on by maturity. But the most powerful things are fleeting—a flash of lightning, a shooting star, a spark. And their kiss too fell to such cruel brevity.

He tucked a wave of her hair behind her ear. "See you, half-breed."

"See you, half-breed."

She turned toward the van, but Johnny clung to her fingers, pulling her back to him.

"I need you to know... I have to tell you that I—"

Paris put a finger to his lips before he could finish. "Tell me in California, and I'll say it too."

Johnny nodded. She stroked his face a final time, each of them staring long enough that the other would be a memory that would never fade. He escorted her to the van and helped her inside.

"I'll be seeing you," he said.

Paris nodded, holding onto his hands with a sure grip.

The van struggled to life and, with a change of gear, it pulled ahead and down the road, disappearing into the setting sun and taking with it the only people left who gave a damn about Johnny.

Cold Breeze

In some ways, it took the van hours to drive down the street, but Johnny's final glimpse of Paris only lasted a second. His drive back into Chicago was serene. The open windows assuaged the heat, and the open road and corresponding silence allowed him to process his many thoughts. But since accepting those truths, dismissing the lies, and answering the questions, they were powerless. But nothing is more alienating than to be utterly alone in a city of millions. To pass skipping children holding their parents' hands, young lovers conversing arm-in-arm, or a group of friends sharing a laugh and never experience that feeling of belonging.

Johnny parked across from Goma's Burial Service and left the keys in the car. He removed his M1911 and set it on the passenger seat. Mere weeks ago, he had been parked in the very spot with Hotsy and Tomato, waiting in a baking car for Al. Now, it was only him—the only one left. As soon as he stepped out of the car, the heat trapped between the Chicago skyscrapers swarmed him like mosquitoes. The glass windows of Goma's Burial Service were pristine. Al was inside finishing up his day job and preparing for the business of the nightlife underground when Johnny knocked on the glass door. Al's eyes widened, then darted to the calendar hanging behind his desk. It wasn't Tuesday, and he breathed a deep sigh of relief before opening the door.

"Johnny... what a surprise," he said.

"Al, I need your help," Johnny said.

"Okay..."

"I need help planning a funeral... Hotsy's gone..."

He kept his eyes levelled at Al, not daring to look at any of the coffins and caskets. But their effect on him had diminished.

I'm never going to end up in one of those.

"I'm so sorry to hear that," Al said.

His words were genuine, but considering their line of work, Johnny wouldn't have faulted him had they not been so. But everyone liked Hotsy. He was like a playful puppy. The fact that he had destroyed Al's shop, and Al still liked him was a testament to Hotsy's infectious spirit.

"Please, take a seat. Can I get you something to drink?" Al asked, offering the chair in front of his desk.

"I'd take an Old Fashioned, Al," Johnny said.

"Of course. I'll ask that we take this business downstairs then, if you don't mind," he answered.

Johnny had zero gripes about that. To him, those coffins and caskets were filled with the ghosts of men he had failed.

He followed Al downstairs. In less than an hour, the place would be packed with people, damp with sweat and deafened by music. Al wobbled behind the bar and mixed Johnny's drink.

"That's a damn good drink, Al," Johnny said, after taking a sip.

Al thanked him, then organized his stack of papers and readied his pen. "Never easy going through this, I find it best to just read them... Burial or cremation?"

"Cremation."

Johnny sipped his Old Fashioned, going over the details and confronting the mortality of men. He paid Al handsomely, for the funeral arrangement, his Old Fashioned, and a bottle of Moscato. Al wanted to say something on their way up the stairs and to the door, but Johnny patted his back and left before he could summon the words.

Lauer's Bakery was a few blocks away, and in a city dominated by Italians and Irish, it provided a taste of Germany by selling German pastries—chiefly *kringles*. The older woman at the counter greeted him in a strong German accent. Johnny replied to her greeting in German, which made her smile. He sampled different flavors of *kringle*. But he settled on ordering a loaf of French bread and left the change with the old woman.

Johnny strolled the Magnificent Mile before heading into Grant Park. The winds off the lake squeezed through the trees with a hushed whistle. He came to an unfinished fountain, grand in scale. The outer wall and first two-tiers of the fountain had been completed, showcasing what a spectacle it would be when it was finished sometime next year. He sat on the outer wall, his back to the fountain and his eyes on the glowing city.

He yanked the cork out of the wine bottle and tore a chunk of the baguette. Thankfully, the wine had stayed cold on the walk from Al's to the fountain. He drank half before taking his first bite. The bread crust was crispy, but the body was light and fluffy. Sight and sound powered a person's senses in the here and now. But smell is a sense that takes a person back and induces a palpable nostalgia. The smell of the bread brought him back to his night in Paris, and a shiver ran down his arms at the horrors he had experienced hours later.

He ate as much bread as he could until the expanding dough filled his stomach. He checked his watch and then finished the rest of his wine. From his pack of Chesterfields, he drew a joint Paris had given him. He lit it and took a long, smooth drag and released the musky cloud into the city air.

The half-moon illuminated the tranquil park, painting the trees in shades of gray and black. With the city behind him and nothing in front of him but the black marble lake and the prism of angelic white light reflecting off it, Johnny was back in Wisconsin. Paris filled his thoughts, fueling what the next few minutes would bring. Having a vivid memory had mostly been a curse, but being able to recall every moment of his embrace with Paris was worth all the deleterious visions he had suffered his whole life.

And then, he was back in that field in France, gazing at the stars, mesmerized by their cosmic beauty. It was where his mind always brought him back to. The view of heaven never lasted, always replaced by Hell. The artillery smoke blanketing the atmosphere in a cloud like volcanic ash, blocking the stars, moon, and even the sun. The birds chirping, singing their morning songs, were replaced with the cries of damned men. Johnny would always return there, but Paris had given him the gift of being able to go someplace else first. But in the end, she couldn't bring him back.

"Mr. De Luca," a raspy voice cut through the silence.

Johnny didn't break his gaze trained on the stars. Not yet. They gave him strength. He finished another drag and flicked the joint to the ground, grinding it out with his heel. He turned to the voice, his hands held wide at his sides.

Mickey Diamond stood twelve feet away, his hands folded in front of him, surrounded by his posse of hyenas. To call them wolves would have been a disgrace to wolves. Wolves hunted, fought. Hyenas feasted on the dying, scavenging the spoils of another animal's hunt.

O'Malley was impossible to miss, standing almost as tall as the lamppost nearby. Arthur Nash was amongst the ten men, trying to hide in the shadows, foolishly forgetting the entire lit city betrayed his cowardice.

"I get a call from my prohee saying he sees you leaving a burial place. Is that for the kid Hotsy? You should've told me you were going there, I would've let you set your affairs in order too. Maybe you could've got a two-for-one deal," Diamond said.

Diamond's men branched out, covering the distance should Johnny decide to flee, their guns held at their sides. Johnny would have no shot at Diamond. Two men stood directly in front of him, off to the side, but would be used as shields if necessary. Even if he had his gun, Johnny would be hit with ten bullets before he was able to even raise it.

"Search him," Diamond ordered.

O'Malley stepped forward, patting Johnny's body to check for a weapon.

"Clean," he said.

Diamond nodded his satisfaction. O'Malley waited for his next order. It came with a nod. O'Malley drove his boulder of a fist into Johnny's ribs. Hunched over, Johnny tried gulping in air, but he could only sip. The impact stopped his lungs from pumping. It was like a plastic bag had been shoved over his nose and mouth. O'Malley pushed down on Johnny's shoulders. When the air finally surged back into Johnny's lungs, O'Malley drove his fist across Johnny's face, each knuckle a hammer on its own.

Diamond cracked a disgusting, yellow-toothed smile. "You were a hard man to track down. Rat-like in your ability to scamper and disappear. Capuano, well, he was a man, I'll give him that. He faced the music. Quite a bit of music I might add. Hotsy or Holesy as he should be called, at least he got to die thinking he was going to get laid. But you... you are out here all alone."

O'Malley yanked Johnny upright.

"I thought for sure that once I prettied up that nigger bitch of yours, you would come for me. Paris, right? Well, I can assure you Paris was invaded and conquered by a foreign force. But I was wrong about you. You go to the park to gaze upon an unfinished fountain, drink some cheap wine, and eat bread," Diamond said, nodding to the bottle and the bread.

Johnny had no idea how many fibers the human body had. All but one, one with Paris's voice, demanded he charge forward and kill Mickey Diamond. Johnny's soul was torn, battered, and bruised. Paris wouldn't have him destroy what remained by seeking vengeance on her behalf.

"Nothing? Give him another greeting," Diamond said.

O'Malley sent a meteorite crashing into Johnny's face. Blood splattered into the air. Mickey Diamond stepped forward and hurled the next punch. He was an overweight shark, lazy after years of no competition. The only shark in a sea of seals. His early-twenties had been filled with amateur boxing bouts, and his fists reacted out of memory, sending hooks, uppercuts, and jabs. And like his amateur days, Diamond threw plenty of kidney and rabbit punches.

O'Malley and another man forced Johnny to his feet. Diamond stood close, his foul breath crawling out of his mouth like a locust. He sniffed his fingers.

"I can still smell her stench," he said.

He dug his grubby fingers into Johnny's nostrils. Johnny tried to resist, but O'Malley held his head in place like it was a grapefruit.

"Oh, come on, don't act like you don't like that stench," Diamond said, playing for his audience.

Johnny looked at Nash, piercing him with his eyes. Nash looked away.

"I am going to find her," Diamond whispered. "And I am going to have every man on my payroll—gangster, judge, prohee, cop, and councilman—force themselves inside her day after day after day until she can't take dick no more. And then, when she is of no more use to me, I am going to kill her. The pain, the embarrassment she felt before and will feel is all because of you. I want you to know that. You brought this on her."

With that, Diamond drove his ring-covered knuckles into Johnny's still-injured side. The wound split open. Crimson blood stained his gray vest. A sharp pain ripped through his ribs.

"The wound my brother-in-law gave," Diamond commented, nodding at Johnny's bleeding side. "You got him back though, did you not? Four shots to the chest. You're owed three… but I'm not going to shoot you. You deserve something better. Something I can tell my sister to give her some peace knowing how much you suffered. I'm going to carve your heart out."

What's a little pain before the end?

Johnny was on his knees, but he had no intention of staying there. He pushed himself to his feet. A searing pain erupted in his side. His ribs were broken, how many he couldn't say. But with each deep breath his ribs threatened to pierce his lung.

Johnny raised his head, bringing his gaze to the stars. Their cosmic light powered him. That field in France had showed him how courageous men die, and that beach in Wisconsin had given him a reason to.

"I like to write poems for my victims. I think it is a classy thing to do. I would like you to hear yours," Diamond said.

He cleared his throat and read:

Here stands Giovanni De Luca, half-Kraut, half-Wop
I scampered to Wisconsin and to a cabin
Then returned to Chicago where my life comes to a stop
My best friends were shot
But I am scheduled for a stabbing
I lived for the business of booze
But now the time has come
For the eternal snooze

Diamond radiated pride. His posse laughed, as if on cue.

A rational thinker would have thrown Johnny in the back of a car and taken him on a one-way ride. But Mickey Diamond wasn't a rational thinker. He was victim to impulse. He pulled a knife from underneath his pant leg. Old with a dull blade, it was most likely the same one he had had when he was a child.

"In a few minutes, you'll be nothing. Who you were won't matter. Who you were born to won't matter. What you did won't matter. The fact you existed won't matter. You. Won't. Matter. You'll fade into history without a trace."

Johnny let out a broken, half-hearted chuckle. "We all go the way of the dodo bird."

Johnny was tired, but a tiredness that could not be staved off with sleep. He was tired of the attacks. He was tired of the worry, tired of his haunting past and uncertain future, tired of the dark place he'd been in for so long. He longed for it all to end. In France, he had feared death. But now, he welcomed it. That dull blade wouldn't bring pain, it would end it.

Johnny breathed deeply, looking at the majestic night sky. He wouldn't let Mickey Diamond's grotesque face be the last thing he would ever see. The alcohol and cannabis trickled through his veins, reducing the terror he should have experienced. But in combination with the plant and drink was the relief death would bring. In Greek myth, Charon was the ferryman who chartered souls across the rivers Styx and Acheron that divided the world of the living and the world of the dead. Johnny was half-way there. He'd been half-way there for a long time.

Diamond plunged the knife into Johnny's chest, splitting flesh, piercing muscle, cracking bone. He carved and twisted the knife with a perverse smile on his face. Then he wrenched the blade out. Johnny's strength went with it. He fell to his knees and then collapsed onto his back. Blood poured from his body like a prisoner fleeing its captor. The feeling in his hands and feet went first, then the numbness slithered up his arms and legs like a cold-blooded serpent. The stars he gazed at multiplied in number, but their clarity diminished.

"Mickey Diamond, you're under arrest for murder!" Nash shouted out, but his voice grew too distorted for Johnny to make out.

A gunshot rang out. One of Diamond's men fell. Nash wasn't alone. Cops poured in from Michigan Avenue and converged on their location.

Diamond was wrestled to the ground and thrashed like an alligator. O'Malley fell to his knees, knowing full well his size meant the policemen would take no chances. Diamond was read his rights, but the sound didn't reach Johnny. There was commotion all around—men fled, shots were fired, curses and threats were yelled out from both sides. Diamond spat out every curse word known to man as he was handcuffed.

Johnny lay on the pavement, his hands on his chest, too weak to try to contain the outpouring of blood. He gazed upon the magnificent half-moon. The numbness spread further, reaching his thighs and chest. And for the first time since summer had arrived, Johnny was cold. Death was frigid, glacial even. It crept toward him, but he couldn't deny how refreshing the coldness was. The heat, which had attacked him ferociously and relentlessly for two months was now powerless. He had been caressed by death once before in a field in France.

It had been a fading embrace, but now, death wrapped its hands around him and would never let him go. He would never have to endure another ship ride home.

"It's suffering…"

His father's words came to him, distant and distorted as if through a radio.

Johnny's eyes opened and closed rapidly. He was back in that truck on that upstate New York country road, approaching the injured deer. The memory shifted. He was back in France now. Staring at the same moon, bleeding in No Man's Land. The men around him were deer, all injured, all pleading for help, the flares and artillery exploding in flashes of light so that not even the darkness could hide them. Pleading for a salvation that would never come.

Back inside the truck, approaching the deer. Seconds away from flattening it and ending its life. But again, the dream, the memory, the hallucination changed. It was Johnny standing in the middle of the road, the truck speeding toward him. Feet away… inches away.

But something pulled him away from that road and back to Chicago and Grant Park. He turned his head. Paris was there, lying beside him. Her fierce brown eyes stared into his. He smiled, blood trickling out of the corners of his mouth. All a man can ask for when death comes is to have something or someone to ease that cold embrace. Hundreds of thousands hadn't lived long enough to have that mercy. They had died young and unfulfilled. Johnny had his someone to ease the coldness and the fear of the unknown of what came next. Her face, which he had traced onto his mind, wasn't a dream. It was too real. Her skin was palpable, her fingertips cold to the touch, her hair blowing into his face from the breeze. It was enough to give him peace. He was back on that road, the truck speeding at him, waiting for the mercy it would deliver. His eyes blinked one final time.

Johnny was back in that trench, covered in dirt, grime, and blood, standing in front of a ladder, summoning his courage with each deep breath, waiting. A whistle blew. He stormed out of the trench, bracing himself for the gunfire, the thundering and lightning of artillery, the glue-like mud to grab his boots, the thick smoke to hinder his vision, barbed wire to rip his uniform and for the poisonous gas to tear his lungs like paper. But there was no gunfire. Only fireflies flew by, flashing their blue-white and yellow-green lights. The fields were covered in luscious, forest-green grass. There was no smoke, just a cloudless, full moon, star-cast sky—the very same that had made such a lasting impact. No barbed wire or hedgehogs stopped him from advancing, no bodies filled No Man's Land, only thousands of red poppies. Shadows lined the distance ahead. All standing in a row, staring at him. It was too dark, and he too far away, to decipher any faces. He squeezed his M1903 Springfield rifle. He was alone. No other troops had stormed out of the trench. He cautiously continued his approach. The figures in the distance stood there. With each step, faces formed. Johnny stopped, a smile on his lips. He recognized them all, some by both appearance and name, others only by appearance. Soldiers he had served with, bled with, fought with. Hotsy and Tomato were there, silently telling him to continue. In the center were his parents and grandmother gazing upon him with pride. The way he had come was filled with the dead and dying, the mud and dirt, the explosions of artillery and the torrential onslaught of gunfire. It was only the trench that waited for him back there. A trench that had imprisoned him, defined him. Johnny took one last look at it, turned and left the trench and the maze behind forever.

Somewhere

Sunlight poured in through the tall awning-windows overlooking the expansive Pacific Ocean. The soft waves washed along the sandy shore. The kitchen table was bare save for a bowl of lemons and a folded sheet of stationary paper. The interior was painted cotton white with a pineapple yellow trim dancing horizontally midway up the colossal wall, stretching over fifteen feet before connecting with the ceiling.

Car doors clunked shut. The French patio entry doors opened. Wally jogged in, removing his newsboy cap and gawking at the height of the ceiling and taking in his new home. Cilly and Paris helped Clarence inside and to a leather armchair overlooking the beach. It was a view that warranted a person's undivided attention, and Clarence would give it that.

It had been a long ride. They had stopped to stretch every four or five hours but, to Paris, she had been folded in half and packed into a suitcase. It seemed like the bruising on her face would go away before she regained full feeling in her backside.

The Midwest states had made for a boring drive. It was impossible to decipher Iowa from Nebraska. During a stretch of the drive that lasted hours, it appeared as if they had covered no ground because it was nothing but a long line of unbroken corn fields. But Colorado and its Rocky Mountains had taken her breath away. It was impossible not to be overcome with the feeling of joy when they reached Southern California, a sense that this place offered something better that Paris had always hoped to find. The sun was always shining, and not in the attacking way it had in Chicago. The beach was a perfect seventy-three degrees and seemed incapable of producing a cloudy day.

"Can we go out to the beach, mom?" Wally asked, his legs bouncing like loaded springs.

Only a kid could get out of a car after a brutally long drive and want to go swimming immediately.

"Come on dad, we'll get you set up right along the water. I did some reading, and salt water is good for your body," Wally said, grabbing his father's hand and helping him out of the chair.

Cilly rushed after them, fresh water was nerve wracking enough for a parent. Salt water brought about a whole new spectrum of fears and worries. Most of all sharks.

They strolled to the sky-blue water, leaving their shoes in the sand. Paris smiled fondly at them before turning to look at her new home. It was spacious, and there would be no need to worry about lack of privacy. The staircase led to an unknown number of rooms behind the mezzanine. The living room was open, the kitchen too, with enough light pouring in that darkness had no place to breed.

The long, rectangular dining room table had been hand-crafted from thick redwood. The whole house was ready for living. Johnny had thought of everything.

Her eyes caught the bowl of lemons and the note in front of it. The white of the letter blended perfectly with the white bowl, but the black letterhead of Provident Hospital and the Chicago address on it caught her attention. To her, it was a loaded gun pointing right at her. Summoning her courage, she took the letter in her hand and opened it. Her heart receded deeper into her ribcage at the sight of Johnny's writing, like an animal that knew it was about to be attacked.

Paris,

If you're reading this, then it was all worth it. That some good has come from everything that has happened. It also means that I won't be able to keep my promise, and for that, I'm sorry. I've been doing a lot of thinking over the last few weeks. I was forced to confront things I had tried to bury deep in the center of this maze I had created, where I caged and buried all the truths and lies, questions and answers, and memories that haunted me. My maze kept people out. And for a long time it was impenetrable. But then you came, and you walked a straight line, right into the center of it. Over these last few weeks, I've answered questions and accepted truths, and once I did that, I could never live the lies again.

I never expected to live this long. I was twenty-three when I left for France. Like so many, I had illusions of what war was. I believed the newspaper ads and songs on the radio. But after my first night there, seeing the dead and dying carted off in the back of trucks, seeing the look of sheer exhaustion and indifference on the faces of those who had been in the trench, I never expected to make it home. And after what I did, I never wanted to.

When I was bleeding out on that field, my father's words came to me. It's suffering. I thought of that deer in the middle of the road. Every day since, that memory has come back to me. For a long time, I wondered what it meant. It was only after I met you did I accept a truth I think I had known for a long time. The truth that I never made it out of that trench, Paris. Not all of me. Not the best parts. I'm that deer. Suffering in the road, unable to go back or move on. And you're me in that passenger seat, naive enough to think I could be saved. I thank you for that. I love you for that. Mickey Diamond... he's just the truck that will end the suffering.

When I was in France, I thought there had to be someplace better, someplace that would fix what was broken in me. But when I got back, my life was nothing but bullets and booze. But then you came along. I like to think I showed you glimpses of the man I wanted to be. In Wisconsin, on that beach, there were moments when the emptiness went away. But even in this heat, cold hard truths get to you. The pain, the guilt, the emptiness, the remorse, the sadness, I carried all that. It never went away. It never lessened, never faded. Life is attrition. We lose people and things that matter. Pieces of ourselves. Life changes us. Alters who we are and who we were meant to be.

You had said we all go the way of the dodo bird. We all go into extinction. We were all dodo birds over there, Paris.

The dodo bird went extinct before we even knew why it was here. And the same was true of millions of young men. Gone before they could show the world why they were here. Fading away into history to be forgotten.

I am a dodo bird because I couldn't find my place in this world. It was never anything that was broken in me, it wasn't anything anyone could fix or replace or fill. Somewhere inside of me, something is missing. A void that can never be filled. The past never let go of me. It never tapped me on the shoulder, it dug its claws in me and forced me to confront it. And the future abandoned me long ago.

You had said that maybe you were missing too. But you're wrong. You're not missing. You're broken, but you have pulled yourself out of your trench in a way I never could. I know you can do it again. You're stronger than me. Stronger than any person I have ever met. I know you won't let your *trench define you like it did me. I know you'll rise from it and find where you belong.*

Gone the way of the Dodo Bird,

Giovanni.

Paris held the letter close to her chest, allowing the words Johnny had poured from his heart to soak through her chest and into her own heart. It was only when she brought the letter close to breathe in his scent that she noticed the note scribbled on the back.

Check under the lemons.

Her grief was only stifled by her curiosity. She plucked the lemons from the dish, revealing stacks of cash, bills no smaller than twenties. It was enough money for her and the Nettesheims to live comfortably for years. There would be no worrying about food or unaffordable repairs or doctor visits. No more selling herself to strange men.

Johnny could never identify with the entitled affluent. He was born poor and raised poor. But he had seen the corruption money caused. Maybe, that's why he hadn't spent his money—he never wanted anything in common with them.

The letter in her hand and the money were both just paper. One was invaluable and would get her through the rest of her life. The other could buy her things.

"See you half-breed," Paris whispered.

She folded the note and placed it inside her purse. Her eyes only allowed for a lone tear to stroll down her cheek. She stepped through the back door and out into the strong sun and its promise of better days.

Author Note

I have always had a fascination with history. My main area of interest has always been the Second World War—hence my first novel "Forever Fleeting." While reading for leisure and research, I learned about how the treaty that ended the Great War greatly impacted the Second World War. But the Great War had always been the preamble—a necessity in order to understand the cause of the Second World War. I'm ashamed to say I never gave the event the respect it deserves. That changed when I discovered Dan Carlin's podcast and his series "Blueprint to Armageddon." The facts laid before me were harrowing and life-changing. Battles where fifty thousand men were killed in fifteen minutes. Listening, reading, and watching events (or recreations of those events) from the Great War revealed just how truly awful life in the trench had been.

And while today, we have become desensitized to violence, blood, and gore through realistic portrayals of war in film and television, the men who served in the Great War had never seen such images, couldn't fathom the horrors that awaited them.

The genesis of this novel was a story about prohibition. But in writing and crafting the character of Johnny, the story changed. The body of the story was the battle of booze. But the soul of the novel came to be a broken man. What happens when a broken man goes to war? I wanted, *needed* to showcase the trauma these soldiers returned home with. Ernest Hemingway wrote about the "Lost Generation." The men and women who served during the Second World War were dubbed the greatest generation—a moniker certainly earned and deserved. But the veterans of the Great War have been widely forgotten. My hope is that this story helps rekindle their stories in our collective memory.

They stormed blackened earth
They fell under ashen sky
Men of courage, men of worth
By the thousands they die
Beneath green fields they rest
Under blue skies they lie

Author Bio

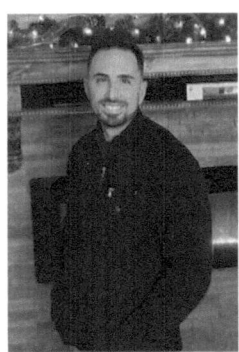

Gone the Way of the Dodo Bird is the second novel written by Bret Kissinger. His first novel was the heralded World War II historical fiction *Forever Fleeting*. He enjoys combing fact and fiction to give readers the chance to experience life throughout different periods of history. He resides in Wisconsin.

Praise for Forever Fleeting

"Forever Fleeting tugs at the heartstrings of each of us that wonders how the life of someone of past romantic significance played out. We all have a Hannah or Wilhelm out there somewhere. The story line of Forever Fleeting was 'can't put it down' excellent."—*Amazon* Review

"This is one of the best books I have read in a long time. It was a page turner from beginning to end. Anyone looking for a good comfortable read should read this one. War. Love story. People at their worst and best... What more could you ask for?"—*Amazon* Review

"My Mom reads approximately 3-5 books a week! With the volume of books she has read in her lifetime, she said "this is one of the best books I have ever read!" The history facts, the story line, and such characteristic details...she couldn't put it down."—*Amazon* Review

"This book has become easily my favorite historical fiction novel. The characters are written beautifully and take the reader on an incredible, albeit painful journey. The atrocities of war not only in the physical sense but the emotional turmoil war provides is evident throughout. This novel is an incredible journey all should experience."—*Amazon* Review

If you enjoyed this book, please consider leaving a review on Amazon.com

www.ingramcontent.com/pod-product-compliance
Lightning Source LLC
Chambersburg PA
CBHW051317250626